# Pediatric Surgery

*Guest Editors*

KENNETH S. AZAROW, MD
ROBERT A. CUSICK, MD

# SURGICAL CLINICS
# OF NORTH AMERICA

www.surgical.theclinics.com

*Consulting Editor*
RONALD F. MARTIN, MD

June 2012 • Volume 92 • Number 3

SAUNDERS an imprint of ELSEVIER, Inc.

**W.B. SAUNDERS COMPANY**

*A Division of Elsevier Inc.*

1600 John F. Kennedy Blvd., Suite 1800, Philadelphia, PA 19103-2899

http://www.surgical.theclinics.com

**SURGICAL CLINICS OF NORTH AMERICA Volume 92, Number 3**
**June 2012 ISSN 0039–6109, ISBN-13: 978-1-4557-3939-4**

Editor: John Vassallo, j.vassallo@elsevier.com
Developmental Editor: Teia Stone

**Photocopying**

Single photocopies of single articles may be made for personal use as allowed by national copyright laws. Permission of the Publisher and payment of a fee is required for all other photocopying, including multiple or systematic copying, copying for advertising or promotional purposes, resale, and all forms of document delivery. Special rates are available for educational institutions that wish to make photocopies for non-profit educational classroom use. For information on how to seek permission visit www.elsevier.com/permissions or call: (+44) 1865 843830 (UK)/(+1) 215 239 3804 (USA).

**Derivative Works**

Subscribers may reproduce tables of contents or prepare lists of articles including abstracts for internal circulation within their institutions. Permission of the Publisher is required for resale or distribution outside the institution. Permission of the Publisher is required for all other derivative works, including compilations and translations (please consult www.elsevier.com/permissions).

**Electronic Storage or Usage**

Permission of the Publisher is required to store or use electronically any material contained in this journal, including any article or part of an article (please consult www.elsevier.com/permissions). Except as outlined above, no part of this publication may be reproduced, stored in a retrieval system or transmitted in any form or by any means, electronic, mechanical, photocopying, recording or otherwise, without prior written permission of the Publisher.

**Notice**

No responsibility is assumed by the Publisher for any injury and/or damage to persons or property as a matter of products liability, negligence or otherwise, or from any use or operation of any methods, products, instructions or ideas contained in the material herein. Because of rapid advances in the medical sciences, in particular, independent verification of diagnoses and drug dosages should be made.

Although all advertising material is expected to conform to ethical (medical) standards, inclusion in this publication does not constitute a guarantee or endorsement of the quality or value of such product or of the claims made of it by its manufacturer.

*Surgical Clinics of North America* (ISSN 0039–6109) is published bimonthly by Elsevier Inc., 360 Park Avenue South, New York, NY 10010-1710. Months of publication are February, April, June, August, October, and December. Business and Editorial Offices: 1600 John F. Kennedy Blvd., Suite 1800, Philadelphia, PA 19103-2899. Periodicals postage paid at New York, NY and additional mailing offices. Subscription prices are $339.00 per year for US individuals, $575.00 per year for US institutions, $166.00 per year for US students and residents, $415.00 per year for Canadian individuals, $714.00 per year for Canadian institutions, $468.00 for international individuals, $714.00 per year for international institutions and $229.00 per year for Canadian and foreign students/residents. To receive student/resident rate, orders must be accompanied by name of affiliated institution, date of term, and the *signature* of program/residency coordinator on institution letterhead. Orders will be billed at individual rate until proof of status is received. Foreign air speed delivery is included in all *Clinics* subscription prices. All prices are subject to change without notice. POSTMASTER: Send address changes to *Surgical Clinics*, Elsevier Health Sciences Division, Subscription Customer Service, 3251 Riverport Lane, Maryland Heights, MO 63043. **Customer Service (orders, claims, online, change of address): Telephone: 1-800-654-2452 (U.S. and Canada); 314-447-8871 (outside U.S. and Canada). Fax: 314-447-8029. E-mail: journalscustomerservice-usa@elsevier.com (for print support); journalsonline support-usa@elsevier.com (for online support).**

*Reprints.* For copies of 100 or more, of articles in this publication, please contact the Commercial Reprints Department, Elsevier Inc., 360 Park Avenue South, New York, New York 10010-1710. Tel. (212) 633-3812, Fax: (212) 462-1935, e-mail: reprints@elsevier.com.

*The Surgical Clinics of North America* is also published in Spanish by McGraw-Hill Interamericana Editores S.A., P.O. Box 5-237 06500 Mexico D.F. Mexico; and in Portuguese by Interlivros Edicoes Ltda., Rua Comandante Coelho 1085, CEP 21250, Rio de Janeiro, Brazil; and in Greek by Paschalidis Medical Publications, Athens Greece.

*The Surgical Clinics of North America* is covered in *MEDLINE/PubMed (Index Medicus), EMBASE/Excerpta Medica, Current Contents/Clinical Medicine, Current Contents/Life Sciences, Science Citation Index,* and *ISI/BIOMED.*

Printed and bound by CPI Group (UK) Ltd, Croydon, CR0 4YY

Transferred to digital print 2012

# Contributors

## CONSULTING EDITOR

**RONALD F. MARTIN, MD**
Staff Surgeon, Department of Surgery, Marshfield Clinic, Marshfield, Wisconsin; Clinical Associate Professor, University of Wisconsin School of Medicine and Public Health, Madison, Wisconsin; Colonel, Medical Corps, United States Army Reserve

## GUEST EDITORS

**KENNETH S. AZAROW, MD, FACS, FAAP**
Alton S.K. Wong Distinguished Professor of Surgery & Program Director, Pediatric Surgery Fellowship, University of Nebraska College of Medicine & Children's Hospital & Medical Center, Omaha, Nebraska

**ROBERT A. CUSICK, MD, FACS, FAAP**
Associate Professor of Surgery, University of Nebraska College of Medicine & Children's Hospital & Medical Center, Omaha, Nebraska

## AUTHORS

**ANNE-MARIE E. AMIES OELSCHLAGER, MD**
Associate Professor and Director, Pediatric and Adolescent Gynecology, Department of Obstetrics and Gynecology, University of Washington School of Medicine, Seattle Children's Hospital, Seattle Children's, Seattle, Washington

**FELIX C. BLANCO, MD**
Surgical Research Fellow, Sheikh Zayed Institute for Pediatric Surgical Innovation, Children's National Medical Center, Washington, DC

**ALLEN F. BROWNE, MD**
Division of Pediatric Surgery, Children's Hospital of Illinois, Order of St. Francis Medical Center, University of Illinois College of Medicine-Peoria, Peoria, Illinois

**ROBERT A. CUSICK, MD, FACS, FAAP**
Associate Professor of Surgery, University of Nebraska College of Medicine & Children's Hospital & Medical Center, Omaha, Nebraska

**KATHERINE P. DAVENPORT, MD**
Joseph E. Robert Jr. Fellow, Sheikh Zayed Institute for Pediatric Surgical Innovation, Children's National Medical Center, Washington, DC

**R. DAWN FEVURLY, MD**
Stuart and Jane Weitzman Fellow of Vascular Anomalies, Department of Surgery, Vascular Anomalies Center, Children's Hospital Boston, Boston, Massachusetts

**STEVEN J. FISHMAN, MD**
Associate Professor of Surgery, Department of Surgery, Vascular Anomalies Center, Children's Hospital Boston, Harvard Medical School, Boston, Massachusetts

**ROBERT J. FITZGIBBONS Jr, MD, FACS**
Harry E. Stuckenhoff Professor of Surgery, Chief of the Division of General Surgery and Associate Chairman, Department of Surgery, Creighton University School of Medicine, Omaha, Nebraska

**ALEJANDRO GARCIA, MD**
Post-Doctoral Clinical Research Fellow, Division of Pediatric Surgery, Columbia University College of Physicians and Surgeons, New York, New York

**MICHAEL J. GORETSKY, MD**
Associate Professor of Clinical Surgery and Pediatrics, Eastern Virginia Medical School; Pediatric Surgery, Children's Hospital of The King's Daughters, Norfolk, Virginia

**CHRISTOPHER GUIDRY, MD**
Resident in General Surgery, Department of General Surgery, University of Virginia Health System, Charlottesville, Virginia

**KURT HEISS, MD**
Division of Pediatric Surgery, Children's Healthcare of Atlanta; Associate Professor of Surgery and Pediatrics, Emory University School of Medicine, Atlanta, Georgia

**MARK J. HOLTERMAN, MD, PhD**
Professor, Division of Pediatric Surgery, Children's Hospital of Illinois, Order of St. Francis Medical Center, University of Illinois College of Medicine-Peoria, Peoria, Illinois

**TOM JAKSIC, MD, PhD**
W. Hardy Hendren Professor of Surgery, Harvard Medical School; Vice-Chairman of Pediatric General Surgery, Children's Hospital Boston; Surgical Director, Center for Advanced Intestinal Rehabilitation (CAIR), Boston, Massachusetts

**DAVID JUANG, MD**
Director of Trauma, Critical Care & Burns, Children's Mercy Hospital; Assistant Professor of Surgery, University of Missouri–Kansas City, Kansas City, Missouri

**TIMOTHY D. KANE, MD, FACS**
Professor of Surgery and Pediatrics, The George Washington University School of Medicine & Health Sciences; Principal Investigator, Department of Surgery, Sheikh Zayed Institute for Pediatric Surgical Innovation, Children's National Medical Center, Washington, DC

**OLIVER B. LAO, MD, MPH**
Department of Pediatric Surgery, Children's Hospital and Regional Medical Center, Pediatric Surgical Fellow, University of Nebraska College of Medicine, Omaha, Nebraska

**CABRINI A. LARIVIERE, MD, MPH**
Clinical Research Fellow, Department of Surgery, Seattle Children's Hospital, University of Washington School of Medicine, Seattle, Washington

**AI-XUAN LE HOLTERMAN, MD**
Professor, Division of Pediatric Surgery, Children's Hospital of Illinois, Order of St. Francis Medical Center, University of Illinois College of Medicine-Peoria, Peoria, Illinois

**DANIEL J. LEDBETTER, MD**
Associate Professor, Department of Surgery, University of Washington; Attending Surgeon, Seattle Children's Hospital, Seattle, Washington

**EUGENE D. MCGAHREN, MD**
Professor of Pediatric Surgery and Pediatrics, Division of Pediatric Surgery, University of Virginia Children's Hospital, University of Virginia Health System, Charlottesville, Virginia

**BIREN P. MODI, MD**
Instructor in Surgery, Harvard Medical School; Assistant in Surgery, Children's Hospital Boston; Staff Surgeon, Center for Advanced Intestinal Rehabilitation (CAIR), Boston, Massachusetts

**ROBERT J. OBERMEYER, MD**
Assistant Professor of Clinical Surgery and Pediatrics, Eastern Virginia Medical School; Pediatric Surgery, Children's Hospital of The King's Daughters, Norfolk, Virginia

**SAMIR PANDYA, MD**
Division of Pediatric Surgery, Maria Fareri Children's Hospital; Assistant Professor of Surgery and Pediatrics, New York Medical College, Valhalla, New York

**RICHARD H. PEARL, MD**
Surgeon-in-Chief, Professor of Surgery and Pediatrics, Section of Pediatric Surgery, Department of Surgery, University of Illinois College of Medicine at Peoria, Children's Hospital of Illinois, Peoria, Illinois

**VICTORIA K. PEPPER, MD**
Resident Surgeon, Associate/Surgical Resident, Section of General Surgery, Department of Surgery, Children's Hospital of Illinois, University of Illinois College of Medicine at Peoria, Peoria, Illinois

**ROBIN PETROZE, MD**
Resident in General Surgery, Department of General Surgery, University of Virginia Health System, Charlottesville, Virginia

**ANTHONY D. SANDLER, MD**
The Joseph E. Robert, Jr. Center for Surgical Care, Chief of Pediatric Surgery, Principal Investigator for Immunology Initiative, Department of Surgery, Sheikh Zayed Institute for Pediatric Surgical Innovation, Children's National Medical Center, Washington, DC

**ROBERT SAWIN, MD**
Herbert E. Coe Professor of Surgery, University of Washington School of Medicine, Seattle Children's Hospital, Seattle, Washington

**CHARLES L. SNYDER, MD**
Chief, Department of Surgery, Children's Mercy Hospital; Professor of Surgery, University of Missouri–Kansas City, Kansas City, Missouri

**VANCE Y. SOHN, MD**
Department of Surgery, Madigan Army Medical Center, Tacoma, Washington

**AMY B. STANFILL, MD**
Attending Surgeon, Clinical Assistant Professor of Surgery and Pediatrics, Section of General Surgery, Department of Surgery, Children's Hospital of Illinois, University of Illinois College of Medicine at Peoria, Peoria, Illinois

**SCOTT R. STEELE, MD, FACS, FASCRS**
Department of Surgery, Madigan Army Medical Center, Tacoma, Washington

**CHARLES J.H. STOLAR, MD**
Professor of Surgery and Pediatrics, Division of Pediatric Surgery, Columbia University College of Physicians and Surgeons, New York, New York

**JOHN H.T. WALDHAUSEN, MD**
Professor of Surgery, Division Chief Pediatric General and Thoracic Surgery, Department of Surgery, Seattle Children's Hospital, University of Washington School of Medicine, Seattle, Washington

**DAVID ZENGER, MD**
Department of Anesthesia, Madigan Army Medical Center, Tacoma, Washington

# Contents

> Surgeons performing painful, invasive procedures in pediatric patients must be cognizant of both the potential short- and long-term detrimental effects of inadequate analgesia. This article reviews the available tools, sedation procedures, the management of intraoperative, postoperative, and postprocedural pain, and the issues surrounding neonatal addiction.

> Pediatric inguinal hernias are extremely common, and can usually be diagnosed by simple history taking and physical examination. Repair is elective, unless there is incarceration or strangulation. Hydroceles are also quite common, and in infancy many will resolve without operative intervention. Undescended testicles harbor an increased risk of infertility and malignancy, and require orchiopexy in early childhood.

> Three of the most common causes of surgical abdominal pain in pediatric patients include appendicitis, Meckel diverticulum, and intussusception. All 3 can present with right lower quadrant pain, and can lead to significant morbidity and even mortality. Although ultrasound is the preferred method of diagnosis with appendicitis and intussusception, considerable variety exists in the modalities needed in the diagnosis of Meckel diverticulum. This article discusses the pathways to diagnosis, the modes of treatment, and the continued areas of controversy.

> Pyloric stenosis is a common pediatric surgical problem that requires a combination of both medical and surgical attention. This article reviews the classical elements necessary to care for the patient in a safe and effective manner. A well-tested management approach that can be applied to the general surgical environment is described. Perioperative management of the patient is discussed and the currently used techniques are reviewed. Current recommendations include the routine use of ultrasonography for

diagnosis, attention to the preoperative correction of electrolytes, and the use of minimally invasive techniques for treatment.

Thoracic tumors are rare in children, and metastatic or malignant conditions must be excluded during the diagnostic evaluation. The majority of primary pulmonary neoplasms in children are malignant; this article primarily addresses benign tumors. Surgical resection is the standard treatment for benign thoracic tumors in children. Thoracotomy is a traditional approach, but the thoracoscopic technique for diagnosis and treatment of thoracic tumors is well established. The term benign tumors can be a misnomer in that although their histology is not malignant, these tumors can be locally aggressive with significant associated morbidity and potential for mortality.

Infants affected with congenital diaphragmatic hernias (CDH) suffer from some degree of respiratory insufficiency arising from a combination of pulmonary hypoplasia and pulmonary hypertension. Respiratory care strategies to optimize blood gasses lead to significant barotrauma, increased morbidity, and overuse of extracorporeal membrane oxygenation (ECMO). Newer permissive hypercapnia/spontaneous ventilation protocols geared to accept moderate hypercapnia at lower peak airway pressures have led to improved outcomes. High-frequency oscillatory ventilation can be used in infants who continue to have persistent respiratory distress despite conventional ventilation. ECMO can be used successfully as a resuscitative strategy to minimize further barotrauma in carefully selected patients.

Chest wall deformities can be divided into 2 main categories, congenital and acquired. Congenital chest wall deformities may present any time between birth and early adolescence. Acquired chest wall deformities typically follow prior chest surgery or a posterolateral diaphragmatic hernia repair (Bochdalek). The most common chest wall deformities are congenital pectus excavatum (88%) and pectus carinatum (5%). This article addresses the etiology, pathophysiology, clinical evaluation, diagnosis, and management of these deformities.

Newborn intestinal obstructions are a common reason for admission to neonatal ICUs. The incidence is estimated to be approximately 1 in 2000 live births. There are 4 cardinal signs of intestinal obstruction in newborns: (1) maternal polyhydramnios, (2) bilious emesis, (3) failure to pass meconium in the first day of life, and (4) abdominal distention. The presentation may vary from subtle and easily overlooked findings on physical examination to massive abdominal distention with respiratory distress and cardiovascular collapse. A careful history and physical examination often identify

# SURGICAL CLINICS
# OF NORTH AMERICA

DOWNLOAD
Free App!

*Review Articles*
THE CLINICS

**NOW AVAILABLE FOR YOUR iPhone and iPad**

# Foreword

# Pediatric Surgery

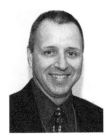

Ronald F. Martin, MD
*Consulting Editor*

The last time we produced an issue of the *Surgical Clinics of North America* on the topic of surgical diseases of children was in 2006. In that issue I wrote about the problems of logistics in trying to care for children closer to their homes and the economic concerns that further complicate the delivery of care to these young people. Now six years later I find that the very same problems remain equally problematic. I am left wondering whether I am failing to recognize progress or whether we really aren't making headway.

Shortly before the writing of this foreword, the Accreditation Council for Graduate Medical Education met for its annual education meeting. Over 2000 people attended the meeting. The two topics of particular merit were the Next Accreditation System (NAS) and the keynote session on workforce and needs. The NAS is a system that will change the way training programs are reviewed and evaluated. I don't plan to discuss the NAS at this time but if you haven't heard of it I would suggest you look it up. The keynote session though is worth a bit of consideration here.

The keynote speakers were two well-known and accomplished gentlemen, Drs Richard "Buzz" Cooper and Fitzhugh Mullan. The main topics were: "Do we have enough doctors?" and "Are we producing enough doctors to meet the needs of our communities?" While there was much agreement in that there are many places without enough doctors, there was some disagreement about whether it is that we have too few physicians or are the physicians we have just mal-distributed.

According to the Association of American Medical Colleges (AAMC) Center for Workforce Studies, in 2010, there were 258.7 active physicians per 100,000 population in the United States, ranging from a high of 415.5 in Massachusetts to a low of 176.4 in Mississippi (*2011 State Physician Workforce Data Book,* www.aamc.org/workforce). Now, by almost anyone's standards, that is a pretty big discrepancy in doctor density per population. Many arguments have been made over the reasons for these differences. Most of them revolve around money and the access it buys in health care.

Surg Clin N Am 92 (2012) xiii–xv
doi:10.1016/j.suc.2012.03.019
0039-6109/12/$ – see front matter © 2012 Elsevier Inc. All rights reserved.

surgical.theclinics.com

Certainly, communities with more resources can afford to attract more physicians, particularly if there are higher volume consumers of medical care living in these areas. Even better if there are higher numbers of commercially insured consumers of health care. Also, areas of greater affluence may offer other nonmonetary enticements that draw physicians for lifestyle and other reasons. Of course, the corollary holds true that some less affluent areas are attractive to some physicians for different lifestyle concerns. At the end of the day, though, there is some significant effect of market force on the distribution of physicians that goes beyond the "supply" of physicians and the "demand" of patients. One of the forces is the effect of "local retention" as well. According to the same report by the AAMC, if a person were to attend undergraduate medical education (UME) and graduate medical education (GME) in the same state, that person would have a two-thirds chance of practicing in that state. Just slightly below 50% of graduates who perform GME in a state remain in that state and the same is true for those who perform UME in a state. So medical practice placement and medical education are both a bit similar to real estate—it's all about location. In particular how the location and distribution of training facilities will generate final practice geographic distribution.

I think it would be disingenuous to suggest that these observations are completely independent or singularly important. People obviously choose the location of medical schools and residencies based on some of the same criteria they would use to choose any other place to live and work. Many of these decisions are based on unrelated topics such as family or climate or cultural similarity as well. No matter how the choice is being made, the net result is marked variation. And the multi-trillion dollar question is: is that nearly three-fold variation in physician force per capita between states justifiable or not?

Part of the variation stems from the fact that we maintain an existing system of GME that largely relies on federal funding to pay for training our future partners and colleagues. The monies from the federal government go predominantly to hospitals and then are distributed to offset the costs of training. The system we have now is large, unwieldy, immobile, and not at all well suited to reflect the dynamic needs of the population.

Most people in the GME business are very frightened that the money from the government will go away and that will cause big trouble. I am not so sure it would be all that bad. After all, government money comes with government rules. And government rules are not always that nimble when you need them to be.

An alternate method might be to consider funding GME training within the health care system. The government contributes somewhere between $10.5 billion and $13.5 billion toward GME. That seems like a lot of money and in some respects it is. As a country we spend over $2.5 trillion annually on health care. That puts the fraction of money spent on GME at just about 0.5% of our annual expenditures for health care in the United States. If we were to give contracts for training that included the costs of training with some plan for the trainee (or her employer) paying the cost off after the physician enters the workforce, the places that train physicians would have to consider their economic model for training quality physicians to essentially get their money back. This would force those of us who provide education to rethink how we deliver a quality education product. It would also force prospective trainees to consider just what kind of education they were "buying." And it would force future employers to develop relationships and investment in quality educational environments, as they would eventually be the ones likely to pay off the contracts in order to secure their workforce. In the end, the cost would be more evenly distributed over the private and public sectors because the revenues to pay off the contract costs would come from all sources.

I am fully aware that such a scheme is a pretty unlikely thing to occur but it is a thought. What we are doing now is not matching the resource of physicians with the populations of the country. If anything, the problem seems to be worsening. We could try to pour more doctors on and hope that they will disperse to less well-served areas—that will be very expensive. We could continue to accept markedly different physician-to-patient ratios but that will lead to (or maintain) either inequitable reimbursement schemes or unjustified variations in utilization. We could realize that we are using a barely modified version of a century old training system to deal with 21st century health care and really rethink what we are doing—but that will take leadership and follower-ship and political will. Not real likely. Most likely we will keep doing the same thing in much the same way and keep expecting different results. And six years hence, perhaps I'll write about this again.

At least you, dear reader, can read this valuable information from Drs Azarow and Cusick and the contributors. And with that knowledge you can do more and better things with the system we have. Perhaps the children who are helped by this knowledge will grow up to do a better job of fixing the system than we. With luck, some of them will become well versed in geriatric surgery. We may need them.

Ronald F. Martin, MD
Department of Surgery
Marshfield Clinic
1000 North Oak Avenue
Marshfield, WI 54449, USA

E-mail address:
martin.ronald@marshfieldclinic.org

# Preface

# Pediatric Surgery

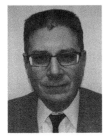 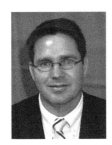

Kenneth S. Azarow, MD    Robert A. Cusick, MD
*Guest Editors*

We feel privileged and honored to be guest editors of this edition of the *Surgical Clinics of North America*. It has been 6 years since the last pediatric surgery edition of *Surgical Clinics of North America* was published with Dr Mike Chen as guest editor. Given the new era of residency training with decreased work hours, increased postgraduate fellowships, and a redefined scope of general surgical practice, we have dedicated this issue to the graduating chief resident in general surgery. It has been said that to be an accomplished pediatric surgeon, one first must be an accomplished general surgeon. Each article is written with the intention of providing newly practicing general surgeons a synopsis of what they should be aware of regarding each of the pediatric conditions discussed. We realize that many of these conditions will not be part of the general surgeon's operative practice; however, it is anticipated that the general surgeon will likely come across or be referred to the disease entities discussed in this edition and thus will need to be prepared.

We have dedicated an entire article to the management of pain in the pediatric population. We felt very strongly about leading off with this article since pain is often underappreciated in this population. Furthermore, we wanted to capture the significant advances that have been made in the last two decades. This is also the only article not authored or coauthored by a pediatric surgeon. These accomplished authors demonstrate that this topic is something that you do not have to be a pediatric surgeon to appreciate or understand. As for the rest of the articles, we feel that we have gathered a cadre of some of the leading experts in the world on a variety of pediatric surgical topics.

The article describing the most common operations we do in children, hernias, hydroceles, and undescended testicles, is coauthored by one of the true hernia masters of our generation, Dr Robert Fitzgibbons, who will add his particular expertise in discussing adolescent hernia repair. This is perhaps the most common arena for general surgeons and pediatric surgeons to overlap and frequently their approaches to these patients are quite divergent. It is important for us as editors and pediatric surgeons to convey that pediatric hernias, especially in the premature and ex-premature population,

Surg Clin N Am 92 (2012) xvii–xix
doi:10.1016/j.suc.2012.03.018
0039-6109/12/$ – see front matter © 2012 Elsevier Inc. All rights reserved.

**surgical.theclinics.com**

can be among the most technically demanding we do. In addition, parents and the lay public consider hernia repairs among the most routine of procedures; thus, there is little tolerance for poor outcome.

The next two articles (intussusception/appendectomy/Meckel's and pyloric stenosis) represent those procedures classically done and taught to general surgeons. Of all the procedures we discuss, these are still most likely present in the community general surgeon's practice today. As with all our articles, there is an emphasis on understanding resuscitation as well as pre- and postoperative management. Surely, if there is a problem that develops in these patients, it is most often associated with the pre- and postoperative care and less likely with the technical aspects of the procedure.

Gastroesophageal reflux disease and obesity surgery are very common entities in both adults and children. General and pediatric surgeons both commonly perform antireflux procedures and obesity surgery is becoming another area where crossover exists between minimally invasive general and pediatric surgeons. These articles emphasize the differences in evaluation and expected outcomes in these two very different age groups. The unique feature about gastroesophageal reflux disease in infants as opposed to adults is that they all have it and they almost all outgrow it. When to intervene is a skill that can only be gained with experience in many cases. Childhood obesity represents perhaps the most important public health concern of our generation. We recognize that most pediatric surgeons will not do bariatric surgery; however, we also recognize that as pediatric surgeons we cannot turn our backs on the disease that is likely to dominate our society's adolescent age group for the next one to two decades.

The next major area where crossover between specialties occurs is with congenital head and neck lesions, and ovarian lesions. Head and neck lesions in children, including the thyroid, are commonly done by pediatric surgeons, general surgeons, and otolaryngologists. We hope you will enjoy this comprehensive overview. Pediatric surgeons also act as gynecologists for the pediatric age group. Since teratomas and ovarian masses are often dealt with by gynecologists and occasionally encountered by general surgeons as unexpected masses at laparotomy, we feel this article has particular interest.

Pediatric surgeons are also thoracic surgeons. The ability to surgically address congenital and acquired thoracic disease is a common part of every pediatric surgeon's practice. There are still several disease processes that are still more commonly managed by general surgeons as well as other specialists: diseases such as spontaneous pneumothorax, empyema, and esophageal and airway foreign bodies, to name a few. In addition, the operation which perhaps defines our specialty more than any other, tracheal-esophageal fistula, will be reviewed. With that in mind, an entire article is devoted to the management of congenital diaphragmatic hernia. Perhaps no other disease entity other than appendicitis has had as much literature devoted to it. The concept of gentle ventilation has been adopted widely and the use of extracorporeal oxygenation has decreased significantly. The overall result is an expected survival of approximately 70% as opposed to the 50% we were classically taught in medical school 20 to 25 years ago. Preventing lung injury is a theme that all providers who take care of critical care patients can utilize.

One of the most popular advances within the specialty of pediatric surgery has been the development of minimally invasive chest wall reconstruction. It is not unusual for the general or thoracic surgeon to be consulted on a pectus patient. Counseling these patients is done by a variety of providers on a very large scale. While an excellent source of information, the Internet is often biased and does not tailor its information to the individual patient. This article reports just how significant the recent advances in the field have been. Whether a surgeon does these procedures or not, knowing the correct information based on all of the recent advances in the field is paramount to advising these patients.

The next group of articles is those that comprise another group of diseases that partly define pediatric surgery as a specialty: neonatal bowel obstruction to include Hirschsprungs, meconium ileus, imperforate anus, atresias, necrotizing enterocolitis, abdominal wall defects, and the devastating complication of these disease processes—short gut. The nuances of these diagnoses need to be understood by anyone undertaking the surgical care of one of these infants. The follow-up article to neonatal bowel obstruction refers to short gut and vascular access. Specifically, this article relates to the prior article by reemphasizing the principles to be followed at the first laparotomy in order to prevent short-gut physiology. Due to the appearance of gastroschisis and omphalocele at delivery, the article on abdominal wall reconstruction of congenital and secondary defects is another topic that defines pediatric surgery. The critical care principles of abdominal hypertension and compartment syndrome are applicable to all surgeons who take care of large abdominal wall hernias, see abdominal trauma, and deal with complex abdominal wounds. It is our hope that this article will give the general surgeon an appreciation for the complexity and severity of the illnesses that pediatric surgeons deal with on a daily basis.

Finally, some of the greatest advances in oncologic care have occurred in the pediatric population. Wilm's tumor, for example, has served as a model to treat a variety of solid tumors over the years. The article on pediatric malignancies should demonstrate the dedication and scientific commitment toward children that we all share. In addition, we have dedicated a separate article to a group of lesions that one can encounter at any stage of life: congenital vascular and lymphatic malformations. The Boston Children's Vascular Group provides a worldwide referral service and has personally offered very valuable opinions on our patients here in Omaha. During the past 30 years our understanding, nomenclature, and management of these lesions, based on their research, have developed considerably.

We would like to thank all of the faculty and residents we trained with at Walter Reed Army Medical Center, University of Cincinnati, Toronto's Hospital for Sick Children, and Seattle Children's Hospital and Medical Center for teaching us more than we ever gave back. To all the residents for whom we have played a small role in their surgical training (either general or pediatric surgical)—we truly dedicate this edition to you. Finally, we would like to thank our wives, Judy and Julie, for all of their love and support as we have progressed in our careers.

Kenneth S. Azarow, MD
University of Nebraska College of Medicine &
Children's Hospital & Medical Center
8200 Dodge Street
Omaha, NE 68114, USA

Robert A. Cusick, MD
University of Nebraska College of Medicine &
Children's Hospital & Medical Center
8200 Dodge Street
Omaha, NE 68114, USA

E-mail addresses:
kazarow@childrensomaha.org (K.S. Azarow)
rcusick@childrensomaha.org (R.A. Cusick)

# Pain Management in the Pediatric Surgical Patient

Vance Y. Sohn, MD[a], David Zenger, MD[b], Scott R. Steele, MD[a],*

## KEYWORDS

- Pediatric • Anesthesia • PCA • Pain • Analgesia

## KEY POINTS

- Inadequate anesthesia, even in neonates and children has found to have deleterious effects.
- Anatomic factors ranging from high oxygen consumption and low alveolar volume, to a larger occiput and tongue can result in more rapid oxygen desaturation during sedation and should be assessed periprocedural.
- The liberal use of local anesthetics during painful procedures and intraoperatively can be helpful in preventing and managing pain both during and postoperatively in the pediatric population.
- A combination of opioid and nonopioid classes of medications are useful in managing pain after major surgery in children.
- Treating postoperative pain in pediatric surgical patients is similar to that of adults, and may include successful use of patient controlled analgesia and epidural catheters.
- Neonatal abstinence syndrome refers to withdrawal symptoms from noxious stimuli that neonates experience in utero exposures, and at-risk patients should be followed for signs that may require intervention.

Before the current appreciation of the potential adverse effects of unabated painful stimuli in pediatric patients, preterm and term infants often underwent procedures and operations with inadequate analgesia. This practice was partly perpetuated by the false notion that neonates cannot sense pain or that the periprocedural side effects

Financial Disclosure: The authors have no financial disclosures pertinent to this manuscript.

[a] Department of Surgery, Madigan Army Medical Center, 9040A Fitzsimmons Drive, Tacoma, WA 98431, USA; [b] Department of Anesthesia, Madigan Army Medical Center, 9040A Fitzsimmons Drive, Tacoma, WA 98431, USA
* 9606 Piperhill Drive SE Olympia, WA 98513.
*E-mail address:* harkersteele@mac.com

Surg Clin N Am 92 (2012) 471–485
doi:10.1016/j.suc.2012.03.002
0039-6109/12/$ – see front matter Published by Elsevier Inc.

of anesthesia were worse than the actual procedure. It is now generally accepted that the neonatal stage of life is characterized by a high sensitivity to pain, and that even a developing fetus can mount a stress response to noxious stimuli at an age as early as 8 to 10 weeks of gestation.[1,2] Pain, according to the International Association for the Study of Pain, is always subjective and is learned through experiences related to injury in early life.[3] Exposing neonatal and pediatric patients to increasing and unneeded painful stimuli does not necessarily translate into a higher tolerance or an improved pain threshold in later years. In fact, it may be more likely to be counterproductive.

In both the inpatient and outpatient settings, inadequate analgesia has been studied and found to have deleterious effects.[4–7] For instance, preterm infants undergoing anesthesia with only nitrous oxide and muscle relaxants were found to have a significantly increased stress response when compared with those receiving fentanyl as the primary anethestic.[8] In another study, infants who had undergone circumcision responded more intensely to subsequent immunization injections than did their uncircumcised peers, indicating an adverse hyperresponsive effect to painful stimuli.[6] Although the ramifications of inadequate pain control, such as future pain hypersensitivity or altered development of neuroanatomy, have yet to be fully understood, the early adverse effects are obvious and favor the use of appropriate procedure-based analgesia. Even beyond the neonatal period, these problems can persist despite the ability of the patient to express their concerns. This may lead to difficulties that extend beyond the noxious stimulus itself, and manifest in psychological or relationship troubles. Often, parents and providers either diminish or do not believe a child's self-report of pain; instead improperly believing the child is exaggerating their suffering, or focus inappropriately on their own frustrations of dealing with a "fussy" child.[9,10] These false assumptions and mischaracterizations may ultimately lead to minor, or even major, issues of a complex nature stemming from a lack of trust or miscommunication. Therefore, for all surgeons dealing with pediatric patients, it is imperative to recognize the importance of periprocedural pain management and the various methods available to evaluate and optimize results. This article focuses on the appropriate pain management of pediatric surgical patients before, during, and after their hospitalization, and outlines strategies to assess pain levels while avoiding common pitfalls of improper treatment.

## PAIN ASSESSMENT

The ideal pain assessment scale is simple, cheap, reproducible, accurately assesses various pain surrogates, and applies to both verbal and nonverbal pediatric patients. Although a multitude of age-specific pain assessment scales currently exist, a single widely accepted, easily administered universal tool remains lacking. The importance of proper identification and treatment of pain cannot be understated; therefore, a basic understanding of the tools available to the surgeon is essential. The various components of these tools are briefly reviewed.

The accurate clinical assessment of pain relies on different formats and tools, including self-reporting, behavior observational pain scales, physiologic measures of pain, and multidimensional pain assessments.[4] Self-reporting relies on the cognitive ability of the patient to effectively convey their discomfort. Although neonates may express pain through crying or physical gestures/grimacing, toddlers generally begin to articulate words for pain by 18 months of age. However, sufficient development to accurately report degrees of pain can take up to 3 to 4 years of age.[11] This format is considered the "most reliable indicator of the existence and intensity of pain," in contradiction to the previously discussed parental and provider assessments.[4,12]

In contrast, observational pain assessments are perhaps the most variable and subjective in nature, although when trying to assess pain severity in nonverbal patients, they can be a valuable measure. In this method, secondary evaluation using cues from the patient are assessed to provide a score. This tool, often performed by nurses or parents, is most effective when combined with the other assessment techniques because of the aforementioned subjective weaknesses inherent to this type of scale. When using observational assessments, one must be aware that other signs of distress (ie, strangers, unfamiliar environment, fear of needles) can confound the clinical picture through mimicking the same behaviors elicited by the pain response. Similarly, when dealing with physiologic measures of pain, the same limitation exists. For example, tachycardia, hypertension, and diaphoresis can be clinical derangements observed with both pain and anxiety, or may be secondary to an underlying organic problem in the perioperative period. The inherent limitations of these assessment tools, therefore, make the multidimensional assessment the most effective and clinically relevant method compared with single-parameter measurements.[13,14] As the name implies, multiple parameters are assessed to determine the overall pain burden. Generally, younger infants and toddlers (up to 3 or 4 years of age) are assessed using a combination of physiologic and observational scales, whereas self-reporting and physiologic or observational scales are effective in older children. As a rule of thumb, neurologically normal children can start using the standard adult pain assessment scales around 7 to 8 years of age.

Numerous one- and multiple-dimensional pediatric pain assessment tools are currently available. A discussion of these is beyond the scope of this summary, but Franck and colleagues[4] provide a more comprehensive list and description of each. Age-appropriate scales are institution-specific and the surgeon should become familiar with what is available and commonly used by their ancillary staff. More helpful to surgeons is the familiarity with normal developmental milestones and responses to pain of pediatric patients. Infants younger than 6 months have no expression of anticipatory fear. Rather, social cues are obtained from parents and caregivers. Between 6 and 18 months of age is when anticipatory fear of painful experiences begins developing. The next age group, 18 to 24 months of age, is when children begin expressing words of pain, but again, not until approximately 3 years of age do they have the cognitive ability to localize and identify the painful sources. By this age, children can more reliably assess their pain but continue to depend on visual cues for localization. Finally, by 5 to 7 years of age, children have improved understanding of pain and the ability to localize and cooperate.[15]

## NONPHARMACOLOGIC PAIN CONTROL

Methods of nonpharmacologic pain control are well described and, although frequently underused, are often recommended to improve overall pain management.[16–18] These categories include cognitive, behavioral, and physical interventions. For the surgeon treating patients in acute pain, these interventions should be used to augment, rather than supplant, other methods to provide superior analgesia. On the downside, although these methods are effective, they can be costly and time- and resource-prohibitive. Furthermore, extensive education of providers and patients, and, most importantly, a willing and mentally developed patient are required for optimal success.

The goal of cognitive and behavioral therapies is to distract the patient and shift the focus from the pain-inducing source to something else. Examples of cognitive interventions include music, guided imagery, distraction, and hypnosis.[19–21] With programs involving the use of these agents, several studies have noted improved pain control over standard therapies.[4,18] Behavioral techniques include breathing, biofeedback exercises, and relaxation techniques.[22–24] These methods have been shown to not only decrease the levels of pain but also improve physiologic parameters, such as blood pressure and tachycardia. Nonpharmacologic physical interventions include pet therapy, heat and cold application, massage or touch, and acupuncture.[25] The essence of each of these methods involves off-setting the sole reliance on more traditional methods of pain control through incorporation of these alternative techniques.

## PROCEDURAL ANESTHESIA

For surgeons who do not routinely care for children, having to perform an invasive procedure on a child already in distress outside the more controlled setting of an operating room can be anxiety-provoking. The surgeon has to be concerned with not only the intended medical procedure but also a multitude of factors, such as patient maturity, existing pain, previous pain exposures, and the parent-child dynamic. These factors must be rapidly assessed to decide whether to perform the procedure in the operating room or elsewhere, most commonly the emergency department. This complex dynamic, in addition to the simple fact that surgeons typically perform painful invasive procedures, normally mandates that sedation is used along with analgesia. In the authors' experience, sedation provides relief to the patient, surgeon, and parents, and usually allows the procedure to be performed faster, easier, and ultimately more safely.

The technical requirements and certifications necessary to provide conscious sedation are beyond the scope of this article. However, one must remember that, wherever the procedure is performed, at a minimum, appropriately trained medical personnel, continuous hemodynamic and respiratory monitoring, and the capability to rapidly establish a definitive airway must be immediately available. To provide optimal patient care, surgeons must also be educated and experienced in proper pediatric procedural sedation. When administering sedation, the surgeon must be aware of some key differences between children and adults. Among the numerous anatomic and physiologic differences, the most relevant difference during sedation involves the relatively high oxygen consumption combined with the low functional residual capacity of supine sedated children. Clinically, this manifests as a more rapid oxygen desaturation during periods of apnea compared with adults.[26] Other notable distinctions include the disproportionately larger head compared with body size. The larger occiput can act as a fulcrum and lead to upper airway obstruction. This mandates careful positioning of the head to avoid inadvertent airway collapse. Additionally, the tongue is larger in the oropharynx, and can be another source of upper airway obstruction, especially when children are heavily sedated. All of these factors must be assessed during a preprocedural physical examination to anticipate any problems, and be constantly reevaluated during the intervention despite what may seem to be stable vital signs.

Some of the most commonly used sedatives are listed in **Table 1**. When administering these medications, the use of concomitant parenteral analgesia must be considered. Also, no single medication concoction or regimen is always more effective than the other, because clinical effect depends on prior exposure, dosing, and physiologic differences, such as volume of distribution and drug clearance. Surgeons should be aware of the drugs available at their own institution, and if any clinical practice guidelines are in place that would normally require the use of a particular class of medication over another. For periprocedural sedation, in the absence of anesthesia support, the authors prefer ketamine in conjunction with local anesthetics for children. Advantages of ketamine include a rapid onset of anesthesia, minimal respiratory depression, maintenance of or an increase in cardiac output, bronchodilation, and

| Table 1 Commonly used sedatives | | | | |
|---|---|---|---|---|
| Name | Route | Dose (mg/kg) | Onset | Indications |
| *Barbiturates* | | | | |
| Methohexital | IV | 1–2 | 1 min | Sedation |
| | IM | 5–10 | 2–10 min | |
| | PR | 18–25 | 5–15 min | |
| Pentobarbital | IV | 1–3 | 1 min | Sedation |
| | IM | 2–6 | 10–15 min | |
| *Benzodiazepines* | | | | |
| Midazolam | PO | 0.3–0.7 | 10–20 min | Anxiolysis, sedation, amnesia |
| | IV | 0.05–0.2 | 1–5 min | |
| | IM | 0.1–0.15 | <5 min | |
| Lorazepam | PO | 0.05 | 60 min | Anxiolysis, sedation, amnesia |
| | IV | 0.05 | 15–30 min | |
| | IM | 0.05 | 30–60 min | |
| *Other Sedatives* | | | | |
| Chloral hydrate | PR | 25–50 | 10–20 min | Sedation |
| Etomidate | IV | 0.1–0.3 | 30–60 s | Induction agent, sedation |
| Ketamine | IV | 0.05–2 | 30 s | Dissociative state, analgesia |
| | IM | 3–7 | 3–4 min | |
| Propofol | IV | 2–2.5 | 30 s | Induction agent, sedation |

*Abbreviations:* IM, intramuscular; IV, intravenous; PR, per rectum.
*Data from* Refs.[15,25,28,33,42]

inherent analgesic properties. Its availability in intramuscular form can obviate the need for intravenous access. On the downside, the surgeon should keep in mind that any negative effect as a result of ketamine administration cannot be reversed, because no specific reversal agent is available.

Ketamine is a dissociative anesthetic that acts through direct action on the cortex and limbic system. The well-known side effect of an emergence reaction, which can manifest as vivid dreams, hallucinations, or frank delirium, occurs in up to 12% of adults, but less frequently in children. These reactions can often be thwarted by pretreatment with benzodiazepines. Relative contraindications to the use of ketamine include the presence of suspected closed head injury (elevated intracranial pressure), uncontrolled hypertension, psychosis, and thyrotoxicosis.[27–29]

Of the commercially available benzodiazepines, midazolam is most often used because of the short half-life necessary for procedural sedation. Midazolam provides anxiolysis, sedation, and amnesia. Because of its versatility in both adult and pediatric patients, it tends to be readily available in most emergency departments and nursing units. In addition to the usual intramuscular, intravenous, and oral forms, midazolam is also available for intranasal and rectal administration. The dosing of midazolam is variable and depends on the age and weight of the child. Caution should be exercised with the intravenous administration in neonates because of the reported risk of severe hypotension and seizures. These effects may be compounded if used in conjunction with a narcotic such as fentanyl. Besides the adverse effects observed in neonates, another potentially dangerous side effect of all benzodiazepines is the risk of respiratory depression through centrally mediated effects. Flumazenil is the reversal agent for benzodiazepine-induced respiratory depression (**Table 2**).

**Table 2**
**Reversal agents**

| Name | Reversal of | Route | Dose | Onset (min) | Duration |
|------|-------------|-------|------|-------------|----------|
| Flumazenil[a] | Benzodiazepines | IV | 0.01 mg/kg | 1–3 | <1 h |
| Naloxone[b] | Narcotics | | | | |
| Birth to 5 y | | IV | 0.01 mg/kg | <2 | 20–60 min |
| >5 y | | IV | 2 mg | <2 | 20–60 min |

*Abbreviations:* IM, intramuscular; IV, intravenous.
   [a] For flumazenil, can readminister every 1 min at maximum dose of 0.2 mg/min for a total of 1 mg.
   [b] For naloxone, consider starting continuous infusion, because half-life is shorter than narcotics.
   *Data from* Taketomo CK, Hodding JH, Kraus DM. Pediatric dosage handbook. 15th edition. Hudson (OH): Lexi-Comp; 2008. p. 753–5, 1228–30.

Other popular alternatives include the use of barbiturates, such as pentobarbital or methohexital.[25] However, barbiturates are more likely than benzodiazepines to produce potentially lethal side effects of respiratory depression or hypotension. Therefore, as with all of these cases, proper monitoring and vigilance is mandatory. The authors have found that barbiturates are useful for the occasional pediatric patient who experiences paradoxic agitation and disinhibition with a low dose of benzodiazepines. Propofol is another commonly used sedative that may be selected in ventilated patients, although it can be used effectively in nonintubated patients by experienced anesthesia providers. Its rapid onset and recovery, along with its intrinsic amnestic properties, make it an appealing sedative. In conclusion, except for ketamine, one should keep in mind that all of the sedatives discussed contain no intrinsic analgesic property.

## PHARMACOLOGIC PAIN CONTROL
### Local Anesthetics

The liberal use of local anesthetics during painful procedures and intraoperatively can help prevent and manage pain in the pediatric population. Local anesthetics block action potentials along the nerve axon and prevent depolarization of the nerve. The indications and uses are often provider-dependent and too broad to summarize here; however, use may significantly decrease the pain experienced, especially in noncommunicative pediatric patients. Typical dosage and other important properties of commonly selected local anesthetics are listed in **Table 3**.

**Table 3**
**Local anesthetics**

| Name | Maximum Dose (mg/kg) | Onset of Action | Duration (min) |
|------|----------------------|-----------------|----------------|
| Chloroprocaine | 60 | Fast | 30–60 |
| Lidocaine | 5 | Intermediate | 60–90 |
| Lidocaine with epinephrine | 7 | Intermediate | 60–90 |
| Bupivacaine | 2.5 | Slow | 150–360 |
| Ropivacaine | 2.5–4 | Slow | 150–360 |

*Data from* Taketomo CK, Hodding JH, Kraus DM. Pediatric dosage handbook. 15th edition. Hudson (OH): Lexi-Comp; 2008. p. 990–1, and Wilder RT. Local anesthetics for the pediatric patient. Pediatr Clin North Am 2000;47(3):545–58.

A limitation of local anesthetics in nonsedated patients is the pain associated during initial infiltration. Minimizing the pain can be achieved in several ways. One author encourages the following techniques: using the smallest possible needle to form a skin wheal (30-gauge), injecting the subcutaneous tissue first before raising the skin wheal, neutralizing the pH of the local anesthetic using sodium bicarbonate (0.1–0.2 mEq per 1 mL of 1% or 2% lidocaine, 0.1 mEq per 2.9 mL of bupivacaine), using warmed solution, and slowly injecting the medication.[15,30,31] Another helpful tip includes using the initial site of skin infiltration as the starting point for further advancement. This technique is particularly useful when performing field blocks.

When injecting local anesthetic, central nervous system or cardiovascular toxicity can occur from exceeding the maximum recommended dosage (see **Table 3**) or through inadvertent direct intravascular injection. Providers who use local anesthetic should be aware of the signs and symptoms of toxicity and the treatment. In the awake patient, the first signs of toxicity can include a metallic taste, ringing of the ears, auditory disturbances, muscular twitching, or tingling around the mouth or lips. Eventually, this can progress to seizures and ultimately cardiovascular collapse. These symptoms may not clinically present progressively; for instance, a sufficiently toxic dose can lead to cardiovascular collapse without causing seizures. More concerning, in intubated patients cardiovascular collapse may often be the first sign of toxicity. Treatment involves immediate cessation of anesthetic injection and appropriate supportive care that may require advanced cardiac life support protocols. Cardiac toxicity from local anesthetic overdose, especially bupivacaine, may be responsive to the use of intravenous intralipids.[32] This situation is best avoided altogether by accurately calculating the maximum dose based on the patients weight and not exceeding this amount. Toxicity more often occurs with inadvertent intravascular injection. If performing a field block, continuous movement of the needle should avoid a large bolus dose. If performing a single isolated injection, one must first aspirate before injection to ensure the needle is not unintentionally located intravascular.

Topical anesthetics are commonly used and are excellent forms of anesthesia before painful procedures, such as establishing intravenous access, lumbar punctures, and port access. Different topical solutions exist for specifically intact skin, violated skin, and mucous membranes. Examples include EMLA (eutectic mixture of local anesthetics, containing 2.5% each of lidocaine and prilocaine; APP Pharmaceuticals, Schaumburg, IL, USA), LET (lidocaine, epinephrine, tetracaine), or TAC (tetracaine, adrenaline, cocaine) creams/ointments. For surgical patients, these topical anesthetics have little role in routine pain control. In older children, they may minimize pain associated with initial skin puncture if placed on the skin before injection of local anesthesia.[4,25]

### Opioid and Nonopioid Analgesia

Determining the amount and type of appropriate analgesia after painful stimuli is primarily based on the degree of insult, the expected duration of pain, and prior use of medications. Just like in adults, nonopioids may be preferable over opioids; however, in surgical patients, a combination of the two is usually used. This section briefly reviews commonly used narcotics and nonsteroidal anti-inflammatory drugs (NSAIDs) in pediatrics (**Table 4**).

The adverse effects of narcotics are well known and include respiratory depression, constipation, central nervous system depression, sedation, and the possibility of dependence. Narcotics should be administered to neonates cautiously, because these patients are often more sensitive to narcotic effects and resultant respiratory depression.[25] Commonly used parenteral opioids include morphine, hydromorphone,

**Table 4**
**Commonly used analgesics and dose equivalence**

| Name | Route | Dose | Morphine Equivalence Ratio | Onset (min) | Duration (h) |
|---|---|---|---|---|---|
| *Opioid analgesics* | | | | | |
| Morphine | IV | 0.05–0.1 mg/kg | 1 | 5–10 | 3–4 |
| | IM/SC | 0.1–0.2 mg/kg | | 10–30 | 4–5 |
| | PO | 0.3–0.5 mg/kg | | 30–60 | 4–5 |
| Fentanyl | IV | 1 µg/kg | 80–100 | 1–2 | 0.5–1 |
| | PO (oralet) | 10–15 µg/kg | | 15 | |
| Hydromorphone | IV | 0.015 mg/kg | 5–7 | 5–10 | 3–4 |
| Methadone | IV | 0.1 mg/kg | 0.25–1 | 5–10 | 4–24 |
| | PO, IM, SC | 0.1 mg/kg | | 30–60 | 4–24 |
| Meperidine | IV | 1–1.5 mg/kg | 0.1 | 5–10 | 3–4 |
| | PO | 1.5–2 mg/kg | | 30–60 | 2–4 |
| Oxycodone | PO | 0.05–0.015 mg/kg | | 30–60 | 3–4 |
| Codeine | PO | 0.5–1 mg/kg | | 30–60 | 3–4 |
| *Non-opioid analgesics* | | | | | |
| Ketoralac | IV | 0.5 mg/kg | | 30 | 4–6 |
| Acetaminophen | PO | 10–15 mg/kg | | 10–60 | 2–5 |
| | PR | 10–20 mg/kg | | 10–60 | 2–5 |
| Ibuprofen | PO | 4–10 mg/kg | | 50–90 | 6–8 |
| Naproxen | PO | 5–7 mg/kg | | 60–120 | 8–10 |

*Abbreviations:* IM, intramuscular; IV, intravenous; SC, subcutaneous; PR, per rectum.
*Data from* Refs.[15,28,41,42]

and fentanyl. Of these, morphine is the most versatile and readily available in the oral, intravenous, and intramuscular Forms. Its notable adverse effects include seizures in neonates and histamine release, which may clinically mimic allergic reactions. It should be used with caution in patients with renal insufficiency, because toxic metabolites can accumulate in these patients.

Hydromorphone is a more potent narcotic that also acts on the opiate receptors of the central nervous system and is available in intravenous and oral forms. It can be used as an antitussive medication, although not routinely recommended as a first-line agent. Hydromorphone may cause less sedation, nausea, and pruritis compared with morphine, because of its reduced histamine effect. Finally, fentanyl is useful for short procedures because of its rapid onset and short duration of action. It is available for intravenous, transdermal (patch), and transmucosal (oralet) administration.

Like the other narcotics, fentanyl has a high potential for dependence with prolonged use. If using the intravenous form, large rapid boluses should be avoided because of the risk of skeletal muscle and chest wall rigidity, resulting in impaired ventilation, respiratory distress, apnea, bronchoconstriction, and laryngospasm. The transmucosal preparation is useful in children undergoing frequent painful procedures, such as daily dressing changes after burn injury.[33]

All of these narcotics can be used to address postoperative pain in patient-controlled analgesia (PCA) and discussed in the following section.

Common oral opiates include codeine, oxycodone, methadone, and meperidine. The latter two are also available in intravenous forms. Codeine's side effects are notable for possible severe nausea and emesis. Like morphine, it can cause histamine release with resultant allergic-like reactions or even hypotension. Furthermore, dose adjustments for renal insufficiency must be performed. Finally, codeine is ineffective in 10% of the American population because of the lack of enzymatic intrahepatic conversion to its active form. In these patients, alternatives should be sought, such as oxycodone. Oxycodone tends to be much less nauseating than codeine, with similar onset and duration of action. It is available in sustained-release tablet form for 24-hour pain control; however, it is not approved for patients younger than 18 years of age.

Methadone can be prescribed for moderate to severe pain unresponsive to non-narcotics, but is often reserved for the treatment of narcotic dependence. Its duration of action is much longer than other members of this class (4–24 hours), and increased duration is noted with repeat dosing. Methadone is commonly used for the treatment of neonatal abstinence syndrome (discussed later). Dosing for both intravenous and oral methadone are the same. Intravenously, it is given as 0.1 mg/kg every 4 hours for the first two to three doses. After this, doses can be repeated every 6 to 12 hours, for a total maximum dose of 10 mg.[28] Because of the accumulative effect of methadone, decreases in dose or frequency may be required 2 to 5 days after initial therapy. Finally, meperidine is less frequently used because of its toxicity profile and the availability of other suitable alternatives. It is not recommended for prolonged use or in PCA because of the metabolite (normeperidine) buildup that decreases the seizure threshold. It also has known catastrophic interactions when used in patients taking monoamine oxidase inhibitors. At low doses (0.1–0.25 mg/kg), it can be used to stop shivering.

The final class of medications briefly reviewed here is the nonopioid analgesics. Commonly used medications in this category include acetaminophen, ibuprofen, ketorolac, and naproxen. Despite its almost universal use in adults as an analgesic or for its platelet-inhibiting effects, aspirin should be avoided in children because of the risk of Reye syndrome. Ibuprofen and acetaminophen are appropriate alternatives. Ketorolac, a parenteral NSAID, is a potent analgesic commonly used to treat pediatric pain. Intravenous ketorolac at 1 mg/kg is comparable to 0.1 mg/kg of intravenous morphine. Perioperatively, ketorolac should be used cautiously, because it inhibits platelet aggregation and may prolong bleeding time. Because of this, ketorolac is contraindicated in patients with suspected or confirmed intracerebral bleeding, hemorrhagic diathesis, or incomplete hemostasis, or at high risk of bleeding. Furthermore, ketorolac is not approved for use in children younger than 2 years and those with renal disease. Single-bolus dosing for children between 2 and 16 years of age is 0.5 mg/kg, up to a maximum dose of 15 mg. For multiple dose treatment, dosing is less clear, but the usual accepted dose is 0.5 mg/kg every 6 hours.[34]

## ISSUES IN POSTOPERATIVE CARE

Similarities exist when treating postoperative pain in pediatric surgical patients and in adults. If the gastrointestinal tract is intact or not compromised, oral analgesics are often preferred. Parenteral analgesia can then be reserved for breakthrough pain refractory to standard therapy, or if other methods cannot provide adequate pain control. Pediatric surgery–specific topics are discussed in the next section.

Epidural analgesia has become an indispensable tool for managing severe postoperative pain in neonates, infants, and children after a wide variety of painful surgical procedures. Its use has been found to reduce the surgical stress response and hospitalization time, and may improve outcomes in certain pediatric populations.[35] In these patients, besides cardiac conditions, thoracic procedures in which patients might benefit from epidural analgesia include resection of malignant or congenital malformations within the lung, tracheobronchial tree, or esophagus. A procedure often unique to pediatric surgeons is the treatment of chest wall deformities, specifically pectus excavatum.[36,37] Although an effective procedure, the necessary chest wall alteration to correct the depression often results in significant pain. Two prospective, randomized trials evaluating postoperative pain management in children undergoing repair for this condition, along with other trials, highlight the potential benefits of improved pain control using epidural catheters in older children undergoing any major thoracic procedure.

Both randomized studies, published in 2007, examined the efficacy of morphine or fentanyl PCA versus fentanyl and local anesthetic epidural analgesia in patients undergoing pectus repair. The first trial randomized 28 children to fentanyl PCA versus a fentanyl/bupivacaine epidural treatment and found no significant difference in pain scores or complication rates.[38] The second study randomized 40 children also undergoing pectus excavatum repair to morphine PCA versus a fentanyl/ropivacaine epidural.[39] Unlike the first, this study found superior pain control with use of the epidural. More recently, a larger, single-institution, retrospective review was published of 117 patients undergoing Nuss bar placement for pectus excavatum.[40] Most patients had epidurals infusing a combination of narcotic and local anesthetic. Excellent pain control was observed with use of the epidural in this patient cohort.

These data suggest that epidurals for painful thoracic procedures may be effectively used for not only the treatment of pectus excavatum but also other invasive thoracic procedures. An important component of this care, however, is the involvement of a pediatric acute pain service.[41] It is the authors' belief that having dedicated providers with experience placing and monitoring the efficacy of epidurals, and identifying and managing their inherent complications, leads to successful patient outcomes. In their experience, properly adjusting dosages or composition of infused epidural medication, or altogether changing analgesic modalities because of suboptimal placement of the catheter or inadequate pain resolution, are notable benefits of dedicated teams.

As the name implies, PCAs allow patients to manage their own pain control and are often used in the postoperative setting after major thoracoabdominal surgery. In pediatrics, their use is limited to patients who have the cognitive ability to determine the presence of pain and activate the mechanism for narcotic administration, which typically occurs around 5 or 6 years of age. This limitation means that for younger children, postoperative pain control is highly reliant on nurses and other caregivers who need to understand the nature of the procedure performed and age-based pain manifestation. Standard dosing for PCA is listed in **Table 5**. Besides "as needed" bolus doses of narcotics, orders for longer-acting medication to cover baseline pain should be administered to the patients. Based on clinician discretion, baseline coverage can be achieved by setting a basal rate for continuous intravenous infusion of narcotic

**Table 5**
**Patient controlled analgesia dosing**

| Drug | Basal Rate (mcg/kg/h) | Bolus Dose (μg/kg) | Lockout Period (min) | Maximum Dose (h) | Intravenous Rescue Dose (μg/kg) |
|---|---|---|---|---|---|
| Morphine | 10–30 | 10–30 | 6–10 | 100–150 | 50 |
| Hydromorphone | 3–5 | 3–5 | 6–10 | 15–24 | 10 |
| Fentanyl | 0.5–1 | 0.5–1 | 6–8 | 2–4 | 0.5–1 |

*Data from* Refs.[15,41,44]

via the PCA. However, in children, basal infusion has not been found to decrease pain scores or demand dosing compared with no basal infusion.[42,43] Regardless, providers must be aware and remain vigilant for the potentially catastrophic complication of narcotic-induced respiratory depression, especially when continuous basal infusion is added to bolus PCA dosing. When a continuous infusion is used, as in the case of small children and neonates, the authors prefer a morphine infusion at a variable rate between 10 and 25 μg/kg/min (which is less than half the dose known to cause respiratory depression).

One concern with patients on longstanding or high-dose narcotics is the onset of withdrawal symptoms if narcotics are inappropriately discontinued. For the treating surgeon, prevention entails correctly transitioning between intravenous and oral dose equivalents, and, less frequently, having to manage the sequela of narcotic addiction. **Table 4** lists the dose equivalents between various opioids. The topic of chronic pain management and neonatal addiction is covered in later sections. Regardless, proper tapering or weaning of narcotic dosing is a concept that every practitioner should be familiar with.

For patients recovering from gastrointestinal manipulation, transition to oral analgesics should preferentially be performed as bowel function returns. If the gastrointestinal tract is intact, an enteral-based pain regimen is preferred, with intravenous medication given only for baseline or breakthrough pain coverage. In either case, the intravenous to oral transition occurs rapidly, and should ensure adequate pain control based on a strictly oral regimen. However, clinicians must consider opioid tapering in any patient who has received frequent opioid analgesics for more than 5 to 10 days.

General guidelines for tapering include four steps.[15,44] The first step is conversion of all drugs to a single equipotent medication in the same family. Second, the PCA must be weaned off. If a basal rate was selected, an equipotent PO dose should be given and the basal rate turned off while maintaining bolus intravenous dosing. Furthermore, intravenous boluses should be weaned 25% to 50% as the patient can tolerate. Adjunctive measures to help wean off the PCA may include increasing the oral dose or adding an adjuvant analgesic, such as NSAIDs. The rate of the narcotic wean should be approximately 10% to 20% of consumed narcotic every 1 to 2 days. For example, if the 24-hour consumption of morphine is 40 mg, the goal should be to decrease the daily dose 4 to 8 mg every 1 to 2 days. The final step is then to ensure the patient can tolerate the oral regimen before discharge.[15]

## NEONATAL ADDICTION

Neonatal abstinence syndrome (NAS) refers to a generalized disorder of withdrawal symptoms after cessation of in utero toxin exposure. Maternal dependence on and abuse of opiates, heroin, or cocaine during pregnancy lead to a 55% to 94% incidence of NAS.[45–47] Clinical features of newborns with NAS include neurologic hyperexcitability (insomnia, irritability, hypertonia, hyperreflexia, tremors, and seizures), gastrointestinal symptoms (vomiting, diarrhea, feeding disturbances), and autonomic system dysfunction (sweating, fever, tachypnea, and congestion).[48–51] Although milder forms of withdrawal can be treated without medication, severe or progressive forms of NAS require more-intensive intervention.

Fortunately, surgeons rarely are required to deal with these complicated patients without the assistance of neonatologists. Despite their counterparts' expertise and support, surgeons must be aware of this syndrome and the current treatments to determine how postoperative management may be impacted in these newborns. The basis of pharmacologic treatment in these patients is opioid replacement. For initial therapy, most neonatology services use methadone (20%) and opioids other than methadone (63%), most commonly morphine (0.4 mg/mL).[52,53] Extreme variability exists among institutions, however, with no standard medication regimen having been found to be superior.[54] Besides morphine and methadone, dilute tincture of opium (DTO) and buprenorphine have also been used.[55]

As an adjunct, the concomitant use of centrally acting agents and sedatives has been studied.[56,57] In 2009, Agthe and colleagues[48] published their results of a prospective, double-blind, randomized, controlled trial of 80 newborns afflicted with NAS who were randomized to a combination of clonidine with DTO versus placebo and DTO. The placebo group showed higher doses of opium required, longer length of therapy, and higher rates of treatment failure.

Somewhat unique to the syndrome, the treatment algorithm for infants with NAS uses a symptom-based rather than weight-based protocol because of the highly variable presentation and spectrum of symptoms.[58] Therefore, frequent assessments based on the individual institution's preferred scoring system (ie, the Finnegan Neonatal Abstinence Scoring System) are performed to titrate opioid dosing.[59] If no further dose escalation is needed and stabilization occurs for 48 hours, the infant can then be gradually weaned from the medication.

No study on either the effects of NAS on surgical outcomes or the treatment of postoperative NAS seems to have been performed. Based on the authors' limited experience, the treatment of these complicated surgical patients differs primarily in the amount of narcotics consumed compared with their opioid-naïve counterparts. Again, the principle of postoperative pain control in this select group of patients is symptom-centered and not weight-based therapy, which may mean more-intensive assessments by the primary nurse, with frequent medication dosing changes and hourly assessment score variation. The authors prefer to wait until acute symptoms resolve, or at least the patients are physiologically stable, to perform the intended procedure in the operating room with dedicated anesthesia personnel, if possible. Unfortunately, surgery in these neonatal patients is often performed emergently.

Similar to NAS, narcotic dependence among the neonatal population is a growing concern. In the authors' experience, this can result from an iatrogenic problem, arising from frequent painful stimuli, which then leads to more administered analgesics and, over time, physical dependence. Implementation of a narcotic taper should be considered in all patients receiving frequent narcotics for more than 5 days. The four-step guideline for proper tapering of narcotics also applies to the neonatal population. The long-term effects of extensive early narcotic exposure have not been studied, although some reports have suggested that children exposed to opiates in utero may be at risk for neurodevelopmental impairment.[60,61] Whether this finding translates to postnatal opioid exposure is currently unknown.

## SUMMARY

Surgeons performing painful, invasive procedures in pediatric patients must be cognizant of both the short- and long-term detrimental effects of insufficient analgesia. Providers must remain vigilant and knowledgeable of objective age-based signs of pain. Although numerous tools and pain scales are available, clinicians should become familiar with their own institutional preference, and ensure strict adherence among the caretakers to ensure objective documentation and treatment. For minor procedures not requiring intubation, sedation should be strongly considered for patient, parent, and provider comfort. The authors favor ketamine and local anesthesia for most office- or emergency department–based procedures. Overall, the management of postoperative or postprocedural pain is similar to that for adults. Notable differences include using weight-based dosing, rapidly transitioning to oral regimen, and remembering the use of NSAIDs to decrease the narcotic burden. Although narcotic abstinence and addiction continue to be growing problems, often requiring multidisciplinary treatment, surgeons should be aware of common symptoms and signs to provoke a proper evaluation and implementation of treatment strategy.

## REFERENCES

1. Anand KJ, Hall RW. Pharmacological therapy for analgesia and sedation in the newborn. Arch Dis Child Fetal Neonatal Ed 2006;91:448–53.
2. Fitzgerald M. The development of nociceptive circuits. Nat Rev Neurosci 2005; 6(7):507–20.
3. Merskey H, Albe-Fessard DG, Bonica JJ, et al. Pain terms: a list with definitions and notes on usage: recommended by the IASP Subcommittee on Taxonomy. Pain 1979;6:249.
4. Franck LS, Greenberg CS, Stevens B. Pain assessment in infants and children. Pediatr Clin North Am 2000;47(3):487–512.
5. Anand KJS, Plotsky PM. Neonatal pain alters weight gain and pain threshold during development. Pediatr Res 1995;4:57.
6. Taddio A, Goldbach M, Ipp M, et al. Effect of neonatal circumcision on pain responses during vaccination in boys. Lancet 1995;345:291.
7. Gunnar M, Porter FL, Wolf CM, et al. Neonatal stress activity: predictions to later emotional temperament. Child Dev 1995;66(1):1–13.
8. Anand KJ, Hickey PR. Halothane-morphine compared with high-dose sufentanil for anesthesia and postoperative analgesia in neonatal cardiac surgery. N Engl J Med 1992;326:1–9.
9. McGrath PJ, Craig KD. Developmental and psychological factors in children's pain. Pediatr Clin North Am 1989;36:823–36.
10. Hammond D. Unnecessary suffering: pain and the doctor-patient relationship. Perspect Biol Med 1979;23:152–60.
11. Harbeck C, Peterson L. Elephants dancing in my head: a developmental approach to children's concept of specific pains. Child Dev 1992;63:138–49.
12. Acute Pain Management Guideline Panel. Acute pain management: operative or medical procedures and trauma: clinical practice guideline. Washington, DC: US Department of Health and Human Services; 1992.
13. Beyer JE, McGrath PJ, Berde CB. Discordance between self-report and behavioral pain measures in children aged 3-7 years after surgery. J Pain Symptom Manage 1990;5:350.
14. Stevens B. Composite measures of pain. Progress in Pain Research and Measurement 1998;10:161–78.
15. Yang K. Analgesia and sedation. In: Roberton J, Shilkofski N, editors. The Harriet Lane handbook. 17th edition. Philadelphia: Elsevier Mosby; 2005. p. 1011–30.
16. Golden BA. A multidisciplinary approach to nonpharmacologic pain management. J Am Osteopath Assoc 2002;102(Suppl):S1–5.
17. Kennedy RM, Luhmann JD. The "ouchless emergency department." Getting closer: advances in decreasing distress during painful procedures in the emergency department. Pediatr Clin North Am 1999;46(6):1215–47.
18. Doody SB, Smith C, Webb J. Nonpharmacologic interventions for pain management: pain and post anesthesia management. Crit Care Nurs Clin North Am 1991; 3(1):69–75.

19. Standley JM, Hanser SB. Music therapy research and applications in pediatric oncology. J Pediatr Oncol Nurs 1995;12:3–8.
20. McCaffery M. Nursing approaches to nonpharmacological pain control. Int J Nurs Stud 1990;27:1–5.
21. Chaves J. Recent advances in the application of hypnosis to pain management. Am J Clin Hypn 1994;37(2):117–29.
22. French GM, Painter EC, Coury DL. Blowing away a shot pain: a technique for pain management during immunization. Pediatrics 1994;93:384–8.
23. Alcock DS, Feldman W, Goodman JT. Evaluation of child life intervention in emergency department suturing. Pediatr Emerg Care 1985;1:111–5.
24. Manne SL, Backerman R, Jacobsen PB. An analysis of behavioral intervention for children undergoing venipuncture. Health Psychol 1994;13:556–66.
25. Bauman BH, McManus JG. Pediatric pain management in the emergency department. Emerg Med Clin North Am 2005;23:393–414.
26. Benumof JL, Dagg R, Benumof R. Critical hemoglobin desaturation will occur before return to an unparalyzed state following 1 mg/kg intravenous succinylcholine. Anesthesiology 1997;87:979–82.
27. Gutstein HB, Johnson KL, Hear MB, et al. Oral ketamine preanesthetic medication in children. Anesthesiology 1992;76:28.
28. Taketomo CK, Hodding JH, Kraus DM. Pediatric dosage handbook. 15th edition. Hudson (OH): Lexi-Comp; 2008. p. 990–1;1135–8.
29. Grant IS, Nimmo WS, Clements JA. Pharmacokinetics and analgesic effects of IM and oral ketamine. Br J Anaesth 1981;53:807.
30. Serour F, Mandelberg A, Mori J. Slow injection of local anesthetic will decrease pain during dorsal penile nerve block. Acta Anaesthesiol Scand 1998;42: 926–8.
31. Wilder RT. Local anesthetics for the pediatric patient. Pediatr Clin North Am 2000; 47(3):545–58.
32. Weinberg GL. Lipid infusion therapy: translation to clinical practice. Anesth Analg 2008;106(5):1340–2.
33. Henry DB, Foster RL. Burn pain management in children. Pediatr Clin North Am 2000;47(3):681–98.
34. Buck ML. Clinical experience with ketoralac in children. Ann Pharmacother 1994; 28(9):1009–13.
35. Berde CB, Sethna NF. Analgesics for the treatment of pain in children. N Engl J Med 2002;347:1094–103.
36. Kelly RE Jr, Lawson ML, Paidas CN, et al. Pectus excavatum in a 112-year autopsy series: anatomic findings and the effect on survival. J Pediatr Surg 2005;40:1275–8.
37. Scherer LR, Arn PH, Dressel DA, et al. Surgical management of children and young adults with Marfan syndrome and pectus excavatum. J Pediatr Surg 1988;23:1169–72.
38. Butkovic D, Kralik S, Matolic M, et al. Postoperative analgesia with intravenous fentanyl PCA vs epidural block after thoracoscopic pectus excavatum repair in children. Br J Anaesth 2007;98:677–81.
39. Weber T, Matzl J, Rokitansky A, et al. Superior postoperative pain relief with thoracic epidural analgesia versus intravenous patient-controlled analgesia after minimally invasive pectus excavatum repair. J Thorac Cardiovasc Surg 2007;134: 865–70.
40. Densmore JC, Peterson DB, Stahovic LL, et al. Initial surgical and pain management outcomes after Nuss procedure. J Pediatr Surg 2010;45:1767–71.

41. Kraemer FW, Rose JB. Pharmacologic management of acute pediatric pain. Anesthesiol Clin 2009;27:241–68.
42. Doyle E, Robinson D, Morton NS. Comparison of patient-controlled analgesia with and without background infusion after lower abdominal surgery in children. Br J Anaesth 1993;71:670–3.
43. Voepel-Lewis T, Marinkovic A, Kostrzewa A, et al. The prevalence of and risk factors for adverse events in children receiving patient-controlled analgesia by proxy or patient controlled analgesia after surgery. Anesth Analg 2008; 107:70–5.
44. Yaster M, Maxwell LG. Pediatric regional anesthesia. Anesthesiology 1989;70: 324–38.
45. Harper RG, Solish GI, Purow HM, et al. The effect of a methadone treatment program upon pregnant heroin addicts and their newborn infants. Pediatrics 1974;54(3):300–5.
46. Fricker HS, Segal S. Narcotic addiction, pregnancy, and the newborn. Am J Dis Child 1978;132(4):360–6.
47. Lester BM, Lagasse LL. Children of addicted women. J Addict Dis 2010;29: 259–76.
48. Agthe AG, Kim GR, Mathas KB, et al. Clonidine as an adjunct therapy to opioids for neonatal abstinence syndrome: a randomized, control, trial. Pediatrics 2009; 123:e849–56.
49. Blinick G, Wallach RC, Jerez E, et al. Drug addiction in pregnancy and the neonate. Am J Obstet Gynecol 1976;125(2):135–42.
50. Finnegan LP. Discussion: dilemmas in research in perinatal addiction- intervention issues. NIDA Res Monogr 1992;117:344–8.
51. Levy M, Spino M. Neonatal withdrawal syndrome: associated drugs and pharmacologic management. Pharmacotherapy 1993;13(3):202–11.
52. Sarkar S, Donn S. Management of neonatal abstinence syndrome in neonatal intensive care units: a national survey. J Perinatol 2006;26:15–7.
53. Colombini N, Elias R, Busuttil M, et al. Hospital morphine preparation for abstinence syndrome in newborns exposed to buprenorphine or methadone. Pharm World Sci 2008;3:227–34.
54. Osborn DA, Jeffery HE, Cole MJ. Opiate treatment for opiate withdrawal in newborn infants. Cochrane Database Syst Rev 2010;10:CD002059.
55. Kraft WK, Gibson E, Dysart K, et al. Sublingual buprenorphine for treatment of neonatal abstinence syndrome: a randomized trial. Pediatrics 2008;122(3): e601–7.
56. Osborn DA, Jeffrey HA, Cole MJ. Sedatives for opiate withdrawal in newborn infants. Cochrane Database Syst Rev 2010;10:CD002053.
57. Esmaelli A, Keinhorst AK, Schuster T, et al. Treatment of neonatal abstinence syndrome with clonidine and chloral hydrate. Acta Paediatr 2010;99:209–14.
58. Jansson LM, Velez M, Harrow C. The opioid exposed newborn: assessment and pharmacologic management. J Opioid Manag 2009;5(1):47–55.
59. Finnegan L, Connaughton J, Kron R, et al. Neonatal abstinence syndrome: assessment and management. Addict Dis 1975;2:141–58.
60. Ornoy A, Segal J, Bar-Hamburger R, et al. Developmental outcome of school-age children born to mothers with heroin dependency: importance of environmental factors. Dev Med Child Neurol 2001;43:668–75.
61. Hunt RW, Tzioumi D, Collins E, et al. Adverse neurodevelopmental outcome of infants exposed to opiate in-utero. Early Hum Dev 2008;84:29–35.

# Pediatric Inguinal Hernias, Hydroceles, and Undescended Testicles

Oliver B. Lao, MD, MPH[a], Robert J. Fitzgibbons Jr, MD[b],
Robert A. Cusick, MD[c],*

## KEYWORDS

- Hernia • Adolescent hernia repair • Hydrocele • Undescended testicle • Orchiopexy

## KEY POINTS

- Asymptomatic inguinal hernias in children require elective repair.
- Incarcerated inguinal hernias require reduction and urgent repair, whereas strangulated inguinal hernias require emergent repair.
- Noncommunicating hydroceles may be observed up to 24 months of life, as they may spontaneously resolve.
- Communicating hydroceles should be treated as inguinal hernias.
- Undescended testes that are palpable in the inguinal canal should be operated on at 6 to 12 months.
- Testicles that are not palpable should undergo ultrasonography and possibly laparoscopy to define their location.

## PEDIATRIC INGUINAL HERNIA

### Introduction

Pediatric inguinal hernia repair is one of the most common procedures performed by pediatric surgeons, and has historically been considered an "intern case"; however, it can be one of the most difficult procedures a surgeon will perform. In experienced hands, repair can often be performed rapidly and with a low complication rate. The American College of Surgery, in their Maintenance of Certification program, recognizes 3 distinct age groups of inguinal hernia repairs: age less than 6 months, 6 months to 5 years, and 5 years and older. This scale reflects the increasing difficulty of this procedure with decreasing age. Age less than 6 months increases the likelihood of

The authors have nothing to disclose.
[a] Department of Pediatric Surgery, Children's Hospital and Regional Medical Center, University of Nebraska College of Medicine, 8200 Dodge, Omaha, NE 68114, USA; [b] University of Nebraska College of Medicine & Children's Hospital & Medical Center, 8200 Dodge Street, Omaha, NE 68114, USA; [c] Department of Surgery, Children's Hospital and Regional Medical Center, University of Nebraska College of Medicine, 8200 Dodge, Omaha, NE 68114, USA
* Corresponding author.
*E-mail address:* rcusick@childrensomaha.org

Surg Clin N Am 92 (2012) 487–504
doi:10.1016/j.suc.2012.03.017
0039-6109/12/$ – see front matter © 2012 Elsevier Inc. All rights reserved.

comorbidities including prematurity, complicating the decisions on timing of surgery. In this population a surgeon also more likely needs to perform a concomitant repair of the floor or an orchiopexy. To maintain a low complication rate, a thorough knowledge of the anatomy and surgical techniques of the area is crucial.

## Epidemiology

Inguinal hernia repair is the most frequently performed pediatric surgical operation, with an incidence ranging from 0.8% to 4%.[1] The incidence is nearly 10 times more common in boys than in girls, and is much more common in premature babies (13% of babies born before 32 weeks and nearly 30% of babies weighing less than 1 kg). Inguinal hernias are much more common on the right side (75%) than on the left (25%), primarily because of the later descent of the right testicle. Nearly one-third of cases will present before 6 months of age, and bilaterality occurs in 15% to 20% of children.[2,3] As a result of these epidemiologic findings, clinicians should be cognizant of the possibility of a contralateral hernia in children presenting unilaterally, and this should be discussed with the parents. Risk factors for bilateral disease include females, babies with left-sided inguinal hernias, premature babies, young age at presentation (<1 year), and history of an undescended testicle.

## Embryology of Testicular Descent

Gonads descend from the urogenital ridge, in the upper abdomen near the developing kidneys, to the internal ring at 3 months' gestation. The processus vaginalis then develops from the peritoneal lining.[4] At 6 to 7 months' gestation, descent through the inguinal canal follows the course of the gubernaculum, likely following the genito-femoral nerve.[5] Over the next 2 months, the testes come to rest in the scrotum with a gradual obliteration of the processus vaginalis that subsequently becomes the tunica vaginalis.[6] Incomplete obliteration of the processus vaginalis is the underlying feature of pediatric inguinal hernias and hydroceles, and their incidence is inversely proportional to the age of the child.[1,7,8] When there is complete failure of obliteration, the result is both an inguinal and scrotal hernia. When the distal processus is obliterated but the proximal one remains patent, an inguinal hernia results. Narrowing but incomplete closure of the proximal processus results in a communicating hydrocele. Complete obliteration of the proximal portion but partial patency of the processus leads to a noncommunicating hydrocele (**Fig. 1**). Closure of the patent processus is

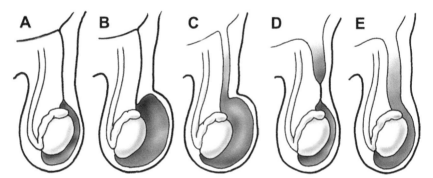

Fig. 1. Configurations of hydrocele and hernia in relation to patency of the processus vaginalis. (A) Normal; (B) hydrocele; (C) communicating hydrocele; (D) inguinal hernia; (E) complete inguinal hernia. (From Snyder CL. Inguinal hernias and hydroceles. In: Holcomb GW III, Murphy JP, editors. Ashcraft's pediatric surgery, 5th edition. Philadelphia: WB Saunders; 2010. p. 670; with permission.)

asymmetric, with the left closing earlier than the right. This asymmetry explains the higher prevalence of right-sided hernias, hydroceles, and undescended testicles.

In females, the round ligament represents the analogous processus vaginalis. The canal of Nuck is an outpouching of peritoneum anterior to the round ligament, and is the location of most inguinal hernias in females, although the floor may be weak as well.

### Anatomic Considerations in Children

The inguinal canal in children is much shorter than that of an adult, with resultant overlapping of the internal and external rings. Passage of the testicle through the canal is at an angle from the superior and lateral internal ring to the more medially located external ring. Because the inguinal canal is short in infants, with the internal and external rings overlapping, some surgeons believe that opening the external oblique in infants is unnecessary during a pediatric hernia repair. Because most childhood hernias are related to the processus vaginalis, the floor rarely requires repair.

### Diagnosis and Examination

Inguinal hernias may be asymptomatic or symptomatic. Most inguinal hernias are minimally symptomatic and present as intermittent bulges in the groin, scrotum, or labia, made worse by activities that cause increased intra-abdominal pressure (crying or straining). Other children may present with vague pain in the inguinal area. Symptomatic hernias may also present with incarceration (unable to be reduced) or strangulation (loss of blood supply) with a resultant bowel obstruction. Although the swelling from the hernia may not be noticed for many years, hernias in children represent congenital defects and have been present since birth.

The examination in a child should focus on the external ring just lateral to the pubic tubercle. Standing on one side and palpating along the contralateral inguinal canal at the external ring is the best way to examine the canal for hernias. This maneuver, referred to as the silk glove sign, will demonstrate thickening of the cord (representing the hernia sac) in comparison with that on the contralateral side. Although the diagnostic accuracy of the silk glove sign has previously been called into question, the use of the findings of this physical examination to support the diagnosis may be useful.[8,9] If the hernia is difficult to appreciate, provocative maneuvers should be undertaken such as standing, straining, or the performance of an age-appropriate Valsalva maneuver (jumping). Ultrasonography of a hernia that is difficult to palpate may help with diagnosis as well.[10,11]

The examination of the child with a possible hernia should (in the male) include an examination of the testicles and scrotum. Occluding the external ring with one hand and palpating the testicle should prevent it from ascending into the inguinal canal. Absence of the testicle suggests an undescended or retractile testicle (see later discussion) and likely makes the repair more difficult. In the infant female, the ovary is the most common structure to be palpated in a hernia, and may become incarcerated. Bilateral hernias in a female should raise the concern of an abnormality with sexual differentiation, the evaluation of which is beyond the scope of this article.

If the hernia is complicated by incarceration the child will present with pain, abdominal distension, and emesis. The incidence of incarceration in the pediatric population is reported at 5% to 15% but is much higher in infants (30%).[12] After an incarcerated hernia is diagnosed, all attempts should be made at reduction of the hernia. Appropriate pain medication and sedation along with the Trendelenburg position may assist in reduction. These maneuvers are successful 70% to 85% of the time.[12–14] If the hernia is easily reduced, an elective hernia repair may be scheduled on an outpatient basis. If it is reduced with difficulty, there are some who would advocate admitting and repairing within 24 hours. If the hernia is not reducible (incarcerated) or there is concern for strangulation (fever, tachycardia, leukocytosis, emesis, severe pain, prolonged history of bulge and erythema), immediate surgery is warranted. The caveat that dead bowel cannot be reduced must be borne in mind.

### Differential Diagnosis

The differential for groin pain is substantial. However, swelling in the groin extending into the scrotum is a limited differential. Scrotal swelling that will not reduce is either an incarcerated hernia that is an emergency, or a noncommunicating hydrocele that can be managed electively. An incarcerated hernia is usually erythematous, swollen, and exquisitely tender. The rest of the history and examination are also consistent with a bowel obstruction: vomiting and abdominal distension. If the clinical picture is unclear, which is more common in infants, an abdominal radiograph may show the typical findings of a bowel obstruction (**Fig. 2**). In this setting, ultrasonography can also be helpful.[10,11] Other entities that may mimic a hernia include testicular torsion and torsion of the appendix testes; however, both present with the acute onset of pain. Torsion of the testicle should have an associated scrotal mass that is not contiguous with the inguinal canal. Torsion of the appendix testes often has a blue-dot sign representing the torsed, necrotic appendix testes at the superior pole of the testicle. Enlarged inguinal lymph nodes are also on the differential.

### Treatment

Although there is some variability in technique, high dissection and high ligation of the hernia sac at the level of the internal ring remains the gold standard for repair.[15,16] As previously mentioned, this may or may not involve opening the external oblique to obtain adequate exposure of the internal ring. Before ligation, the sac is opened to ensure there are no contents within the sac. The distal sac is not resected because of concern about damage to the testicle. The distal sac is instead widely opened to prevent a postoperative hydrocele. A transient postoperative hydrocele is common and can be very large in neonates with large hernias. In this setting, parents should

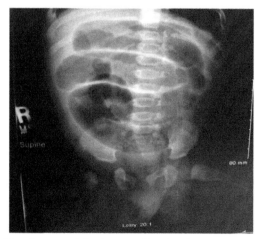

**Fig. 2.** Abdominal film from an infant presenting to the emergency room with scrotal swelling. Differential included an incarcerated hernia and a hydrocele on physical examination. The film is consistent with a bowel obstruction from an incarcerated inguinal hernia. Note the air in the right scrotal sac.

be counseled preoperatively. Once the sac has been ligated and the distal sac opened, the floor of the canal is examined. In neonates with large hernias the floor can be quite weak. In this setting, some clinicians advocate interrupted sutures to approximate the conjoined tendon and the shelving edge of the inguinal ligament with interrupted sutures (**Figs. 3** and **4**). It should be noted that mesh is rarely used because of the historically low recurrence rates.

In girls, the hernia sac follows the round ligament. Again, the sac is opened and then ligated at the level of the internal ring. The internal ring is then closed with interrupted sutures by approximating the conjoined tendon and the inguinal ligament.

### Timing of Repair

The timing of inguinal hernia repair is debatable, and is dependent on age and comorbidities. Because most hernias are asymptomatic, the principal concern is risk of incarceration. In older children and adolescents, in whom risk of incarceration is low, the hernia repair can be performed electively.[15] The timing of infant hernia repair is more complicated. Compared with older children, Term infants are at increased risk of incarceration and therefore repair should be undertaken without delay.[13,17] For older term infants who are otherwise healthy, hernia repairs can be done on an outpatient basis.

Preterm infants have a higher incidence of inguinal hernias (20%–30%) as well as rates of incarceration.[18–20] For preterm infants with hernias, the timing of repair is controversial.[21–27] For those infants hospitalized for prematurity, the surgeon may choose to monitor the baby in the neonatal intensive care unit (NICU) and delay repair until ready for discharge.[19,25–29] Alternatively, the surgeon may opt to perform the hernia repair shortly after discharge from the NICU.[19,28] In this population there is concern about apnea after a general anesthetic, therefore these patients require apnea and bradycardia monitors overnight.[30,31] Determination of which patients require admission is based on gestational age at birth, comorbidities, and postconceptual age (ranging from 46 to 60 weeks), and varies among hospitals. Comorbidities associated with an increased risk of apnea include lung disease, home apnea monitoring, anemia, and use of supplemental oxygen, as well as use of narcotics and muscle relaxants during the operation.[30,32,33] The question of whether to repair the hernia before discharge from the newborn nursery or to wait until the anesthetic risk of apnea subsides does not have a clear answer in the literature.[25,27,28,31,32]

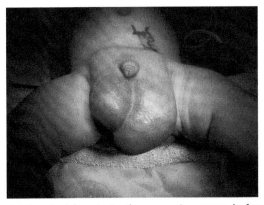

**Fig. 3.** Giant neonatal inguinal hernia in the operating room before reduction of the hernia.

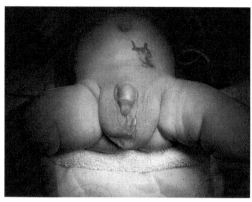

**Fig. 4.** After reduction of the hernia. The floor of the canal was quite weak and required reinforcement with sutures. The patient also required an orchiopexy at the same time for an undescended testicle diagnosed at the time of surgery.

### Contralateral Groin

The question of whether to explore or repair the contralateral groin was raised by a report in 1955 citing the rate of bilateral hernias as 100% in infants and 60% in children.[34] Other reports have similarly noted the presence of a patent processus vaginalis on routine exploration of the contralateral side as well as the risk of a metachronous contralateral hernia after unilateral repair. These findings led many surgeons to recommended routine, bilateral groin exploration in all children with unilateral hernias.[35,36] Other surgeons have pointed to the risk of injuring the vas deferens and testes bilaterally, and questioned the true incidence of bilaterality as reasons for not exploring both groins.[37–40] The clinical question is whether a patent processus vaginalis always becomes an inguinal hernia. The percentage of children with a patent processus on the contralateral side was studied with bilateral exploration, and was found to range from 40% to 60% with apparent decline with increasing age.[7,41] The percentage of children that develops a metachronous hernia was found to be anywhere from 10% to 30% in a group observed following a unilateral hernia repair.[41–43] An autopsy study has suggested that adults who die without a clinical hernia will have a patent processus vaginalis 15% to 30% of the time.[44] Taken together, the aggregate of these studies points toward roughly 50% of infants having a patent processus vaginalis, with slightly fewer (~20%–40%) children having a patent processus as they progress to adulthood.

Another option is to perform routine laparoscopic evaluation of the contralateral groin through the hernia sac.[1,8,45–47] A recent study by Lazar and colleagues[45] reported that 30% to 40% of children with clinically relevant unilateral inguinal hernias will have a contralateral patent processus vaginalis when studied laparoscopically. It is still unclear as to what percentage of those patent processi, visualized laparoscopically, will progress to clinical hernias. A meta-analysis of more than 13,000 unilateral inguinal hernia repairs in children demonstrated a 7% rate of metachronous hernia, although a rate of 8% to 20% has been reported elsewhere.[1–3,6,37,43,48,49] In an effort to reduce the number of negative explorations of the contralateral groin, additional patient characteristics such as age, sex, side, and underlying disease process have been considered.[7] Risk factors for contralateral disease are infants with left hernias, early age at presentation, and females. Also, patients with unique underlying conditions such as cystic fibrosis, ventriculoperitoneal shunts, peritoneal dialysis catheters, or connective tissue disorders are at increased risk for contralateral hernias.[50] Additional testing such as ultrasonography should be considered in these patients.[10,51]

In their practice, the authors do not routinely offer contralateral exploration. Selective contralateral exploration is offered after consultation with the parents of patients who fall into the following categories: girls younger than 5 years with a unilateral hernia, and premature infants. In boys with a question of bilateral disease, the authors recommend laparoscopy through the umbilicus to evaluate the contralateral side (**Fig. 5**).

### Laparoscopic Repair

Laparoscopic inguinal hernia repair in children was first described in females in 1997 and in males in 1999.[27,43,49] Multiple techniques have been described to replicate the open repair. Most of these techniques begin with access through the umbilicus, and both internal rings are evaluated. Hernia repair begins with passage of a needle through a stab incision over the internal ring. The needle is passed superficial to the peritoneum around the internal ring, taking care to avoid cord structures. A modification includes making a second pass of the needle to bisect the sac and to further ligate the sac, similar to what is done with open repairs. This procedure is performed with a permanent suture to decrease the recurrence rate (**Figs. 6–8**).[52]

Most laparoscopic series to date have documented an increased recurrence rate in comparison with the open repair. With increasing experience, the recurrence rate has approached that of open repair in some series.[53–58] Proponents of the laparoscopic method tout cosmesis, ease of evaluation of the contralateral side, and visualization of the vas and vessels, perhaps making the repair less traumatic.[59–61] One study found decreased pain along with parental perception of a faster recovery and better wound cosmesis compared with open repair. Another study found similar recovery and outcomes but worse pain in the laparoscopic group.[57,62] Subjective outcomes such as pain and cosmesis are difficult to quantify and even more difficult to compare between the two groups.[63] Although this is a safe and effective alternative to open repair, it cannot yet be considered the gold standard because long-term data are still lacking.

### Outcomes

Overall, pediatric inguinal hernia repairs have a low complication rate. Complications include recurrence, testicular atrophy, injury to the vas, and infection. The largest

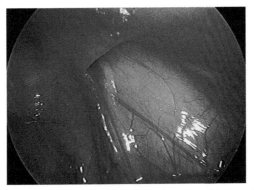

**Fig. 5.** Male presenting with an umbilical hernia and a vague history of intermittent right scrotal swelling. During the umbilical hernia repair, a 5-mm trocar was placed in the umbilicus and confirmed a right-sided hernia.

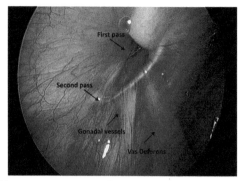

**Fig. 6.** Technique of laparoscopic repair of an inguinal hernia in a boy. A second pass has been used to bisect the hernia sac. (Photo *courtesy of* Dr Matias Bruzoni.)

single-surgeon series including 6361 patients describes a 1.2% recurrence rate and a 0.3% rate of testicular atrophy.[3] The recurrence rate of 1% is mirrored in a survey study.[31] Although there is evidence of transient changes in the vascularity of the testes immediately postoperatively, these nearly all resolve with time.[64] In preterm infants the complication rate may be higher.[44,65] The long-term effects of pediatric inguinal hernia repair have recently been reported over an average 49-year follow-up. The data demonstrated an 8.4% reexploration for a hernia on the ipsilateral side presenting at an average of 38.4 years postoperatively. The majority of these cases were "new" direct hernias rather than recurrences of an indirect hernia (2.8% recurrence rate).[66]

## ADOLESCENT INGUINAL HERNIA
### Principles of Inguinal Hernia Surgery in Adults

There is overwhelming evidence in the literature that a mesh-based inguinal herniorrhaphy dramatically decreases the recurrence rate in comparison with a pure tissue repair.[67] Mesh-based repairs, as a group, are usually referred to as tension-free repairs (TFR). There are more than 70 named tissue repairs in the literature, but most are simple modifications of operations already illustrated in this article for pediatric patients.[68] The classic Bassini is the prototype operation, and involves reconstruction of the posterior wall by suturing Bassini's famous triple layer (the transversalis fascia, the transversus abdominis muscle, the internal oblique muscle) to the inguinal ligament (**Fig. 9**).

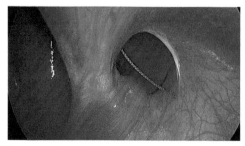

**Fig. 7.** Technique of laparoscopic repair of an inguinal hernia in a girl before tying the suture.

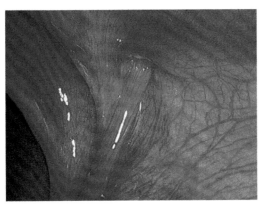

**Fig. 8.** Technique of laparoscopic repair of an inguinal hernia in a girl after tying the suture. (*Courtesy of* Dr Matias Bruzoni.)

Tissue repairs are not be discussed further because they are only used today in exceptional circumstances such as for infected or contaminated wounds. The technique popularized by Liechtenstein is considered the gold-standard TFR operation.[69] In this procedure the groin is initially prepared in a manner similar to a tissue repair. The external oblique is exposed through a transverse groin incision and opened through the external ring. A large space is then created beneath the fascia of the external oblique using blunt dissection from the anterior superior iliac spine laterally to a point 2 cm medial to the pubic tubercle medially. Dissection is continued from lateral to medial along the inferior edge of the external oblique aponeurosis; the so-called shelving edge of the inguinal ligament. The pubic tubercle is exposed and the cord structures are elevated out of the inguinal floor. Indirect inguinal hernia sacs are dissected from

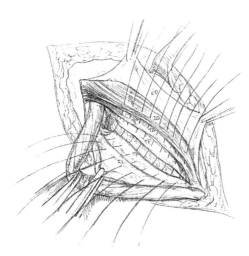

**Fig. 9.** The classic Bassini is the prototype operation and involves reconstruction of the posterior wall by suturing Bassini's famous triple layer (the transversalis fascia, the transversus abdominis muscle, the internal oblique muscle) to the inguinal ligament. (*From* Fitzgibbons RJ Jr, Greenburg AG. Nyhus and Condon's hernia. Philadelphia: Lippincott Williams & Wilkins; 2001. p. 108; with permission.)

the cord and reduced into the preperitoneal space. High ligation is also an option, but is not preferred in deference to the possibility of greater pain because of the incision across the richly innervated peritoneum. An exception is the inguinal scrotal indirect hernia because dissecting out the entire sac, as in pediatric hernias, is associated with an increased rate of testicular complications. Division of the sac with high ligation of the proximal sac and generous opening of the distal sac is recommended. Direct hernias are dissected away from surrounding structures and reduced. Commonly the musculofascial elements that make up the ring of the direct hernia are closed to maintain reduction while the formal repair of the inguinal hernia is accomplished. This action adds little to the ultimate strength of the repair and is more a matter of making the prosthetic repair easier by keeping the hernia sac out of the field, especially if the procedure is being performed under local anesthesia. It is at this point that the procedure begins to differ from a tissue repair. Instead of suturing the triple layer to the inguinal ligament, a prosthesis, which is at least 9 by 12 cm and usually a polypropylene mesh, is sutured to the anterior rectus sheath 2 cm medial to the pubic tubercle. This same suture is continued laterally, securing the inferior edge of the prosthesis to either side of the pubic tubercle and then the inguinal ligament. The suture is tied at the internal ring and the mesh is slit laterally to accommodate the cord structures. The tails created are tucked beneath the fascia of the external oblique aponeurosis to the level of the anterior superior iliac spine, with the superior tail overlapping the inferior tail. A so-called shutter-valve stitch is placed next, which incorporates the inferior edge of the superior tail, the inferior edge of the inferior tail, and the inguinal ligament. This stitch serves to create a new internal ring and also to wrinkle the mesh somewhat medially, which is believed to be important in minimizing tension when the patient is in the upright position. The mesh is then trimmed and secured to the anterior rectus sheath and the internal oblique aponeurosis medially and cranially (**Fig. 10**). The external oblique aponeurosis is closed over the repair, reconstructing the external ring.

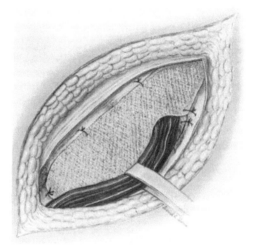

**Fig. 10.** The mesh repair technique popularized by Liechtenstein. The lower edges of the 2 tails are sutured to the inguinal ligament for creation of a new internal ring made of mesh. (*From* Fitzgibbons Jr RJ, Greenburg AG. Nyhus and Condon's Hernia. Philadelphia: Lippincott Williams & Wilkins; 2001. p. 108; with permission.)

An alternative to a TFR is a laparoscopic herniorrhaphy. Unlike the conventional TFR the laparoscopic operation is performed in the preperitoneal space, which may be entered either through the abdomen after a conventional laparoscopy (transabdominal preperitoneal or TAPP) or a totally extraperitoneal technique (TEP) using a dissecting balloon placed between the posterior rectus sheath and the rectus muscle. A pneumo-extraperitoneum is then produced. With either approach, a radical dissection of the preperitoneal space is next accomplished exposing both pubic tubercles, the Cooper ligament, the inferior epigastric vessels, and the cord structures. It is important that the peritoneum over the internal spermatic vessels be dissected well proximally so that a large space is created to prevent roll-up of the prosthesis when the peritoneum is eventually closed. Next, a mesh prosthesis, usually made of polypropylene, is positioned to widely overlap both the direct and indirect spaces, that is, the myopectineal orifice (**Fig. 11**). In addition to the laparoscopic operation there are several conventional operations, such as popularized by Kugel,[70] that take advantage of the preperitoneal space.

### Mesh Repair or High Ligation for Adolescents

The critical question is, when should the principles of adult inguinal hernia surgery be applied to the pediatric population? In other words, when is a child an adult? Clearly there is no high-level evidence in the literature to answer this question. However, most surgical textbooks are consistent in a recommendation that prosthetic material is not

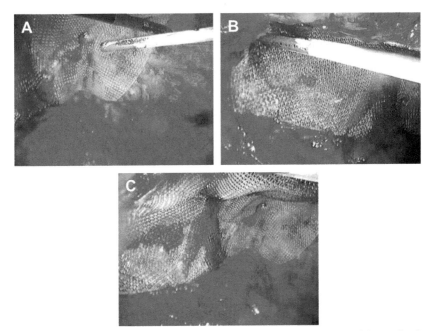

**Fig. 11.** Laparoscopic repair. The mesh prosthesis usually is positioned to widely overlap both the direct and indirect spaces (ie, the myopectineal orifice). (*A*) Medial mesh fixation over a left-sided inguinal hernia defect. (*B*) Lateral mesh fixation over a left-sided inguinal hernia defect, taking care to place the endotack above the iliopubic tract. (*C*) Final orientation of the mesh covering all left-sided myopectineal orifices. (*From* Kim B, Duh QY. Laparoscopic inguinal hernia repair. In: Evans SR, editor. Surgical pitfalls—prevention and management. Philadelphia: Elsevier; 2009. p. 515–21; with permission.)

appropriate in patients younger than 15 years, because of continuing growth considerations. There is another unsettled controversy pertinent to this consideration, which is whether mesh in contact with the cord structures might result in vasal obstruction in a small subset of patients because of an exasperated fibroplastic inflammatory response caused by mesh.[71] Scattered case reports of apparent infertility caused by mesh have surfaced, but alternative explanations for the vasal obstruction have been proposed.[72] Most adult inguinal hernia surgeons will recommend the use of a prosthesis for any patient aged 20 years or older, with appropriate counseling for patients potentially intending to have children. This counseling is particularly important in patients with bilateral operations. For adolescents aged 15 to 19 years this question remains unsettled, with almost no objective scientific evidence to address the question.

## PEDIATRIC HYDROCELE

A hydrocele is a collection of fluid in the tunica vaginalis around the testicle. If there is no connection to the abdominal cavity through a patent processus vaginalis, it is called a noncommunicating hydrocele. If there is a patent processus vaginalis, this is termed a communicating hydrocele. A communicating hydrocele is essentially a hernia. Hydroceles, like hernias, are more common on the right side.

Distinguishing between a communicating and noncommunicating hydrocele is important because they are managed very differently. Hydroceles usually can be differentiated by history and physical examination. A communicating hydrocele will fluctuate throughout the day in size, especially when in the dependent position (standing). A noncommunicating hydrocele will not fluctuate in size but may gradually change in size over weeks. On physical examination a communicating hydrocele can be compressed into the abdomen. A noncommunicating hydrocele will not compress. The differential of scrotal swelling also includes a hernia (incarcerated hernia) or a varicocele.

Treatment for a communicating hydrocele is essentially the same as for a hernia: operative repair once the diagnosis has been confirmed.[15,19] Noncommunicating hydroceles are extremely common at birth and should be considered a normal part of development. Most will resolve spontaneously. If they persist after a period of time (12 to 24 months), they should be repaired.[73] When hydroceles are present at birth, they do not increase the likelihood of a subsequent hernia.[74] However, if the hydrocele develops after birth there is a higher likelihood, by definition, that the patent processus vaginalis will not close.[74] Repair of a hydrocele involves an inguinal approach to make sure there is not a patent processus vaginalis (a hernia). A high ligation of the processus is performed (**Fig. 12**). Once this has been completed, the distal hydrocele is widely opened to prevent recurrence. The hydrocele sac is not completely removed to avoid injury to the testicle.

## UNDESCENDED TESTICLE

The incidence of cryptorchidism is between 1% and 3%. Prematurity is a risk factor because of testicular descent during the seventh month of gestation.[75] Descent of the testicle is limited by the vasculature rather than the vas deferens. An undescended testicle is at increased risk for malignancy and will be unable to properly produce sperm.[76] The testicle requires a cooler environment, such as in the scrotum, to produce sperm.

Although the risk of malignancy is increased in the undescended testicle, it is still relatively rare. Multiple studies suggest a relative risk of 4.0 to 5.7 for testicular cancer

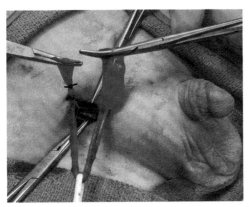

**Fig. 12.** High ligation of a processus vaginalis in a boy presenting with a communicating hydrocele.

in the undescended testicle. This risk also seems to be higher if the testicle is in the abdominal location rather than in the inguinal location. The contralateral side is thought by some to also be at increased risk for malignancy, while others suggest the rate is similar to that in the general population.[77] Orchiopexy does not completely negate the increased risk of malignancy.[78,79] However, performance of orchiopexy at an earlier age has been associated with a decreased relative risk of cancer.[77] Another potential advantage of orchiopexy is improved surveillance and earlier detection.

### Diagnosis

An undescended testicle is often detected at birth on routine examination. An empty hemiscrotum at birth represents either in utero torsion of the testicle or an unde-scended testicle. On physical examination, with the aid of lubricating jelly, an examiner stands on the contralateral side and slides his or her fingers from the anterior superior iliac spine down to the pubic tubercle. The testicle within the canal can be felt with this maneuver, even in a toddler. The size of the testicle should be documented because undescended testicles are generally smaller than the contralateral gonad.

If the testicle can be easily pulled into the scrotum, it is a retractile testicle and needs no additional therapy. If the testicle is palpable but will not descend, it will require orchiopexy. If the testicle is nonpalpable, ultrasonography can be used to identify the testicle. If an ultrasonogram does not identify a testicle, this may indicate that the testicle is intra-abdominal or not present (from in utero testicular torsion). In this setting some advocate the use of magnetic resonance imaging.[80,81] The authors prefer proceeding to laparoscopy to differentiate an intra-abdominal testicle and in utero testicular torsion.

### Treatment

Orchiopexy is performed in the setting of an undescended testicle, and may be per-formed in either the open or laparoscopic fashion.[80,82,83] Timing of orchiopexy is controversial, but most surgeons recommend performing this procedure at 6 to 12 months of age.[83] Waiting 6 months, especially in premature infants, may allow a partially descended testicle to completely descend. Historically, orchiopexy was per-formed in older boys. There is increasing evidence from testicular biopsies that waiting could affect fertility. Cortes and colleagues[81] demonstrated complete loss of germ cells on biopsy as early as 18 months of age. Others have demonstrated progressive loss of not only germ cells but also Leydig cells, and this is more severe in nonpalpable testes.[84] For these reasons the authors prefer to operate before 1 year of age.

In the setting of a palpable testicle, a 1-stage orchiopexy is performed. An inguinal incision is made, slightly larger than a hernia incision, to allow access to the external and internal rings. The external oblique is approached with care because the testicle may reside in a hernia sac that exits the external ring and sits in an ectopic position in the thigh or over the external oblique. Once the external oblique is identified and opened, the hernia sac is mobilized with sharp and blunt dissection from the gubernaculum. The hernia sac is then opened opposite the vas and the vessels (in a minority of cases no hernia sac is identified). The hernia sac is peeled off the cord structures and ligated at the level of the internal ring.[82,83,85] The process of mobilizing the hernia sac and dividing the retroperitoneal attachments to the hernia sac gives the testicle length to reach the scrotum in most cases. An incision is then made in the scrotum, and a pouch is created for the testicle. The testicle is then passed into the scrotum and secured to the median raphe using nonabsorbable sutures.

### Nonpalpable Testis

When the testicle is nonpalpable and not identified on the ultrasonogram, laparoscopic exploration is performed.[82,85] Laparoscopy can distinguish an in utero torsion or an intra-abdominal testicle. Laparoscopy is diagnostic of an in utero torsion if there is a blind-ending vas deferens and spermatic vessels at the level of the internal ring.[80] These remnants can be left because their malignant potential is very low.[77] If the testicle is found to be intra-abdominal on laparoscopic exploration, the first stage of a Fowler-Stephens orchiopexy can be performed. With this procedure the testicular vessels are divided 2 to 3 cm from the testicle laparoscopically during the first operation. The testicle then survives on the peritoneum and the vessel to the vas. In 3 to 6 months the child is returned to the operating room for an open or a laparoscopic orchiopexy. Others report similar results with a 1-stage Fowler-Stevens.[86]

### Outcomes

In terms of testicular salvage, outcomes are excellent for orchiopexy overall. Series report testicular salvage as high as 90% even when using the Fowler-Stevens approach of dividing the testicular vessels, documented by preservation of testicular size on physical examination during long-term follow-up. Fertility for males with unilateral undescended testicles is nearly normal, whereas it drops to 65% with bilateral disease.[87] Studies also demonstrate decreased sperm counts and abnormal hormone levels compared with controls, especially in patients with bilateral disease.

### REFERENCES

1. Manoharan S, Samarakkody U, Kulkarni M, et al. Evidence-based change of practice in the management of unilateral inguinal hernia. J Pediatr Surg 2005; 40(7):1163–6.
2. Brandt ML. Pediatric hernias. Surg Clin North Am 2008;88(1):27–43, vii–viii.
3. Ein SH, Njere I, Ein A. Six thousand three hundred sixty-one pediatric inguinal hernias: a 35-year review. J Pediatr Surg 2006;41(5):980–6.
4. Shrock P. The processus vaginalis and gubernaculum. Their raison d'etre redefined. Surg Clin North Am 1971;51(6):1263–8.
5. Davenport M. ABC of general paediatric surgery. Inguinal hernia, hydrocele, and the undescended testis. BMJ 1996;312(7030):564–7.

6. Toki A, Watanabe Y, Tani M, et al. Adopt a wait-and-see attitude for patent processus vaginalis in neonates. J Pediatr Surg 2003;38(9):1371–3.
7. Rowe MI, Copelson LW, Clatworthy HW. The patent processus vaginalis and the inguinal hernia. J Pediatr Surg 1969;4(1):102–7.
8. Miltenburg DM, Nuchtern JG, Jaksic T, et al. Laparoscopic evaluation of the pediatric inguinal hernia—a meta-analysis. J Pediatr Surg 1998;33(6):874–9.
9. Luo CC, Chao HC. Prevention of unnecessary contralateral exploration using the silk glove sign (SGS) in pediatric patients with unilateral inguinal hernia. Eur J Pediatr 2007;166(7):667–9.
10. Chen KC, Chu CC, Chou TY, et al. Ultrasonography for inguinal hernias in boys. J Pediatr Surg 1998;33(12):1784–7.
11. Erez I, Rathause V, Vacian I, et al. Preoperative ultrasound and intraoperative findings of inguinal hernias in children: a prospective study of 642 children. J Pediatr Surg 2002;37(6):865–8.
12. Grosfeld JL. Current concepts in inguinal hernia in infants and children. World J Surg 1989;13(5):506–15.
13. Stylianos S, Jacir NN, Harris BH. Incarceration of inguinal hernia in infants prior to elective repair. J Pediatr Surg 1993;28(4):582–3.
14. Goldman RD, Balasubramanian S, Wales P, et al. Pediatric surgeons and pediatric emergency physicians' attitudes towards analgesia and sedation for incarcerated inguinal hernia reduction. J Pain 2005;6(10):650–5.
15. Potts WJ, Riker WL, Lewis JE. The treatment of inguinal hernia in infants and children. Ann Surg 1950;132(3):566–76.
16. Levitt MA, Ferraraccio D, Arbesman MC, et al. Variability of inguinal hernia surgical technique: a survey of North American pediatric surgeons. J Pediatr Surg 2002;37(5):745–51.
17. Chen LE, Zamakhshary M, Foglia RP, et al. Impact of wait time on outcome for inguinal hernia repair in infants. Pediatr Surg Int 2009;25(3):223–7.
18. Harper RG, Garcia A, Sia C. Inguinal hernia: a common problem of premature infants weighing 1,000 grams or less at birth. Pediatrics 1975;56(1):112–5.
19. Rescorla FJ, Grosfeld JL. Inguinal hernia repair in the perinatal period and early infancy: clinical considerations. J Pediatr Surg 1984;19(6):832–7.
20. Puri P, Guiney EJ, O'Donnell B. Inguinal hernia in infants: the fate of the testis following incarceration. J Pediatr Surg 1984;19(1):44–6.
21. Gonzalez Santacruz M, Mira Navarro J, Encinas Goenechea A, et al. Low prevalence of complications of delayed herniotomy in the extremely premature infant. Acta Paediatr 2004;93(1):94–8.
22. Krieger NR, Shochat SJ, McGowan V, et al. Early hernia repair in the premature infant: long-term follow-up. J Pediatr Surg 1994;29(8):978–81 [discussion: 981–2].
23. Melone JH, Schwartz MZ, Tyson KR, et al. Outpatient inguinal herniorrhaphy in premature infants: is it safe? J Pediatr Surg 1992;27(2):203–7 [discussion: 207–8].
24. Misra D, Hewitt G, Potts SR, et al. Inguinal herniotomy in young infants, with emphasis on premature neonates. J Pediatr Surg 1994;29(11):1496–8.
25. Misra D. Inguinal hernias in premature babies: wait or operate? Acta Paediatr 2001;90(4):370–1.
26. Rajput A, Gauderer MW, Hack M. Inguinal hernias in very low birth weight infants: incidence and timing of repair. J Pediatr Surg 1992;27(10):1322–4.
27. Uemura S, Woodward AA, Amerena R, et al. Early repair of inguinal hernia in premature babies. Pediatr Surg Int 1999;15(1):36–9.

28. Wiener ES, Touloukian RJ, Rodgers BM, et al. Hernia survey of the Section on Surgery of the American Academy of Pediatrics. J Pediatr Surg 1996;31(8): 1166–9.

29. DeCou JM, Gauderer MW. Inguinal hernia in infants with very low birth weight. Semin Pediatr Surg 2000;9(2):84–7.

30. Warner LO, Teitelbaum DH, Caniano DA, et al. Inguinal herniorrhaphy in young infants: perianesthetic complications and associated preanesthetic risk factors. J Clin Anesth 1992;4(6):455–61.

31. Antonoff MB, Kreykes NS, Saltzman DA, et al. American Academy of Pediatrics Section on Surgery hernia survey revisited. J Pediatr Surg 2005;40(6):1009–14.

32. Walther-Larsen S, Rasmussen LS. The former preterm infant and risk of post-operative apnoea: recommendations for management. Acta Anaesthesiol Scand 2006;50(7):888–93.

33. Allen GS, Cox CS Jr, White N, et al. Postoperative respiratory complications in ex-premature infants after inguinal herniorrhaphy. J Pediatr Surg 1998;33(7):1095–8.

34. Rothenburg R, Barnett T. Bilateral herniotomy in infants and children. Surgery 1955;37:947–50.

35. Zona JZ. The incidence of positive contralateral inguinal exploration among preschool children—a retrospective and prospective study. J Pediatr Surg 1996;31(5):656–60.

36. Rowe MI, Clatworthy HW Jr. The other side of the pediatric inguinal hernia. Surg Clin North Am 1971;51(6):1371–6.

37. Given JP, Rubin SZ. Occurrence of contralateral inguinal hernia following unilat-eral repair in a pediatric hospital. J Pediatr Surg 1989;24(10):963–5.

38. Janik JS, Shandling B. The vulnerability of the vas deferens (II): the case against routine bilateral inguinal exploration. J Pediatr Surg 1982;17(5):585–8.

39. McGregor DB, Halverson K, McVay CB. The unilateral pediatric inguinal hernia: should the contralateral side by explored? J Pediatr Surg 1980;15(3):313–7.

40. Surana R, Puri P. Is contralateral exploration necessary in infants with unilateral inguinal hernia? J Pediatr Surg 1993;28(8):1026–7.

41. Sparkman RS. Bilateral exploration in inguinal hernia in juvenile patients. Review and appraisal. Surgery 1962;51:393–406.

42. Kiesewetter WB, Parenzan L. When should hernia in the infant be treated bilater-ally? J Am Med Assoc 1959;171:287–90.

43. Tackett LD, Breuer CK, Luks FI, et al. Incidence of contralateral inguinal hernia: a prospective analysis. J Pediatr Surg 1999;34(5):684–7 [discussion: 687–8].

44. Rathauser F. Historical overview of the bilateral approach to pediatric inguinal hernias. Am J Surg 1985;150(5):527–32.

45. Lazar DA, Lee TC, Almulhim SI, et al. Transinguinal laparoscopic exploration for identification of contralateral inguinal hernias in pediatric patients. J Pediatr Surg 2011;46(12):2349–52.

46. Wulkan ML, Wiener ES, VanBalen N, et al. Laparoscopy through the open ipsilat-eral sac to evaluate presence of contralateral hernia. J Pediatr Surg 1996;31(8): 1174–6 [discussion: 1176–7].

47. Holcomb GW 3rd, Brock JW 3rd, Morgan WM 3rd. Laparoscopic evaluation for a contralateral patent processus vaginalis. J Pediatr Surg 1994;29(8):970–3 [discussion: 974].

48. Rowe MI, Marchildon MB. Inguinal hernia and hydrocele in infants and children. Surg Clin North Am 1981;61(5):1137–45.

49. Miltenburg DM, Nuchtern JG, Jaksic T, et al. Meta-analysis of the risk of meta-chronous hernia in infants and children. Am J Surg 1997;174(6):741–4.

50. Sozubir S, Ekingen G, Senel U, et al. A continuous debate on contralateral processus vaginalis: evaluation technique and approach to patency. Hernia 2006; 10(1):74–8.
51. Hata S, Takahashi Y, Nakamura T, et al. Preoperative sonographic evaluation is a useful method of detecting contralateral patent processus vaginalis in pediatric patients with unilateral inguinal hernia. J Pediatr Surg 2004;39(9):1396–9.
52. Kastenberg Z, Bruzoni M, Dutta S. A modification of the laparoscopic transcutaneous inguinal hernia repair to achieve transfixation ligature of the hernia sac. J Pediatr Surg 2011;46(8):1658–64.
53. Parelkar SV, Oak S, Gupta R, et al. Laparoscopic inguinal hernia repair in the pediatric age group—experience with 437 children. J Pediatr Surg 2010;45(4): 789–92.
54. Montupet P, Esposito C. Fifteen years experience in laparoscopic inguinal hernia repair in pediatric patients. Results and considerations on a debated procedure. Surg Endosc 2011;25(2):450–3.
55. Sneider EB, Jones S, Danielson PD. Refinements in selection criteria for pediatric laparoscopic inguinal hernia repair. J Laparoendosc Adv Surg Tech A 2009; 19(2):237–40.
56. Becmeur F, Phillipe P, Lemandat-Schultz A, et al. A continuous series of 96 laparoscopic inguinal hernia repairs in children by a new technique. Surg Endosc 2004;18(12):1738–41.
57. Chan KL, Hui WC, Tam PK. Prospective randomized single-center, single-blind comparison of laparoscopic vs open repair of pediatric inguinal hernia. Surg Endosc 2005;19(7):927–32.
58. Spurbeck WW, Prasad R, Lobe TE. Two-year experience with minimally invasive herniorrhaphy in children. Surg Endosc 2005;19(4):551–3.
59. Schier F. Laparoscopic inguinal hernia repair—a prospective personal series of 542 children. J Pediatr Surg 2006;41(6):1081–4.
60. Ozgediz D, Roayaie K, Lee H, et al. Subcutaneous endoscopically assisted ligation (SEAL) of the internal ring for repair of inguinal hernias in children: report of a new technique and early results. Surg Endosc 2007;21(8):1327–31.
61. Dutta S, Albanese C. Transcutaneous laparoscopic hernia repair in children: a prospective review of 275 hernia repairs with minimum 2-year follow-up. Surg Endosc 2009;23(1):103–7.
62. Koivusalo AI, Korpela R, Wirtavuori K, et al. A single-blinded, randomized comparison of laparoscopic versus open hernia repair in children. Pediatrics 2009;123(1):332–7.
63. Saranga Bharathi R, Arora M, Baskaran V. Pediatric inguinal hernia: laparoscopic versus open surgery. JSLS 2008;12(3):277–81.
64. Palabiyik FB, Cimilli T, Kayhan A, et al. Do the manipulations in pediatric inguinal hernia operations affect the vascularization of testes? J Pediatr Surg 2009;44(4): 788–90.
65. Phelps S, Agrawal M. Morbidity after neonatal inguinal herniotomy. J Pediatr Surg 1997;32(3):445–7.
66. Zendejas B, Zarroug AE, Erben YM, et al. Impact of childhood inguinal hernia repair in adulthood: 50 years of follow-up. J Am Coll Surg 2010;211(6):762–8.
67. Repair of groin hernia with synthetic mesh: meta-analysis of randomized controlled trials. Ann Surg 2002;235(3):322–32.
68. Amid PK. Groin hernia repair: open techniques. World J Surg 2005;29(8):1046–51.
69. Amid PK. Lichtenstein tension-free hernioplasty: its inception, evolution, and principles. Hernia 2004;8(1):1–7.

70. Kugel RD. Minimally invasive, nonlaparoscopic, preperitoneal, and sutureless, inguinal herniorrhaphy. Am J Surg 1999;178(4):298–302.
71. Fitzgibbons RJ Jr. Can we be sure polypropylene mesh causes infertility? Ann Surg 2005;241(4):559–61.
72. Shin D, Lipshultz LI, Goldstein M, et al. Herniorrhaphy with polypropylene mesh causing inguinal vasal obstruction: a preventable cause of obstructive azoospermia. Ann Surg 2005;241(4):553–8.
73. Koski ME, Makari JH, Adams MC, et al. Infant communicating hydroceles—do they need immediate repair or might some clinically resolve? J Pediatr Surg 2010;45(3):590–3.
74. Katz DA. Evaluation and management of inguinal and umbilical hernias. Pediatr Ann 2001;30(12):729–35.
75. Cortes D. Cryptorchidism—aspects of pathogenesis, histology and treatment. Scand J Urol Nephrol Suppl 1998;196:1–54.
76. Lee PA. Fertility after cryptorchidism: epidemiology and other outcome studies. Urology 2005;66(2):427–31.
77. Wood HM, Elder JS. Cryptorchidism and testicular cancer: separating fact from fiction. J Urol 2009;181(2):452–61.
78. Swerdlow AJ, Higgins CD, Pike MC. Risk of testicular cancer in cohort of boys with cryptorchidism. BMJ 1997;314(7093):1507–11.
79. Prener A, Engholm G, Jensen OM. Genital anomalies and risk for testicular cancer in Danish men. Epidemiology 1996;7(1):14–9.
80. Jordan GH. Laparoscopic management of the undescended testicle. Urol Clin North Am 2001;28(1):23–9, vii–viii.
81. Cortes D, Thorup JM, Visfeldt J. Cryptorchidism: aspects of fertility and neoplasms. A study including data of 1,335 consecutive boys who underwent testicular biopsy simultaneously with surgery for cryptorchidism. Horm Res 2001;55(1):21–7.
82. Escarcega-Fujigaki P, Rezk GH, Huerta-Murrieta E, et al. Orchiopexy-laparoscopy or traditional surgical technique in patients with an undescended palpable testicle. J Laparoendosc Adv Surg Tech A 2011;21(2):185–7.
83. Hutson JM, Clarke MC. Current management of the undescended testicle. Semin Pediatr Surg 2007;16(1):64–70.
84. Tasian GE, Hittelman AB, Kim GE, et al. Age at orchiopexy and testis palpability predict germ and Leydig cell loss: clinical predictors of adverse histological features of cryptorchidism. J Urol 2009;182(2):704–9.
85. Peters CA. Laparoscopy in pediatric urology. Curr Opin Urol 2004;14(2):67–73.
86. Elyas R, Guerra LA, Pike J, et al. Is staging beneficial for Fowler-Stephens orchiopexy? A systematic review. J Urol 2010;183(5):2012–8.
87. Lee PA, Coughlin MT. Fertility after bilateral cryptorchidism. Evaluation by paternity, hormone, and semen data. Horm Res 2001;55(1):28–32.

# Diagnosis and Management of Pediatric Appendicitis, Intussusception, and Meckel Diverticulum

Victoria K. Pepper, MD, Amy B. Stanfill, MD, Richard H. Pearl, MD*

## KEYWORDS

- Right lower quadrant • Abdominal pain • Appendicitis • Appendectomy
- Meckel diverticulum • Intussusception • Pediatric

## KEY POINTS

- A classic presentation of appendicitis begins with the gradual onset of dull periumbilical pain followed by migration of this pain to the right lower quadrant.
- Initially, the appendiceal lumen becomes obstructed, leading to distention and increased intraluminal pressure.
- An increased white blood cell (WBC) count (>10,000–12,000 cells per cubic millimeter) significantly increases the odds of appendicitis. In the abscence of leukocytosis and fever, appendicitis is unlikely.

## APPENDICITIS

Appendicitis is the most common pediatric abdominal surgical emergency worldwide. It is estimated that 86 cases of appendicitis per 100,000 people occur annually, with an estimated 70,000 pediatric appendectomies performed in the United States each year.[1] In the last several decades, both the diagnosis and management of appendicitis have undergone significant evolution. These changes stem from a variety of causes, including recent advances in laparoscopy, concerns regarding radiation exposure, and advances in pediatric imaging. This article highlights those changes in practice as well as some of the remaining controversies in care regarding pediatric appendicitis.

### Diagnosis

#### Demographics

The peak incidence occurs in the second decade of life with the median age at diagnosis between 10 and 11 years. Male/female ratio is 1.4:1. Appendicitis also seems to have

The authors have nothing to disclose.

Section of Pediatric Surgery, Department of Surgery, University of Illinois College of Medicine at Peoria, Children's Hospital of Illinois, Peoria, IL, USA
* 420 NE Glen Oak Avenue #201, Peoria, IL 61603.
E-mail address: rhpearl@uic.edu

a seasonal variation with increased presentation of appendicitis in the summer months. However, perforated appendicitis occurs more frequently in the fall and winter.[2]

### Symptoms

A classic presentation of appendicitis begins with the gradual onset of dull periumbilical pain followed by migration of this pain to the right lower quadrant. Nausea and vomiting, when they occur, typically follow the onset of pain. Anorexia and fever are also common complaints, with diarrhea occurring less frequently. Classic teaching suggests that perforation occurs at 24 to 36 hours from the onset of the first symptom, which is usually pain. When perforation occurs, the pain may increase greatly and can become more generalized. Because of the increased inflammatory response, perforation is often associated with higher fevers, increased systemic symptoms, and increased laboratory values (WBC count and C-reactive protein [CRP]).

The cause of this progression lies in the physiology of the abdomen and peritoneum. Initially, the appendiceal lumen becomes obstructed, leading to distention and increased intraluminal pressure. This distention causes stimulation of the eighth to tenth visceral afferent thoracic nerves, leading to a mild periumbilical pain. Increasing intraluminal pressure evolves into tissue ischemia, mucosal compromise, and eventual transmural inflammation. This inflammation spreads to the parietal peritoneum, leading to localized somatic pain in the right lower quadrant and constitutional symptoms of fever, nausea, emesis, and anorexia. Necrosis is followed by eventual perforation.

Although this is presented as the classic picture of appendicitis, it occurs in fewer than 50% of children. However, certain findings have been shown to increase or decrease the likelihood of appendicitis. Most significant is the evolution of midabdominal pain migrating to the right lower quadrant (likelihood ratio [LR] 1.9–3.1) and the presence of fever (LR 3.4). The absence of fever lowers the likelihood of appendicitis by two-thirds. This confusion in clinical picture leads to a delay in diagnosis, as well as increasing the rate of perforated appendicitis among pediatric patients. Because of a lack of reliable history, rates of perforation as high as 80% to 100% have been reported in children less than 3 years of age. Children aged 10 to 17 years have a lower rate of perforation at 20%.[3]

### Signs

The signs of appendicitis in the pediatric population are equally difficult to interpret. Up to 44% of children present with multiple atypical clinical findings. Classic physical examination findings include tenderness to palpation and guarding in the right lower quadrant, hypoactive bowel sounds, percussive tenderness, and rebound tenderness. Certain maneuvers can be used to assess for appendicitis. The Rovsing sign involves palpating the left lower quadrant and is considered positive when the patient feels referred pain in the right lower quadrant. A positive obturator sign occurs when pain is elicited with internal rotation of the right lower extremity while it is flexed at the knee and hip. The Psoas sign is elicited while the patient lies on his or her left side and is considered positive if pain occurs with extension at the hip. Of these findings, only rebound tenderness has been shown to correlate with increased likelihood of appendicitis (LR 2.3–3.9). Lack of tenderness in the right lower quadrant reduces the likelihood of appendicitis by half.[4]

### Laboratory studies

Typical studies ordered for suspected appendicitis include a complete blood count (CBC) and a comprehensive metabolic panel (CMP). Although the CMP has little diagnostic usefulness for appendicitis, it allows assessment of electrolyte status as well as evaluation for potential alternative causes of abdominal pain. An increased WBC count (>10,000–12,000 cells per cubic millimeter) significantly increases the odds of appendicitis. Kwan and Nager[5] showed an adjusted odds ratio of 6.5 for a WBC count greater than 12,000 per cubic millimeter. In toddlers (<4 years), a normal WBC count has a negative predictive value of 95.6%, whereas the negative predictive value in children (ages 4–11.9 years) is 89.5%. The negative predictive value of a low or normal WBC count among adolescents is 91.9%.[4] A left shift (increased immature forms of neutrophils) also has a strong association with appendicitis, because only 3.7% of pediatric patients without left shift have appendicitis.

## Scoring systems

Several scoring systems exist for the diagnosis of appendicitis; however, 2 systems have been evaluated in pediatric patients. The first is the Alvarado score, which was initially developed for use in the adult population. The Alvarado score is composed of 8 components with a total score of 10 (**Table 1**). Alvarado scores of 1 to 4 are negative for appendicitis, whereas scores from 9 to 10 are diagnostic of appendicitis. In cases of intermediate scores of 5 to 8, further diagnostic studies are required. Using these specifications, a 93% sensitivity, 100% specificity, 100% positive predictive value (PPV), and 96% negative predictive value (NPV) are obtained.[6]

The Pediatric Appendicitis Score (PAS) is composed of 8 components with a total score of 10 (**Table 2**). A score of 1 to 3 is considered negative for appendicitis, whereas scores from 8 to 10 are considered positive. The intermediate scores of 4 to 7 require further diagnostic testing. With these thresholds, the sensitivity for appendicitis is 97% with a specificity of 97.6%, a PPV of 97.2%, and an NPV of 97.6%.[7,8] Although both of these systems have been shown to be useful in the diagnosis of appendicitis, they do not replace an experienced clinician.

## Differential Diagnosis

The differential diagnosis is varied, but is divided into 5 general categories: inflammatory, infectious, vascular, congenital, and genitourinary conditions. Inflammatory mimickers of appendicitis include mesenteric adenitis (primary or secondary), inflammatory bowel disease, intussusception, omental infarction, or epiploic appendagitis. When CT (computed tomography) scans are performed for right lower quadrant pain, mesenteric adenitis is the most common alternative diagnosis, followed closely by inflammatory bowel diseases. Infectious causes include viral infections, bacterial infections, and parasitic infections. Among vascular causes, Henoch-Schonlein purpura can initially

| Table 1<br>Alvarado score | |
|---|---|
| Migration of pain | 1 |
| Anorexia | 1 |
| Nausea/vomiting | 1 |
| Right lower quadrant tenderness | 2 |
| Rebound pain | 1 |
| Increase in temperature (>37.3°C) | 1 |
| Leukocytosis (>10,000/μL) | 2 |
| Polymorphonuclear neutrophilia (>75%) | 1 |
| Total | 10 |

| Table 2 PAS | |
|---|---|
| Migration of pain | 1 |
| Anorexia | 1 |
| Nausea/vomiting | 1 |
| Right lower quadrant tenderness | 2 |
| Cough/hopping/percussion tenderness in right lower quadrant | 2 |
| Increase in temperature | 1 |
| Leukocytes >10,000/μL | 1 |
| Polymorphonuclear neutrophilia >75% | 1 |
| Total | 10 |

present as severe abdominal pain before the characteristic purpuric rash appears. Congenital causes include Meckel diverticulum, Meckel diverticulitis, and duplication cysts. Genitourinary causes include pyelonephritis, nephrolithiasis, ovarian torsion, ovarian tumors, hemorrhagic ovarian cysts, pelvic inflammatory disease, and infected urachal remnants. Constipation cannot be forgotten when evaluating pediatric patients because it is often a culprit in abdominal pain.

### Imaging

**Radiograph** Radiograph imaging has little usefulness in confirming straightforward appendicitis and should not be performed unless considering alternative diagnoses, such as constipation. Occasionally an appendicolith can be seen on abdominal film, although, without symptoms, it is not an indication for appendectomy.

**Ultrasound** Ultrasound (US) has become an increasingly sophisticated diagnostic modality in the last 20 years with the added bonus of no radiation exposure. US has also allowed improved selection of patients requiring surgery and/or admission from the emergency department, as well as decreasing recurrent emergency room referrals. Multiple studies have focused on the ability of US to be used as an adjunct in the diagnosis of appendicitis in the adult population as well as in the pediatric population. Sonographic criteria for appendicitis include a blind-ending tubular structure with a diameter greater than 6 mm; a wall thicker than 2 mm; or an irregular wall that is rigid, noncompressible, and lacks peristalsis. Other signs that may suggest appendicitis include absence of air in the appendiceal lumen, periappendiceal fat changes, visible appendicolith, complex mass, mesenteric lymph nodes, and free fluid.[9] A wide range of sensitivities and specificities can be found in the literature. Goldin and colleagues[10] showed that increasing the parameters of the diameter to 7 mm and the thickness to 1.7 mm improved the sensitivity to 98.7% and the specificity to 95.4%. Further studies have also shown that surgeon-performed US with clinical evaluation may yield similar accuracy as radiologist-performed US.[11]

One concern regarding US surrounds its use in obese patients. Although some studies state that there is no difference based on weight within the pediatric population, several studies have shown decreased visualization of the appendix with increased obesity or abdominal wall thickness.[12,13] Other studies have revealed an increased need for CT to definitively diagnose appendicitis in obese pediatric patients.[14] Because of the conflicting data on this subject, no firm answer can be provided currently and further prospective studies are needed for evaluation.

**CT** Two types of CT scans can be performed when evaluating for appendicitis. The first protocol consists of oral and intravenous contrast, whereas the second uses rectal and intravenous contrast. Both methods use criteria including nonfilling appendix, appendicolith, fat stranding in the right lower quadrant, appendix diameter greater than 6 mm, appendiceal wall thickening, or arrowhead sign. The sensitivity of CT scan for appendicitis is 97%, with a specificity of 99%, PPV of 98%, and NPV of 98%. The accuracy of CT scan for diagnosing acute appendicitis is 96%.[15,16] Perforated appendicitis is suggested by appendicolith with intraluminal appendiceal air, extraluminal air, bowel wall thickening, ileal wall enhancement, extraluminal appendicolith, abscess, phlegmon, periappendiceal inflammatory stranding, and free fluid. The accuracy of CT scan for perforation is 72%, with a sensitivity of 62% and specificity of 82%. Both the standard prep of Gastrografin and Volumen (1-hour prep) have been shown to be equally efficacious in visualization of the appendix.[17] Nonvisualization of the appendix has been shown to have a high NPV (98.7%).[18]

**US versus CT** Current controversy seems to center around the use of CT versus US. US has the advantage of being low-cost without exposure to dyes and radiation, as well as providing dynamic information. However, it has significant disadvantages including being highly operator dependent and being limited by patient body habitus as well as appendiceal location. In the pediatric population, the sensitivity of US ranges from 78% to 94% and the specificity ranges from 89% to 98%. Accuracy has been reported between 89% and 98%.[1] Another concern regarding US is the potential lack of availability during the night shifts, when CT scan use has been shown to increase.[19] CT scans are not affected by the patient's size, the position of appendix, or availability of experienced technicians.[20] CT scans also have a higher sensitivity (95%–99%) and specificity (83%–100%) throughout the literature. Disadvantages include a prolonged preparation time as well as exposure to both intravenous dyes and radiation. One CT scan of the abdomen in a 5-year-old child increases the lifetime risk of radiation-induced cancer to 26.1 per 100,000 in women and 20.1 per 100,000 in men.[21]

Most of the literature now focuses on a combination of analytical models such as the PAS or Alvarado score with sequential imaging. Most centers first perform an US in the intermediate groups, followed by CT scan or serial examinations if the US is nondiagnostic. This protocol has resulted in a high sensitivity (96%–99%) and specificity (83%–92%) for the diagnosis of appendicitis.[22] These pathways have also shown an improvement in the overall hospital costs, as well as the incremental cost-effectiveness ratios.

When evaluating a patient for appendicitis, the importance of clinical judgment cannot be overstated. Although at many centers there is an increased reliance on CT scans, studies have clearly shown that the diagnosis of appendicitis can be made with history, examination, and selective use of US. Williams and colleagues[23] showed that a pediatric surgeon can differentiate appendicitis from other abdominal disorders with 92% accuracy. Our center's experience and the literature confirm that patients with suspected appendicitis can be successfully evaluated without the use of CT scan in most patients.

## Treatment

### Antibiotics

For more than 30 years, pediatric surgeons used a triple-antibiotic regimen when dealing with appendicitis, consisting of ampicillin, gentamicin, and clindamycin. With the changes in the adult antibiotic regimens, pediatric surgery has evolved from this triple-antibiotic regimen to a simpler single-drug regimen. Bacteriologic epidemiology of appendicitis shows that the most commonly isolated organisms are *Escherichia coli*, *Streptococcus* group *milleri*, anaerobes, and *Pseudomonas aeruginosa*. Both piperacillin/tazobactam and cefoxitin have been shown to be at least as efficacious as the triple-drug regimen, and may also decrease length of stay and pharmaceutical costs.[24] Other studies suggest that metronidazole must be added to a third-generation cephalosporin to cover anaerobic isolates.[25,26]

The length of treatment is determined by presence or lack of perforation. In general, broad-spectrum coverage is recommended before operation. Our center prefers a single dose of cefoxitin (40 mg/kg). In simple appendicitis, the treatment of pediatric patients mirrors that of adults and consists of a single perioperative dose of antibiotics. With perforated appendicitis, at least a 5-day course of broad-spectrum antibiotics, such as piperacillin/tazobactam, is recommended. However, similar results were achieved using a 7-day course that initiated with intravenous antibiotics and finished with oral antibiotics. Total length of antibiotic therapy should be determined by the clinical condition of the patient, including resolution of fever, pain, bowel function, and WBC count.[27]

### Nonoperative management of acute appendicitis

Limited data exist from Europe regarding the management of acute appendicitis with antibiotics alone. One study from Turkey selected outpatients with less than 24 hours of pain and treated them with parenteral antibiotics (ampicillin/sulbactam) with resolution of symptoms within all 16 patients.[28] The experience with nonoperative management in this fashion is limited and it is not recommended.

### Surgical options for acute appendicitis

**Incidental appendectomies** Incidental appendectomy is not advocated except in specific situations, including any surgery that has a right lower quadrant incision such as Meckel diverticulectomy or intussusception reduction. Occasionally a patient is found to have appendicolith while being evaluated for other disorders and this is not, in itself, an indication for appendectomy. Incidental appendectomy has not shown any benefit and usually should not be pursued, particularly if the procedure will be converted from a clean to clean-contaminated case.

**Delayed appendectomy** Although traditional teaching was that appendectomy must be performed emergently, recent studies have challenged this belief. When comparing emergent appendectomy (within 5 hours of admission) to urgent appendectomy (within 17 hours), it has been shown that there is no difference in gangrenous/perforated appendixes, operative length, readmission, postoperative complications, hospital stay, or hospital charges.[29] Most centers think that appendectomy can safely be delayed until morning in patients presenting at night, although it is recommended to start broad-spectrum antibiotics during the delay.

**Open appendectomy** Traditional appendectomy was first described by McBurney[30] and is still used for both acute and perforated appendicitis, although our center has not performed one in more than 10 years. Most surgeons use a transverse or oblique right lower quadrant incision. Dissection is carried down to the muscle, which is split.

The mesoappendix is divided, followed by excision of the appendix at its base. Management of the appendiceal stump can involve simple ligation, ligation and inversion using a purse-string, or pure inversion without ligature. The method used is a matter of physician preference.

**Three-port laparoscopic appendectomy** Traditional laparoscopic appendectomies involve one 10-mm to 12-mm port and two 5-mm ports. Traditionally, the larger port is placed at the umbilicus, although variations exist. The two 5-mm port sites can be placed in the left lower quadrant and in the suprapubic midline, with care taken to avoid injury of the bladder. Once ports are in place, the camera is usually placed in the left lower quadrant port. Laparoscopy allows visualization of the entire abdomen, which provides a significant advantage compared with open appendectomies.

Regarding division of the mesoappendix, several methods are available. Studies have shown than division of the mesoappendix in pediatric patients with electrocautery is safe and cost-effective.[31] Some physicians prefer a US-activated scalpel (Harmonic) for division of the mesoappendix. The advantages include decreased exchanges of instruments as well as preventing theoretic current transmission.[32] With either of these methods, an endoloop can be used to effectively ligate the appendiceal stump, which provides further cost saving measures compared with an endostapling device. Alternatively, endostapling devices can be used to divide both the mesoappendix and the appendix.

**Transumbilical laparoscopic appendectomy** Transumbilical laparoscopic appendectomy provides a middle ground of open and laparoscopic appendectomies. The procedure starts with the placement of a 12-mm umbilical trocar site, through which a working laparoscopic camera with single 5-mm instrument port is inserted. Once the appendix has been grasped, it is withdrawn through the umbilical incision (**Fig. 1**). A traditional appendectomy with division of the mesoappendix and excision of the appendix can then be performed. Multiple studies have shown that transumbilical laparoscopic appendectomies are safe with similar complication rates to traditional laparoscopic appendectomies in both simple and complicated appendicitis. They also provide the benefit of scarless surgery.[33]

**Single-incision laparoscopic appendectomy** Single-incision laparoscopic appendectomies are performed using a 12-mm incision at the umbilicus. Multiple devices

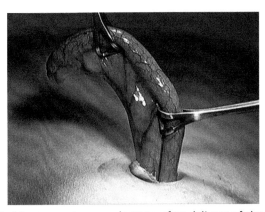

**Fig. 1.** Transumbilical laparoscopic appendectomy after delivery of the appendix through the umbilical incision. The appendix and mesoappendix may be resected at this point using traditional techniques.

have been developed to provide multiple ports through this single-incision including the SILS port (Covidien, Norwalk, CT, USA) and the TriPort Access System (Advanced Surgical Concepts, Wicklow, Ireland). Dissection and transection of the appendix and mesoappendix can proceed similarly to a traditional laparoscopic appendectomy. Safety and efficacy are noted to be the same as with other methods, but operative times are slightly longer, most likely secondary to the learning process.[34]

### Laparoscopic versus open appendectomy

When dealing with either simple or perforated appendicitis, the laparoscopic approach has been found to be safe and efficacious. Overall, laparoscopy leads to decreased length of stay and decreased time to oral intake. Length of stay decreases from an average of 3 days to 2 days for simple appendicitis and 7 to 5 days for complicated appendicitis.[35] In many centers, simple appendectomies can lead to discharge within 24 hours. Complication rates are lower overall for laparoscopic appendectomies, although the postoperative intra-abdominal abscess rate is higher with the laparoscopic approach.[36] For this reason, laparoscopic appendectomy is thought to be a safe option when dealing with appendicitis in any stage of disease.

### Nonoperative versus operative management of perforated appendicitis

Complicated or perforated appendicitis remains an area of significant debate. As discussed earlier, laparoscopic appendectomy can safely be performed when dealing with perforated appendicitis. When dealing with complicated perforated appendicitis with abscess or phlegmon, the treatment can either be antibiotics with or without immediate drainage or surgical intervention. Nonoperative management is most commonly used in patients with symptoms for more than 3 days, absence of diffuse peritonitis, absence of obstruction, and mass on imaging or examination. These patients are placed on broad-spectrum antibiotics (Zosyn, triple-antibiotic therapy, gentamicin, and clindamycin) can undergo drainage of the fluid collections greater than 2 cm in size.[37] Drainage can be performed through US or CT guidance and may be performed via a transabdominal, transgluteal, or transrectal approach. The transvaginal approach is not recommended in pediatric patients unless the patient is a teenager who is postpartum or admits to sexual activity.

A nonoperative approach to appendicitis is traditionally followed by an interval appendectomy. The need for interval appendectomy has been called into question recently. Retrospective studies have shown that up to 80% of children may not require appendectomy and that 3% of patients suffer a complication secondary to interval appendectomy.[38] More recent prospective studies have shown a recurrence rate of 8% to 43%, with an increased rate of reoccurrence among patients with appendicolith.[39,40] This finding suggests that the morbidity of surgery may be avoided by selective surgery in patients with certain criteria, such as the presence of appendicolith.

Another issue under debate is whether these patients with complicated appendicitis should have conservative management or undergo initial operative management. Recent studies have shown improvement in return to normal activity as well as decreased complications when early appendectomy is performed.[41] At our center, we practice selective early intervention depending on patient condition and size or presence of fluid collection.

### Postoperative Care

Postoperative care depends largely on a patient's intraoperative findings. With simple appendicitis, early oral intake and discharge within 24 hours is increasingly seen. With laparoscopic approaches, patients are frequently discharged from the recovery room. Perforated appendicitis requires postoperative antibiotics and more care should be taken with advancement of diet. Routine nasogastric tube placement with perforated appendicitis has been abandoned and should only be performed in cases of ileus or obstruction. Many patients with simple perforated appendicitis tolerate advancement of diet at a similar rate as with nonperforated appendicitis. However, patients with complicated appendicitis often suffer significant ileus. Antibiotic therapy should be continued until the patient's clinical condition improves, as seen by resolution of ileus, abdominal pain, normalization of WBC count, and lack of fever.

### Complications

Postoperative complications include wound infection, deep-space infections, bowel obstruction, and stump appendicitis.[42] Different measures have been advocated to prevent wound infections, including use of wound protectors in perforated appendicitis and Endobag. No benefit has been seen with interrupted closure of wounds or with keeping wounds open. To decrease intra-abdominal abscess formation, many surgeons use peritoneal lavage with saline or sterile water. Drain placement has largely been abandoned.

### SUMMARY

1. Appendicitis most frequently occurs between the ages of 10 to 11 years.
2. The classic signs and symptoms of appendicitis occur in less than half of pediatric patients. The most sensitive symptoms include migrating pain to the right lower quadrant and fever. Rebound tenderness on examination also increases the likelihood of appendicitis.
3. Increased WBC count and left shift are the most accurate laboratory values when assessing for appendicitis.
4. Clinical judgment and judicious studies are the best methods when assessing for appendicitis. Scoring systems such as the Alvarado score and PAS have also been shown to be useful in diagnosis.
5. US is the imaging study of choice and CT scans should be avoided in pediatric patients because of radiation exposure.
6. Although both open and laparoscopic approaches have been shown to be safe and effective with simple or complex appendicitis, laparoscopic appendectomies are recommended.
7. The treatment of complex appendicitis with mass or abscess is still controversial, with support for both operative and conservative management. With nonoperative management, controversy also exists regarding interval appendectomy.

### INTUSSUSCEPTION

The invagination of a proximal intestinal segment into a distal section of bowel is referred to as intussusception. The portion of bowel that invaginates into the distal bowel is referred to as the intussusceptum, whereas the distal segment is referred to as intussuscipiens (**Fig. 2**). Intussusception is one of the most frequent causes of bowel obstruction in the pediatric population. Significant complications including bowel necrosis, perforation, and death can occur if there is a delay in diagnosis. For this reason, there is significant onus on clinicians to accurately and promptly diagnose intussusception.

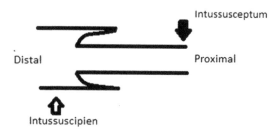

**Fig. 2.** The intussusceptum (*dark arrow*) invaginates into the intussuscipiens (*outlined arrow*). In ileocecal intussusception, the ileum is the intussusceptum and the cecum is the intussuscipiens.

## Diagnosis

### Demographics

Although intussusception can occur at any age, it most frequently occurs before the age of 2 years, with peak incidence between 5 and 10 months.[43] The incidence is reported as 56 children per 100,000 per year. The ratio of males to females is 2:1. There is also a seasonal variation, with increasing incidence in the fall and winter months.

### Classification and pathogenesis

Intussusception is classified by anatomic location or by pathogenesis. Most commonly, intussusceptions are ileocolic, but can also be ileoileal, colocolic, or located at other gastrointestinal tract locations. Intussusceptions can also be divided into idiopathic intussusception and those secondary to a pathologic lead point.

**Idiopathic** As opposed to adult intussusception, intussusception amongst the pediatric population is usually idiopathic because more than 90% of pediatric intussusception is without pathologic lead point. A greater percentage of idiopathic cases occur among patients less than the age of 2 years. Many mechanisms have been proposed for the pathogenesis of idiopathic intussusception. Because of frequent association with current or recent upper respiratory infections or enteritis, viral or bacterial infections have been proposed as a cause. This theory seemed to be supported by both the seasonal variation of intussusception as well as the increased incidence associated with the tetravalent rhesus-human reassortment rotavirus vaccine (RotaShield; Wyeth-Lederle Vaccines, Philadelphia, PA). This vaccine was initially released in 1998, but was subsequently withdrawn from the market when there was shown to be a 20-fold increase in the risk of intussusception during the first 14 days following vaccine administration.[44] Two further vaccines have been developed since that time: RotaTeq (a live oral human-bovine reassortment rotavirus vaccine; Merck and Co, Whitehouse Station, NJ, USA) and Rotarix (live, oral, human attenuated rotavirus vaccine; GlaxoSmithKline, Brentford, Middlesex, United Kingdom). Multiple studies have shown the safety and efficacy of these vaccinations without increased incidence of intussusception. Current recommendations from the American Academy of Pediatrics advise vaccination with either RotaTeq at ages 2,4, and 6 months or with Rotarix at ages 2 and 4 months.[45]

**Secondary to lead point** Although intussusception secondary to a lead point is more often associated with the adult population, approximately 10% of pediatric patients also have a pathologic lead point.[43] There are multiple possible lead points that are divided into anatomic (Meckel diverticulum, appendix, duplication cyst, heterotopic tissues), tumors (lipomas, lymphoma, ganglioneuroma, Kaposi sarcoma), genetic (hamartomas secondary to Peutz-Jeghers syndrome, cystic fibrosis), vascular (Henoch-Schonlein purpura, hemorrhagic edema, blue rubber bleb nevus syndrome), infectious (pseudomembranous colitis, bacterial), traumatic (secondary to hematoma or dysmotility), secondary to a foreign body (enterostomy tube), and postsurgical lead points. After the age of 3 years, the incidence of pathologic lead point increases with the most common pathologies including Meckel diverticulum, lymphoma, and polyps.[46]

Pathologic lead points are often suggested by an irreducible or recurrent intussusception. When a patient fails enema reduction of the intussusception, care must be taken during surgery to assess the bowel for disorders and treat appropriately, if found. Some studies suggest that recurrent intussusception should increase the clinical suspicion for a lead point, prompting further investigation by radiologic means or by laparoscopy.[47] The appropriate number of repeated nonoperative attempts is still subject to debate.

Patients with lead points secondary to Burkitt lymphoma require special consideration. These children present at a higher median age (10 years) than idiopathic intussusception and are almost always ileocolic intussusceptions. These intussusceptions are usually irreducible by enema techniques. Up to 70% present with stage II disease (primary gastrointestinal tract tumor with or without involvement of associated mesenteric nodes) and can undergo curative resection. These patients benefit from a decreased duration and intensity of chemotherapy, along with an increased survival. Surgeons must therefore be alert for this possibility when operating on irreducible intussusception and thoroughly explore all peritoneal surfaces. Consideration should also be given to collection of ascitic fluid and examination of liver, spleen, and retroperitoneal nodes.[48]

Peutz-Jeghers syndrome (PJS) is an autosomal dominant inherited disorder characterized by gastrointestinal hamartomas, mucocutaneous pigmentation, and an increased cancer risk. It requires special attention secondary to the hamartomas that occur in more than 90% of patients with PJS. These hamartomas occur predominantly in the jejunum, and carry up to a 69% risk of intussusception. Hamartomas greater than 15 mm in diameter have been shown to significantly increase the risk of intussusception and some centers recommend polypectomy at greater than or 10 mm diameter. Surveillance for hamartomas can be achieved through a combination of CT enteroclysis, small bowel follow-through, magnetic resonance enteroclysis, video-capsule endoscopy, and endoscopy with balloon-assisted enteroscopy (BAE). Endoscopy with BAE also allows polypectomy.

### Symptoms and signs

The classic symptoms of intussusception include abdominal pain, vomiting, and currant jelly stool. Patients experience episodic abdominal pain and present with calmness interspersed with fussiness. Other less common symptoms include fever, diarrhea, and constipation. The patient's examination may range from completely benign to tenderness in the right lower quadrant, or even frank peritonitis in a patient with perforation. Some patients may have a tubular, sausage-shaped mass on palpation of the abdomen and/or guaiac-positive stool. However, history and physical examination are unreliable in the diagnosis of intussusception and fewer than 25% to 50% of patients have the classic triad of symptoms.[49]

### Laboratory studies

Although it is useful to obtain a CBC and basic metabolic panel when evaluating a patient with abdominal pain, there are no consistent findings among patients with intussusception. However, increased white blood count or bandemia should alert a clinician to the possibility of perforation or gangrenous bowel.

### Imaging

**Abdominal radiograph** Findings consistent with intussusception on plain film include presence of small bowel obstruction, paucity of right lower quadrant gas, presence of an intracolonic mass, and presence of a rim sign. Some studies suggest that plain films are useful only to detect pneumoperitoneum or for the evaluation of other pathologic conditions.[50,51] Other studies suggest that, in combination with an accurate assessment of the clinical scenario, 2-view or 3-view films of the abdomen can yield similar results to US for sensitivity and specificity.[52,53] These studies generally require the availability of an experienced pediatric surgeon or pediatric radiologist to achieve these results. Most centers prefer US for confirmation of diagnosis and only use plain films as an adjunct to diagnosis.

**US** US was first identified as a promising diagnostic modality for intussusception in the 1980s, and has become the primary modality for diagnosis at many centers. Although US is highly operator dependent, skilled technicians can achieve a sensitivity of 97.9% with a specificity of 97.8%.[54] Findings that indicate intussusception include a target or bull's-eye lesion with concentric echogenic layers. Findings that suggest a decreased likelihood of enema reduction include trapped peritoneal fluid, absence of blood flow, enlarged lymph nodes, and intramural gas.[55] US also allows measurement of length and width of these lesions, aiding in differentiation of small bowel intussusceptions from ileocolonic intussusception. Small bowel intussusceptions have a mean diameter of 1.5 cm with a length of 2.5 cm. Ileocolic intussusceptions have a mean diameter of 3.7 cm and a mean length of 8.2 cm.[56] This differentiation is thought to be important because small bowel intussusceptions are often transient and some centers choose to monitor these patients.

**Fluoroscopy** Although many centers prefer diagnosis with US before fluoroscopic studies, some centers progress straight from initial evaluation to diagnostic contrast enema. This progression is beneficial in initial cost to the patient, as well as in decreasing time to reduction. However, studies show that the lifetime cost-effectiveness increases because of radiation exposure and increased risk of radiation-induced malignancy from 59.7 cases per 100,000 to 79.3 cases per 100,000.[57] For this reason, our center prefers an initial screening evaluation with US followed by therapeutic air enema when required.

**CT/magnetic resonance imaging** Although CT and magnetic resonance imaging (MRI) both have high sensitivity and specificity for intussusception, the use of these modalities is limited. CT scans increase the risk of radiation-induced malignancy. Although MRI is lacking in radiation exposure, it is not cost-effective or readily available in many center. As mentioned earlier, CT scans may be useful for identification of lead points in patients with multiple episodes of intussusception.

### Treatment

#### Antibiotics

Before any treatment of intussusception, our center prefers to administer 1 dose of cefoxitin (40 mg/kg). Although perforation is rare, this provides antibiotic coverage should complications arise. In patients with gross peritonitis, coverage with broad-spectrum antibiotics is necessary and length of treatment should be determined once the degree of contamination is determined.

*Therapeutic enemas*

Therapeutic enemas have become the mainstay in treatment of intussusception. Contraindications to therapeutic enema reduction include evidence of peritonitis, perforation, or necrotic bowel. Both fluoroscopic and US-guided reduction have been advocated with the use of different solutions, including barium, Gastrografin, saline, or pneumatic reduction. Although some centers still use Gastrografin or barium, pneumatic reduction has been shown to have a higher rate of success (>90%) without risk of peritoneal exposure to contrast with perforation. This higher rate of reduction with pneumatic reduction may be secondary to the level of experience in those who use pneumatic reduction, as well as the higher intraluminal pressure used with pneumatic reduction. Although Gastrografin is favored more than barium by some because of its water-soluble state and because it does not hold stool in suspension, which causes intra-abdominal abscesses on perforation, it is less favored than pneumatic reduction secondary to the osmotic shifts of fluid and electrolytes that occur with perforation.[58] Fluoroscopic reduction provides visualization of reduction in most cases, but does expose the patient to radiation. Although classically the fluid or air must be visualized refluxing into the ileum, some studies have shown that nonoperative management may be used in patients without reflux into the ileum if there is symptom resolution.[59] US-guided reduction is limited by the operator's experience.

Therapeutic enemas can be performed even with delayed presentation with similar outcome in reduction.[60] Some centers advocate repeated attempts at reduction before operative intervention if there is suspicion of partial reduction.[61] Studies have also shown the benefit of repeating reduction at a tertiary care center after failed attempts at an outlying facility.[62] This aggressive approach with therapeutic enemas is prompted by the vast improvement in patient outcome for length of stay and return to oral intake. For this reason, it is also advocated that recurrent intussusception be treated with repeat therapeutic enema.

*Operative intervention*

Indications for operative intervention include perforation, peritonitis, and failed nonoperative reduction of intussusception. Both open and laparoscopic approaches can be used for this procedure.

**Open** The open approach consists of performing a right lower quadrant incision similar to that used in appendectomy. Once the abdomen is entered, gentle pressure is placed on the intussuscipiens, gently milking it away from the intussusceptum. Pulling the 2 ends apart is classically avoided secondary to the friability of the bowel and possible perforation. It is also important to examine the bowel following reduction to rule out a lead point as well as to determine the viability of the bowel. If there is ischemia of the bowel, resection is necessary. Most surgeons also perform an appendectomy at the time of reduction because of the location of the incision.

**Laparoscopic** Laparoscopic reduction of intussusception can either be performed using a single-trocar or 3-trocar approach. Although traditionally avoided in open approach, laparoscopic reduction has shown that gentle tension on the intussusceptum while applying gentle pressure to the edge of the intussuscipiens is safe and effective (**Fig. 3**). Although some centers previously advocated ileopexy, it has not been shown to be beneficial in reducing reoccurrences.[63] If there is failure of reduction using this technique, bowel resection can proceed transumbilically or via conversion to a right lower quadrant incision. Although initial success rates with laparoscopic reduction were poor, many centers now achieve approximately an 85% success rates with reduction.[64] Laparoscopic reduction has a small but significant decrease in hospital

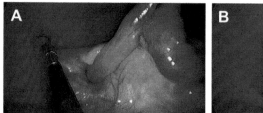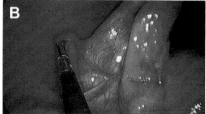

**Fig. 3.** Laparoscopic view of ileocecal intussusception with prereduction view (*A*) and post-reduction view (*B*) of the terminal ileum and cecum.

stay, as well as in time to diet resumption.[65] Whether this is of clinical significance remains controversial.

### Postreduction Management

Most patients who undergo enema reduction can be started immediately on a liquid diet and advanced as tolerated. Some centers advocate reduction and immediate discharge to home. When patients undergo surgical reduction, most can also be rapidly advanced. However, many require a more gradual advancement to general diet. Judgment must be used in patients with significant edema of the bowel and after resection of the bowels.

## SUMMARY

1. A patient presenting with intussusception is usually less than 2 years old. The classic triad of abdominal pain, emesis, and bloody stool is only present in 25% of the population.
2. In older patients (>3 years) with irreducible intussusception or recurrent intussusception, thought should be given to a possible pathologic lead point.[66]
3. After history and physical examination, most patients should undergo US for diagnosis.
4. Therapeutic enema is currently the initial treatment of choice for intussusception and can be used in delayed presentation, recurrent intussusception, and in transferred patients who have had failed reduction attempts at outlying facilities.
5. Patients should be taken to the operating room for gross peritonitis, perforation, or failure of nonoperative reduction techniques. Laparoscopic reduction has been shown to be safe and effective, with reduction in length of stay and return to oral intake.

## MECKEL DIVERTICULUM

Meckel diverticulum is the most common anomaly of the gastrointestinal tract with prevalence from 1% to 4%. Presentation can include gastrointestinal bleed, obstruction, diverticulitis, perforation, and volvulus. Because of this wide range of clinical scenarios, it is important for a clinician to have a high index of suspicion to prevent significant complications.

### Embryology

Meckel diverticula arise through a failure of the omphalomesenteric duct to involute. The omphalomesenteric duct is a connection between the yolk sac and the primitive gut and typically recedes between the fifth and ninth week of gestation. Failure of this obliteration can result in several anomalies including a persistent omphalomesenteric fistula, umbilical cyst, vitelline duct remnant, fibrous bands from the umbilicus to the small bowel, mesodiverticular bands, and Meckel diverticula.[67] Because of the nature of formation, Meckel diverticula are true diverticula involving all layers of the bowel.

## Diagnosis

### Epidemiology

Meckel diverticulum is often referred to by the rule of twos[68]:
- Occurs in 2% of the population (1%–4%)
- Has a 2:1 male/female ratio
- Located within 2 ft (60 cm) of the ileocecal valve on the antimesenteric border
- Commonly 2 cm in diameter
- Commonly 2 in (5 cm) in length
- Can contain 2 types of ectopic tissue (pancreatic and gastric)
- More common before 2 years of age.

### Signs, symptoms, and differential

Meckel diverticulum can present with a wide range of clinical scenarios and can pose a diagnostic challenge. The most common presentations of Meckel diverticula are obstruction and gastrointestinal bleed.

**Gastrointestinal bleed** Heterotopic gastric tissue can be present in up to 50% of symptomatic Meckel diverticula.[69] Because of this active tissue, ulcerations can form at the edge of diverticulum or in the adjoining ileum. These patients present with bloody stool, fatigue, irritability, and abdominal pain. Physical examination is often unremarkable. The bleeding can occur intermittently, causing significant delay in diagnosis.[70] The differential diagnosis includes infectious causes (*Clostridium difficile*, *E coli*), angiodysplasia, malignancy, or upper gastrointestinal bleed.

**Obstruction** Some patients present with an obstructive picture with symptoms including abdominal pain, distention, nausea, and vomiting. Physical examination can include distention, tenderness with palpation, hypoactive bowel sounds, mass, or even peritonitis. Obstruction is often secondary to intussusception of the Meckel into the ileum; however, some Meckel diverticula are attached to the umbilicus by bands of tissue that can lead to internal hernia or volvulus.[71,72] Differential diagnosis includes intussusception, obstruction secondary to adhesions, ileus, gastroenteritis, or tumor with mass effect.

**Diverticulitis/perforation** In some patients, the symptoms that lead to diagnosis of a Meckel diverticulum are similar to those of appendicitis, and can include fever, right lower quadrant abdominal pain, nausea, and vomiting. Physical examination may be indistinguishable from appendicitis, with tenderness to palpation, guarding, and rebound tenderness. The mechanism is thought to be similar to diverticulitis in the colon with obstruction of the lumen leading to inflammation and eventual perforation.[73] The differential diagnosis includes appendicitis, gastroenteritis, mesenteric adenitis, and gynecologic issue (eg, ovarian torsion, pelvic inflammatory disease). When encountering signs of inflammation intra-abdominally with a normal appendix, an exploration for Meckel diverticulitis should be performed.

### Other Presentations

A patent vitelline duct presents as drainage from the umbilicus. Littre hernia is an inguinal hernia containing the Meckel diverticulum and is indistinguishable from any other herniation until operation. Other less common presentations include tumors that form in the Meckel diverticulum. Many of these present at late stages.

### Laboratories

The laboratory testing that should be undertaken with a Meckel diverticulum depends on the presentation. Basic metabolic panel and CBC are a starting point, allowing evaluation for dehydration and anemia. In the case of diverticulitis and/or perforation, a WBC count is also important.

### Imaging

#### Abdominal radiographs

Plain films are of limited use in diagnosing a Meckel diverticulum, but can be used to evaluate for pneumoperitoneum and obstruction.

#### Contrast studies

Both upper gastrointestinal series and enteroclysis have been used to detect Meckel diverticulum. However, these tests have a low sensitivity and are difficult to interpret. The classic finding is a single diverticulum arising from the antimesenteric border of the distal ileum. In instances of intussusception, these studies may also reveal a filling defect with possible obstruction.[74]

#### US

US is often used in evaluation of pediatric patients with abdominal pain. Just as Meckel diverticulitis mimics appendicitis clinically, it may also do so on US with the appearance of a long tubular structure with thickened walls. A Meckel diverticulum may also appear similar to a duplication cyst. Intussusception of a Meckel diverticulum may appear as a double-target sign with a targetlike mass with a central area of hyperechogenicity.[75]

#### CT/MRI

Both CT and MRI are of limited diagnostic value when evaluating for Meckel diverticulum. They may reveal nonspecific signs such as inflammation, calcifications, obstruction, pneumoperitoneum, and free fluid. CT and MRI enteroclysis have been shown to be more effective when identifying Meckel disorders. However, both tests are expensive, with the added risk of contrast and radiation exposure, and should not be used in the diagnosis of Meckel diverticulum.[76,77]

#### Nuclear medicine

For a bleeding diverticulum, the current test of choice is a technetium-99 pertechnetate scan (Meckel scan). Studies have revealed approximately 65% to 85% sensitivity in the pediatric population. This sensitivity can be increased using an H2 antagonist, pentagastrin, and glucagon. However, the NPV is only 74%. Different reasons have been proposed regarding this low value, including rapid loss of blood leading to loss of the tracer, previous inflammation, and postsurgical changes.[78]

#### Other tests

Mesenteric angiography and tagged red blood cell scanning may also be used to evaluate for Meckel diverticulum. These imaging studies allow the identification of bleeding, but require a 0.1 to 0.5 mL per hour blood loss for tagged red blood cell scans or a 1 mL per hour blood loss for mesenteric angiography. Both can be useful to localize the site of bleeding to a Meckel diverticulum that has not been identified on nuclear medicine imaging. Using mesenteric angiography, a persistent vitellointestinal artery may be shown in individuals who are no longer actively bleeding. Endoscopy, both upper and lower, may be used to evaluate for other disorders, but are not directly useful in identifying Meckel diverticula. Capsule endoscopy has been useful in identifying a Meckel diverticulum in several cases, but is not regularly used for this purpose.[74] Although the studies evaluating these methodologies have low power and have not assessed for specificity or sensitivity, these procedures may be used when all other tests have failed to identify the source of occult bleeding.

## Treatment

### Incidental diverticulum

There continues to be significant debate surrounding whether an asymptomatic Meckel diverticula should be excised. In the adult population, most literature agrees that excision is not required unless there is a palpable mass raising concern for cancer. In the pediatric population, the picture is less clear. Many studies conclude that the risk of serious complication exceeds that of the operative risk in children less than 8 years old.[79] A recent study from the University of Pittsburgh urges resection of Meckel diverticulum at all ages because of the risk of cancer as well as the late stage of cancer presentation in most patients.[80] Another study evaluated the increased morbidity with incidental Meckel diverticulum excision compared with the lifetime risk of complication. They concluded that the risk of excision was not worth the increased rate of complications.[81] Because of this debate within the literature, the excision of incidentally noted Meckel diverticula is still highly controversial.

### Symptomatic diverticulum

The treatment of symptomatic diverticulum is resection performed either laparoscopically or open. In a recent survey, more than 75% of resections were still performed open.[82] The traditional open approach is performed through a right lower quadrant incision similarly to an appendectomy. For this reason, most surgeons perform an appendectomy at the same time as diverticulectomy.

Laparoscopic diverticulectomies can be performed via a transumbilical approach or through a 3-port laparoscopic approach similarly to laparoscopic appendectomy. Many studies have shown that a laparoscopic approach is as safe and effective as the open approach. They have also shown a decreased time to oral intake and to discharge.[83,84] The disadvantage of a total laparoscopic approach is the loss of tactile sensation, preventing palpation of the base of the Meckel diverticulum to ensure complete resection and lack of masses. For this reason, some surgeons prefer a transumbilical approach, which provides the cosmetic and postoperative advantages of laparoscopic surgery but also enables a surgeon to palpate the specimen.[85,86] For bleeding diverticula, some centers have reported isolated resection of the diverticula. However, our center still prefers resection of the diverticula as well as the adjoining segment of ileum because of the presence of ulceration in the small bowel.

## SUMMARY

1. A Meckel diverticulum is an embryologic remnant of the omphalomesenteric duct.
2. Rule of twos: 2% of the population, within 2 ft (60 cm) of the ileocecal valve, 2:1 predominance in males/females, before 2 years of age, and 2 types of tissue (gastric and pancreatic).
3. Meckel diverticula can present in multiple ways, but most commonly present with obstruction or gastrointestinal bleeding.

4. Diagnostic testing depends on the presentation.
5. Resection of asymptomatic diverticula remains controversial.
6. Resection can be performed safely either open or laparoscopically. We recommend a laparoscopic approach for its benefits for postoperative recovery.

## REFERENCES

1. Brennan GD. Pediatric appendicitis: pathophysiology and appropriate use of diagnostic imaging. CJEM 2006;8:425–32.
2. Deng Y, Chang DC, Zhang Y, et al. Seasonal and day of the week variations of perforated appendicitis in US children. Pediatr Surg Int 2010;26:691–6.
3. Pearl RH, Hale DA, Molloy M, et al. Pediatric appendectomy. J Pediatr Surg 1995; 30:173–8.
4. Wang LT, Prentiss KA, Simon JZ, et al. The use of white blood cell count and left shift in the diagnosis of appendicitis in children. Pediatr Emerg Care 2007;23: 69–76.
5. Kwan KY, Nager AL. Diagnosing pediatric appendicitis: usefulness of laboratory markers. Am J Emerg Med 2010;28:1009–15.
6. Escriba A, Gamell AM, Fernandez Y, et al. Prospective validation of two systems of classification for the diagnosis of acute appendicitis. Pediatr Emerg Care 2011; 27:165–9.
7. Rezak A, Abbas H, Ajemian MS, et al. Decreased use of computed tomography with a modified scoring system in the diagnosis of pediatric acute appendicitis. Arch Surg 2011;146:64–7.
8. Goldman RD, Carter S, Stephens D. Prospective validation of the Pediatric Appendicitis Score. J Pediatr 2008;153:278–82.
9. Schupp CJ, Klingmuller V, Strauch K, et al. Typical signs of acute appendicitis in ultrasonography mimicked by other diseases? Pediatr Surg Int 2010;26:697–702.
10. Goldin AB, Khanna P, Thapa M, et al. Revised ultrasound criteria for appendicitis in children improve diagnostic accuracy. Pediatr Radiol 2011;41:993–9.
11. Buford JM, Dassinger MS, Smith SD. Surgeon-performed ultrasound as a diagnostic tool in appendicitis. J Pediatr Surg 2011;46:1115–20.
12. Yigiter M, Kanterci M, Yalcin O, et al. Does obesity limit the sonographic diagnosis of appendicitis in children? J Clin Ultrasound 2011;39:187–90.
13. Butler M, Servaes S, Srinivasan A, et al. US depiction of the appendix: role of abdominal wall thickness and appendiceal location. Emerg Radiol 2011;18(6): 525–31.
14. Sulowski C, Doria AS, Langer JC, et al. Clinical outcomes in obese and normal-weight children undergoing ultrasound for suspected appendicitis. Acad Emerg Med 2011;18:167–73.
15. Stephen AE, Segev D, Ryan DP, et al. The diagnosis of acute appendicitis in a pediatric population: to CT or not to CT. J Pediatr Surg 2003;38:367–71.
16. Mullins ME, Kircher MF, Ryan DP, et al. Evaluation of suspected appendicitis in children using limited helical CT and colonic contrast material. Am J Roentgenol 2001;176:37–41.
17. Victoria T, Mahboubi S. Normal appendiceal diameter in children: does choice of CT oral contrast (VoLumen versus Gastrografin) make a difference? Emerg Radiol 2010;17:397–401.
18. Garcia K, Hernanz-Schulman M, Bennett DB, et al. Suspected appendicitis in children: diagnostic importance of normal abdominopelvic CT findings with non-visualized appendix. Radiology 2009;209:531–7.

19. Burr A, Renaud EJ, Manno M, et al. Glowing in the dark: time of day as a determinant of radiographic imaging in the evaluation of abdominal pain in children. J Pediatr Surg 2011;46:188–91.
20. Abo A, Shannon M, Taylor G. The influence of body mass index on the accuracy of ultrasound and computed tomography in diagnosing appendicitis in children. Pediatr Emerg Care 2011;27(8):731–6.
21. Hall EJ. Lessons we have learned from our children: cancer risks from diagnostic radiology. Pediatr Radiol 2002;32:700–6.
22. Hagendorf BA, Clarke JR, Burd RS. The optimal initial management of children with suspected appendicitis: a decision analysis. J Pediatr Surg 2004;39:880–5.
23. Williams RF, Blakely ML, Fischer PE, et al. Diagnosing ruptured appendicitis preoperatively in pediatric patients. J Am Coll Surg 2009;208:819–28.
24. Goldin AB, Sawin RS, Garrison MM, et al. Aminoglycoside-based triple-antibiotic therapy versus monotherapy for children with ruptured appendicitis. Pediatrics 2007;119:905–11.
25. Guillet-Caruba C, Cheikhelard A, Guillet M, et al. Bacteriologic epidemiology and empirical treatment of pediatric complicated appendicitis. Diagn Microbiol Infect Dis 2011;69:376–81.
26. St Peter SD, Little DL, Calkins CM, et al. A simple and more cost-effective antibiotic regimen for perforated appendicitis. J Pediatr Surg 2006;41:1020–4.
27. Lee SL, Islam S, Cassidy LD, et al. Antibiotics and appendicitis in the pediatric population: an American pediatric surgical association outcomes and clinical trials committee systematic review. J Pediatr Surg 2010;45:2181–5.
28. Abes M, Petik B, Kazil S. Nonoperative treatment of acute appendicitis in children. J Pediatr Surg 2007;42:1439–42.
29. Taylor M, Emil S, Nguyen N, et al. Emergent vs urgent appendectomy in children: a study of outcomes. J Pediatr Surg 2005;48:1912–5.
30. McBurney CIV. The incision made in the abdominal wall in cases of appendicitis, with a description of a new method of operating. Ann Surg 1894;20:38–43.
31. Pensky TA, Rothenberg SS. Division of the mesoappendix in children is safe, effective and cost-efficient. J Laparoendosc Adv Surg Tech A 2009;19:S11–3.
32. Bartenstein A, Cholewa D, Boillat C, et al. Dissection of the appendix with ultrasound-activated scalpel: an experimental study in pediatric laparoscopic appendectomy. J Laparoendosc Adv Surg Tech A 2010;20:199–204.
33. Stanfill AB, Matilisky DK, Kalvakuri K, et al. Transumbilical laparoscopically-assisted appendectomy: an alternative minimally invasive technique in pediatric patients. J Laparoendosc Adv Surg Tech A 2010;20:873–6.
34. Chandler NM, Danielson PD. Single-incision laparoscopic appendectomy vs. multiport laparoscopic appendectomy in children: a retrospective comparison. J Pediatr Surg 2010;48:2186–90.
35. Canty T, Collins D, Losanao B, et al. Laparoscopic appendectomy for simple and perforated appendicitis in children: the procedure of choice? J Pediatr Surg 2000;35:1582–5.
36. Vegunta RK, Wallace LJ, Switzer DM, et al. Laparoscopic appendectomy in children: technically feasible and safe in all stages of acute appendicitis. Am Surg 2004;70:198–201.
37. Hogan MJ. Appendiceal abscess drainage. Tech Vasc Interv Radiol 2003;6:205–14.
38. Hall NJ, Jones CE, Eaton S, et al. Is interval appendectomy justified after successful nonoperative treatment of appendix mass in children? A systematic review. J Pediatr Surg 2011;46:767–71.

39. Ein SH, Langer JC, Daneman A. Nonoperative management of pediatric ruptured appendix with inflammatory mass or abscess: presence of an appendicolith predicts recurrent appendicitis. J Pediatr Surg 2005;40:1612–5.

40. Puapong D, Lee SL, Haigh PI, et al. Routine interval appendectomy in children is not indicated. J Pediatr Surg 2007;42:1500–3.

41. Blakely ML, Williams R, Dissinger MS, et al. Early vs interval appendectomy for children with perforated appendicitis. Arch Surg 2011;146:660–5.

42. Hale DA, Molloy M, Pearl RH, et al. Appendectomy: a contemporary appraisal. Ann Surg 1997;225:252–61.

43. Cserni T, Paran S, Puri P. New hypothesis on the pathogenesis of ileocecal intussusception. J Pediatr Surg 2007;42:1515–9.

44. Belongia EA, Irving SA, Shui IM, et al. Real-time surveillance to assess risk of intussusception and other adverse events after pentavalent, bovine-derived rotavirus vaccine. Pediatr Infect Dis J 2010;29:1–5.

45. Committee on Infectious Diseases. Prevention of rotavirus disease: updated guidelines for use of rotavirus vaccine. Pediatrics 2009;123:1412–20.

46. Lehnert T, Sorge I, Till H, et al. Intussusception in children – clinical presentation, diagnosis, and management. Int J Colorectal Dis 2009;24:1187–92.

47. Chang Y, Lee J, Wang J, et al. Early laparoscopy for ileocolic intussusception with multiple recurrences in children. Surg Endosc 2000;23:2001–4.

48. Gupta H, Davidoff AM, Pui C, et al. Clinical implications and surgical management of intussusception in pediatric patients with Burkitt lymphoma. J Pediatr Surg 2007;42:998–1001.

49. Blanch AJ, Perel SB, Acworth JP. Paediatric intussusception: epidemiology and outcome. Emerg Med Australas 2007;19:45–50.

50. Hernandez JA, Swischuk LE, Angel CA. Validity of plain films in intussusception. Emerg Radiol 2004;10:323–6.

51. Morrion J, Lucas N, Gravel J. The role of abdominal radiography in the diagnosis of intussusception when interpreted by pediatric emergency physicians. J Pediatr 2009;155:556–9.

52. Mendez D, Caviness C, Ma L, et al. The diagnostic accuracy of an abdominal radiograph with signs and symptoms of intussusception. Am J Emerg Med 2012;30(3):426–31.

53. Roskind CG, Ruzal-Shapiro CB, Dowd EK, et al. Test characteristics of the 3-view abdominal radiograph series in the diagnosis of intussusception. Pediatr Emerg Care 2007;23:785–9.

54. Hryhorczuk AL, Strouse PJ. Validation of US as a first-line diagnostic test for assessment of pediatric ileocolic intussusception. Pediatr Radiol 2009;39:1075–9.

55. Strazinger E, DiPietro MA, Yarram S, et al. Intramural and subserosal echogenic foci on US in large-bowel intussusceptions: prognostic indicator for reducibility? Pediatr Radiol 2009;39:42–6.

56. Wiersma F, Allema JH, Holscher HC. Ileoileal intussusception in children: ultrasonographic differentiation from ileocolic intussusception. Pediatr Radiol 2006;36:1177–81.

57. Bucher BT, Hall BL, Warner BW, et al. Intussusception in children: cost-effectiveness of ultrasound vs diagnostic contrast enema. J Pediatr Surg 2011;46:1099–105.

58. Applegate KE. Intussusception. In: Slovis TL, editor. Caffey's pediatric diagnostic imaging, vol. 2, 11th edition. Philadelphia: Elsevier; 2008. p. 2177–87.

59. Shekherdimian S, Lee SL, Sydorak RM, et al. Contrast enema for pediatric intussusception: is reflux into the terminal ileum necessary for complete reduction? J Pediatr Surg 2009;44:247–50.

60. Tareen F, Ryan S, Avanzini S, et al. Does length of the history influence the outcome of pneumatic reduction of intussusception in children. Pediatr Surg Int 2011;27:587–9.
61. Pazo A, Hill J, Losek JD. Delayed repeat enema in the management of intussusception. Pediatr Emerg Care 2010;26:640–5.
62. Jen HC, Shew SB. The impact of hospital type and experience on the operative utilization in pediatric intussusception: a nationwide study. J Pediatr Surg 2009; 44:241–6.
63. Koh C, Sheu J, Wang N, et al. Recurrent ileocolic intussusception after different surgical procedures in children. Pediatr Surg Int 2006;22:725–8.
64. Burjonrappa SC. Laparoscopic reduction of intussusception: an evolving therapeutic option. JSLS 2007;1:235–7.
65. Kia KF, Mony VK, Drongowski RA, et al. Laparoscopic vs open surgical approach for intussusception requiring operative intervention. J Pediatr Surg 2004;40: 281–4.
66. Navarro O, Dameman A. Intussusception part 3: diagnosis and management of those with identifiable or predisposing cause and those that reduce spontaneously. Pediatr Radiol 2004;34:305–12.
67. Gandy J, Lees G. Neonatal Meckel's diverticular inflammation with perforation. J Pediatr Surg 1997;32:750–1.
68. Poley JR, Thielen TE, Pence JC. Bleeding Meckel's diverticulum in a 4-month-old infant: treatment with laparoscopic diverticulectomy. A case report and review of the literature. Clin Exp Gastroenterol 2009;2:37–40.
69. Tseng Y, Yang YJ. Clinical and diagnostic relevance of Meckel's diverticulum in children. Eur J Pediatr 2009;168:1519–23.
70. Codrich D, Taddio A, Schleef J, et al. Meckel's diverticulum masked by a long period of intermittent recurrent subocclusive episodes. World J Gastroenterol 2009;15:2809–11.
71. Ko S, Tiao M, Huang F, et al. Internal hernia associated with Meckel's diverticulum in 2 pediatric patients. Am J Emerg Med 2008;26:86–90.
72. Limas C, Seretis K, Soultanidis C, et al. Axial torsion and gangrene of a giant Meckel's diverticulum. J Gastrointestin Liver Dis 2006;15:67–8.
73. Jelenc F, Strlic M, Gvardijanc D. Meckel's diverticulum perforation with intraabdominal hemorrhage. J Pediatr Surg 2002;37:18–9.
74. Thurley PD, Halliday KE, Somers JM, et al. Radiological features of Meckel's diverticulum and its complications. Clin Radiol 2009;64:109–18.
75. Kaste SC. Abdominal walls and its abnormalities. In: Slovis TL, editor. Caffey's pediatric diagnostic imaging, vol. 2, 11th edition. Philadelphia: Elsevier; 2008. p. 1822–5.
76. Olson DE, Kim Y, Donnelly LF. CT findings in children with Meckel diverticulum. Pediatr Radiol 2009;39:659–63.
77. Hegde S, Dillman JR, Gadepalli S, et al. MR enterography of perforated acute Meckel diverticulitis. Pediatr Radiol 2012;42(2):257–62.
78. Swaniker F, Hirschl RB. The utility of technetium 99m pertechnetate scintigraphy in the evaluation of patients with Meckel's diverticulum. J Pediatr Surg 1996;34: 760–5.
79. Onen A, Cigdem MK, Ozturk H, et al. When to resect and when not to resect and asymptomatic Meckel's diverticulum: an ongoing challenge. Pediatr Surg Int 2003;19:57–61.
80. Thirunavukarasu P, Sathaiah M, Sukumar S, et al. Meckel's diverticulum – a high-risk region for malignancy in the ileum. Ann Surg 2011;253:223–30.

81. Sani A, Eaton S, Rees CM, et al. Incidentally detected Meckel diverticulum: to resect or not to resect. Ann Surg 2008;247:276–81.
82. Ruscher KA, Fisher JN, Hughes CD, et al. National trends in surgical management of Meckel's diverticulum. J Pediatr Surg 2011;46:893–6.
83. Shalaby RY, Soliman SM, Fawy M, et al. Laparoscopic management of Meckel's diverticulum in children. J Pediatr Surg 2005;40:562–7.
84. Prasad S, Chui CH, Jacobsen AS. Laparoscopic-assisted resection of Meckel's diverticulum in children. JSLS 2006;10:310–6.
85. Cobellis G, Cruccetti A, Mastroanni L, et al. One-trocar transumbilical laparoscopic-assisted management of Meckel's diverticulum in children. J Laparoendosc Adv Surg Tech A 2007;17:238–41.
86. Clark JM, Koontz CS, Smith LA, et al. Video-assisted transumbilical Meckel's diverticulectomy in children. Am Surg 2008;74:327–9.

# Pyloric Stenosis in Pediatric Surgery

## An Evidence-Based Review

Samir Pandya, MD[a],*, Kurt Heiss, MD[b]

## KEYWORDS

- Pyloric stenosis • Pyloromyotomy • Projectile vomiting • Hypochloremic
- Hypokalemic metabolic alkalosis

## KEY POINTS

- Hypertrophic pyloric stenosis (PS) is a benign condition presenting with projectile, non bilious emesis in the newborn infant. The etiology of this condition is still unclear.
- Ultrasound is the preferred diagnostic study if the history, physical and labs aren't sufficient to make the diagnosis.
- Fluid replacement and electrolyte correction will correct the hypochloremic, hypokalemic metabolic alkalosis, and are necessary to avoid post operative apnea.
- Pyloromyotomy is curative after resuscitation. The laparoscopic approach is becoming increasingly common, and seems to have some advantages over the open method.
- Early post operative feeding is safe and effective, frequently allowing discharge on the first post operative day.

In 1960, Willis J. Potts[1] wrote the following in his classic text on pediatric surgery *The Surgeon and the Child:*

> *"The operation for pyloric stenosis is the most satisfactory procedure in the entire field of pediatric surgery. The sick baby vomits all its feedings, the mother is distraught, a simple operation is performed, the baby thrives, and the mother is happy."*

Pyloric stenosis (PS) is a well-known surgical problem within the pediatric population. The treatment is quickly successful and is very rewarding to both parents and surgeon. The patient swiftly recovers and is returned to normal diet and activity within days.

---

The authors have nothing to disclose.

[a] Division of Pediatric Surgery, Maria Fareri Children's Hospital, New York Medical College, Munger Pavilion, Room 321, Valhalla, NY 10595, USA; [b] Division of Pediatric Surgery, Children's Healthcare of Atlanta, Emory University School of Medicine, 1405 Clifton Road, Atlanta, GA 30322, USA
* Corresponding author.
*E-mail address:* spandya01@yahoo.com

Surg Clin N Am 92 (2012) 527–539
doi:10.1016/j.suc.2012.03.006
surgical.theclinics.com
0039-6109/12/$ – see front matter © 2012 Elsevier Inc. All rights reserved.

This article outlines the classic elements necessary to care for the patient in a safe and effective manner. Because variation in care has been associated with increased levels of error, evidenced-based clinical practice guidelines are set forth, which can be modified easily to work well in a general surgery environment. This article has been crafted specifically with the adult general surgeon in mind.

## HISTORICAL PERSPECTIVE

Although first described by Hildanus in 1627, it was not until Hirschsprung's unequivocal clinical and autopsy description in 1887 the pathologic basis of this disease is understood.[2] After this description, a variety of surgical approaches including the creation of a gastroenterostomy or forceful dilation via gastrostomy were practiced. The results, however, were poor with mortality rates approaching as high as 50%. Fredet in 1908 was the first to suggest a full-thickness incision of the pylorus followed by a transverse closure. Although this was successful, Ramstedt modified the technique and later described the sutureless, extramucosal longitudinal splitting of the pyloric muscle, which left an intact mucosa.[2] This technique continues to be the guiding principle of current surgical approaches for PS to this day.

## EPIDEMIOLOGY AND ETIOLOGY

The incidence of PS varies with geographic and ethnic populations for reasons unclear. For example, PS occurs in approximately 2 to 4 per 1000 live births in the Western population, whereas the incidence has been reported to be approximately 4 times lower in the Southeast Asian and Chinese populations.[3–5] There have been numerous reports in the literature citing a wide variety of etiologic factors, some of which are discussed below.

Although no specific gene has been identified as the cause of PS, genetic syndromes, such as Smith-Lemli-Opitz, Cornelia de Lange, and other chromosomal abnormalities, have been associated with PS.[6] In addition, PS is 4 times more likely to present in boys than girls. The exact reason for the gender bias is still unknown. However, children of affected men are only affected between 3% and 5% of the time, whereas children of affected women are affected between 7% and 20% of the time.[7]

Pharmaceutical agents, hormones, and growth factors have all been linked to PS through small case reports.[6] Erythromycin, through its action as a motilin agonist, induces strong gastric and pyloric contractions that may eventually lead to hypertrophy of the pylorus.[6] SanFilippo[8] deduced that postnatal use of erythromycin estolate in infants might have resulted in a transient increase in the incidence of PS. In those infants, the incidence seemed to normalize after terminating the administration of erythromycin estolate. Since this early description, a few subsequent studies have described a 10-fold increase in the incidence of PS in infants treated with erythromycin, whereas other studies have failed to corroborate the findings.[9] Conversely, in terms of antenatal exposure, erythromycin estolate does not have a positive correlation for developing PS. Exposure of the lactating mother to erythromycin estolate does show increased rates of PS in whom the drug is clearly contraindicated.[6]

Several studies have also implicated higher acid exposure to have a causal effect on the development of PS.[10] A study in canines conducted by Dodge demonstrated that gastrin exposure to either puppies or pregnant female dogs resulted in an increased incidence of PS or duodenal ulcers.[11] This study was not replicated in other species and a definitive link has not been established.[12]

Prostaglandins have also been implicated as causative agents of PS. High levels of prostaglandins have been found to be present in infants with PS, which suggests a positive association. Prostaglandins are often used as part of medical therapy of infants with cyanotic congenital heart conditions. In these patients, emesis secondary to antral hyperplasia and gastric outlet obstruction that mimics PS has been observed. However, other studies have found prostaglandins to have a relaxing effect on circular smooth muscle making it difficult to completely characterize its relationship to PS.[13,14]

In addition to the above, several investigators have attempted to identify the causes of PS. Despite some promising hypotheses and findings, a definitive association has yet to be determined. For an excellent review of all of these studies, please refer to the article by Pantelli.[6]

## CLINICAL PRESENTATION AND EVALUATION

The dominant consideration in the differential diagnosis of PS is given to feeding intolerance in this age group. The differential diagnosis includes overfeeding, gastroesophageal reflux, milk protein allergy, intestinal rotational anomalies, and other forms of obstruction. Gastroesophageal reflux is usually the first consideration and is managed with thickened feeds and the use of histamine blockers or proton pump inhibitors. Infants who do not respond to these interventions may have milk protein allergy. This is usually managed by changing the infant's formula. As is the case in reflux, persistence of symptoms after formula changes should lead the clinician to pursue an alternate diagnosis. It is not uncommon for parents to describe multiple changes in the feeds and addition of antacids or thickeners over the last few days or even weeks without any symptomatic relief. It is at this point that the evaluation for PS is begun.

Babies with PS are commonly term infants who are otherwise healthy. The infant presents with nonbloody, nonbilious emesis, which is often described as projectile in nature. Although the propulsive nature of the emesis can be impressive, focus must be on the color instead. Yellowish/greenish emesis is unlikely to be PS because of the hypertrophied pylorus preventing bile reflux in PS. Emesis resembling the feeds indicates PS. Greenish emesis (ie, bilious) should be presumed to be from a more ominous diagnosis, such as malrotation with volvulus or Hirschsprung disease.[15]

Although PS most likely presents between the second and fourth week of life, there have been reports of PS in the newborn as well as in infants aged 4 months. However, these extremes are uncommon, and most patients present between 3 and 10 weeks. A call from the emergency department about a 4-month-old patient with PS should prompt some caution on the part of the surgical consultant.[2,3,16]

Because of the diminished oral intake and repeated bouts of emesis, the babies are typically not very vigorous on presentation. The hydration status can be judged by inquiring about the voiding pattern as well as assessing the fontanelles, mucous membranes, and skin turgor. The absence of tears when the baby cries and/or a history of dry diapers during the day suggest a need for thoughtful volume replacement. In advanced cases, there is a small amount of weight loss owing to the limited intake, and a gastric peristaltic wave may also be seen in the upper abdomen.

During examination, one must take advantage of the time when the infant is resting or sleeping to palpate the mobile pyloric tumor or olive. The abdominal wall must be completely relaxed or else palpation is nearly impossible. Emptying the stomach with a nasogastric or orogastric tube (OG) can sometimes make the olive more palpable. Giving the infant a pacifier with highly concentrated sucrose solution results in aggressive sucking and relaxation of the abdominal wall. Palpation of the olive can be a time-consuming process (up to 20 minutes) and requires patience on the part of the practitioner and time for the infant to relax and acclimate to the surgeon's hands. Additional maneuvers such as flexing the infant's hips or lifting the infant's legs up in the air in the supine or decubitus positioning may be helpful.[2,17] Younger infants seem to be easier to relax and examine than older infants.

The absence of a palpable olive or negative radiographic evaluation for PS should prompt the surgeon to initiate a more extensive workup to evaluate the suspected intestinal obstruction. A detailed algorithm for the workup of a neonatal intestinal obstruction is beyond the scope of this article but can be found in an excellent review by Ricketts.[15]

## LABORATORY AND RADIOLOGIC STUDIES

Adjuncts to the clinical evaluation include blood chemistries and abdominal ultrasonography (US). Serum sodium, chloride, potassium, and bicarbonate values should be obtained when establishing intravenous (IV) access. An abnormally low chloride and high bicarbonate value is characteristic of a patient with PS.

At present, upper abdominal US is the imaging modality of choice in pediatric centers. The success and reliability of this modality depend somewhat on the user and their experience. This competency may not be available in a community hospital or may be inconsistent. US is done after feeding the infant dextrose solution to dilate the fundus, which improves the image quality. The length of the pyloric channel and thickness of the pyloric muscle are the quantitative parameters derived in the longitudinal view. Although there is some variation among radiologists, a muscle thickness greater than 3 mm and channel length greater than 15 mm is considered to be highly sensitive and specific for PS (**Fig. 1**).[18,19] The classic target sign is seen in the transverse view. Other positive sonographic findings include observation of the lack of opening of the pyloric channel and the lack of visualization of passage of contrast into the duodenum.

In recent times, there has been a shift in practice methods with an increased emphasis on imaging for diagnosis. In a retrospective chart review, Macdessi and Oates[20] determined that over 2 study periods (1974–1977 compared with 1988–1991), the incidence of a palpable olive being reported decreased from 87% to

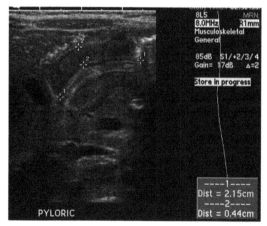

**Fig. 1.** Ultrasonography of pylorus in longitudinal orientation. 1, channel length; 2, muscle thickness.

49%, whereas the use of US increased from 20% to 61%. As such, an abdominal US should be recommended especially in the absence of physical findings or equivocal history.

Most contemporary community hospitals have competent radiology staff who can reliably diagnose PS using US. In a hospital where sonography for PS is not reliable or available, the upper gastrointestinal (UGI) study is a reliable alternative, which confirms the diagnosis of PS by demonstrating poor gastric emptying in the presence of the classic string sign caused by the hypertrophic pyloric muscle (**Fig. 2**). In addition, the pyloric muscle has shoulders that extend into the lumen of the stomach and the duodenum.

## PREOPERATIVE CONSIDERATIONS

The infants are found to have a hypochloremic, hypokalemic, metabolic alkalosis caused by the gastric outlet obstruction. Blood chemistries are evaluated for chloride, bicarbonate, sodium, and potassium. Administration of fluid containing potassium chloride is essential to help resolve the chloride-responsive alkalosis. Although urine is usually alkaline, the body responds to volume contraction and alkalosis by aggressively absorbing $Na^+$. In a patient who is $K^+$ depleted and alkalotic from persistent vomiting of gastric contents, $H^+$ ions are exchanged for $Na^+$ ions, which results in a paradoxic aciduria in the patient who is trying to retain the sodium and water. Giving potassium chloride with the maintenance fluid helps the resolution of the alkalosis quicker, and avoids worsening the hypokalemia to critical levels during resuscitation.

Prompt IV access should be established even though it may prove to be difficult because of the dehydration. Although many algorithms exist, our practice is to administer an initial maintenance rate of 6 mL/kg/h (150% of standard maintenance) of D5.45 normal saline (NS) with 2 mEq of KCl/100 mL should be started until the child's urine output is adequate. An initial goal is 2 mL/kg/h of urine output, which suggests that volume replacement has been reached. Once acceptable urine output is established, decreasing the input of maintenance fluids to 4 mL/kg/h is appropriate. To deal with the electrolyte disorder, the authors administer boluses of 10 to 20 mL/kg 0.9% NS until the chloride level is more than 100 mEq/L and the bicarbonate level is less than 28 mEq/L. Severe comorbidities such as CHD or CHF may require modifications of the resuscitation plan. Correction of the alkalosis in the preoperative period is an important aspect of resuscitation, which prevents the problems of alkalosis-induced apnea in the postoperative period, and prevents the anesthesia staff from having

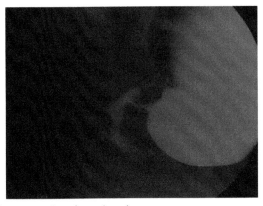

**Fig. 2.** UGI series demonstrating the string sign.

difficulty extubating the patient after the procedure. A persistent alkalosis suppresses respiratory drive and makes a reliable and safe extubation difficult.

Although rarely necessary, a gastric decompression tube may also be inserted for the babies with persistent vomiting. The anesthesia staff may find the presence of an OG tube that drains the stomach reassuring as they prepare the patient for induction.

Approximately 5% of cases may present with an associated hyperbilirubinemia because of a deficiency of the hepatic glucuronyl transferase activity that occurs when oral intake is diminished. The jaundice reverses once the child is feeding regularly after a pyloromyotomy.

## OPERATIVE CARE

Once the patient is properly anesthetized, he/she should be positioned supine on the table, and the bladder and stomach are emptied by the pressure on the bladder and placement of an OG tube in the stomach. The OG tube will be useful later for a leak test to ensure that the submucosa has not been perforated during the myotomy.

There are 3 methods of operative treatment of PS: open, transumbilical, and laparoscopic. Although uncommon in a child in the first 2 months of life, factors such as congenital anomalies or previous abdominal surgeries, such as complicated meconium peritonitis or necrotizing enterocolitis, may influence the choice of operative approach. However, the choice of the approach mostly depends on the comfort level of the provider. The guiding principles of performing a sutureless extramucosal myotomy of adequate length are the same regardless of the approach. The 3 operative methods are described below.

A few comments about the myotomy might be useful before dealing with the 3 operative strategies. An appropriate myotomy extends from the pylorus up onto the antrum, to the circular muscles of the stomach. All general surgeons are heavily scripted during their training to avoid carrying the incision too far down onto the duodenal side of the pylorus to avoid perforating the duodenal mucosa. The vein of Mayo, when present, is a useful boundary to set to keep from continuing the myotomy too far onto the duodenal side, risking a mucosal perforation. Mucosal perforations can be approached in several different ways. Traditionally, general surgeons have been instructed to close the myotomy, rotate the pylorus by 90°, and redo the myotomy. However, because of a limited rotational freedom in some cases, this repair can be a difficult procedure. An easier but equally effective approach is to primarily repair the mucosa with an absorbable stitch followed by placement of an omental patch, which can be done either via an open or laparoscopic approach by experienced hands. Based on the outcomes, infants with mucosal perforation recover just as well as those without with the exception of the feeds being started a day later in the perforation group. Delays in diagnosis of perforation, however, can lead to septic complications.

Similarly, it is common as people are learning to do this procedure to make the myotomy too short on the antral side, thus not making the myotomy sufficient and causing unnecessary postoperative vomiting. The adequacy of myotomy on the antral side is confirmed when the circular fibers of the stomach wall on the proximal side of the incision are seen. The myotomy is carried out until the 2 halves of the pylorus can be moved independently which demonstrates that the myotomy is sufficient. If vomiting persists longer than 5 days, the possibility of an inadequate myotomy is considered. An UGI study would aid in making this diagnosis, however, it is usually very difficult to interpret. Most postoperative UGI tracts show a string sign even when an appropriate myotomy was performed. This string sign is usually secondary to postoperative antral and pyloric spasm, and the treatment of this condition is time. In patients with incomplete myotomy, some can be managed expectantly and in others with more severe scenarios, a redo pyloromyotomy is considered.

The open pyloromyotomy is performed by making a transverse incision on a normally occurring skin line in the right upper quadrant over the rectus muscle (**Fig. 3**). This location is usually about 2 fingerbreadths above the umbilicus. The abdomen is entered with either a muscle splitting or a muscle cutting approach. Once the abdomen is entered the liver edge is gently retracted cephalad, thereby exposing the stomach. The omentum can be grasped with forceps and the greater curve of the stomach pulled up until the pylorus is delivered into the wound. The surgeon should then hold the pyloric olive between thumb and index finger with their nondominant hand and incise/score the anterior surface of the pylorus taking care not score beyond the depth of the beveled blade on the scalpel. At this point, the scalpel handle can be used to press down on the incision, essentially cracking the muscle such that the submucosa is seen. The pyloric spreader can then be placed into the wound and gently spread until the myotomy extends from the distal pylorus to the antrum, a length of about 2 cm. The anesthesiologist can then inflate the stomach using a 14F suction catheter attached to a syringe. Approximately 40 mL is usually sufficient. The distended stomach is then squeezed to make the submucosa in the myotomy wound bulge. The myotomy site is checked for leaks. The 2 sides of the myotomy are then moved in opposite directions, demonstrating the complete disruption of the pyloric ring. Inability to move the 2 halves independently indicates an inadequate myotomy. Alternatively, the patency of the channel can be determined by squeezing the air from the stomach into the duodenum. This operative approach would seem to be most common, reliable, and safe for an adult general surgeon who is not experienced in doing laparoscopy on a 3-kg child.

In the transumbilical approach, a semicircular incision is made along the superior crease of the umbilicus. A skin flap is raised toward the xiphoid along the linea alba for approximately 5 cm. The linea alba is then incised and the abdominal cavity is entered. The pylorus is brought into the wound by gentle retraction on the greater omentum in a caudal direction. Once the pylorus is visualized, a babcock grasper can be used to grasp the stomach and deliver the pylorus into the wound. This must be performed in a gentle rocking motion as the stomach can be fragile. Frequently, depending on the size of the pylorus, the skin incision is extended transversely in both directions and thus making an omega shape to accommodate the pylorus. The

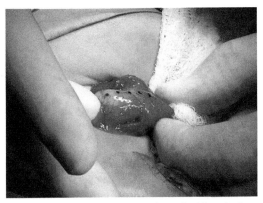

**Fig. 3.** Pylorus delivered through right upper quadrant incision during an open procedure. The inked line is proposed myotomy site. (*Courtesy of* Whitney McBride, MD, Valhalla, NY.)

myotomy, leak, and patency tests are then performed in the same manner as described in the open approach (**Fig. 4**). The pylorus is then replaced back into the abdominal cavity and the fascia and incision are closed.

First described by Alain and colleagues[21] in 1991, the laparoscopic approach has become increasingly popular in many pediatric centers. After the administration of local anesthesia that is appropriately adjusted for the patient's weight, the abdominal cavity is entered via the umbilicus using either the modified Hassan or Veress needle techniques. An intra-abdominal pressure of 8 to 12 mm Hg and flow rate of 2 to 3 liters per minute is usually sufficient. A reusable 3-mm trocar is used in the umbilicus along with a 3-mm 30° lens on the laparoscope. Two stab incisions are made: one in the right hypogastrium and one in the left hypogastrium. The pylorus is grasped with an atraumatic grasper or vascular clamp.[22] Two strategies exist for cutting the pyloric muscle: a nonretractable arthrotomy blade or the long flat electrocautery extender blade. While using the latter, the authors recommend a cautery setting no higher than 8 on the cutting and coagulation currents. The insulated covering of the cautery extender leaves 4 mm of uninsulated blade to the distal tip (**Figs. 5** and **6**). The myotomy is performed in a similar manner to the open procedure, and a laparoscopic pyloric spreader is then used. The tip can be manipulated without cautery to further aid in gauging the depth of the myotomy, as well as creating a space for the pyloric spreader. The leak and patency tests can be done under direct laparoscopic visualization of the submucosa (**Fig. 7**). Variations to the laparoscopic approach include the use of mini laparoscopic instruments and single-incision approaches.[23,24] A myotomy length of 2 cm is the goal to avoid an incomplete myotomy and postoperative vomiting.[25]

Several studies have compared the above 3 approaches using operative time, complication rates, length of stay, time to feeds, and cosmetic appearance as end points.[26–32] In a recent meta-analysis, data from 6 large level 1 or level 2 studies were pooled and analyzed. The investigators, Sola and Neville, found that the laparoscopic approach has a significantly lower incidence of wound infection, shorter length of stay, and decreased time to feeding. The incidence of inadequate pyloromyotomy ranged between 1.4% and 5.6% in this analysis. There was no difference in rates of mucosal perforation.[30] In a retrospective review of all 3 approaches, Kim and colleagues[33] found that in their study, the transumbilical approach had the longest operative time (42 minutes ± 12 minutes) compared with the laparoscopic and open approaches (25 minutes ± 9 minutes and 32 minutes ± 9 minutes, respectively). This

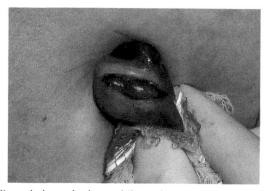

**Fig. 4.** Pylorus delivered through the umbilicus during a transumbilical procedure. The myotomy has been performed and the mucosa visible. (*Courtesy of* Whitney McBride, MD, Valhalla, NY.)

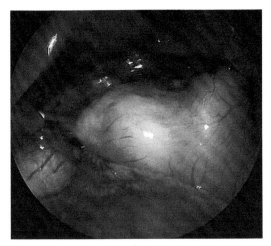

**Fig. 5.** Laparoscopic view of hypertrophic pylorus.

also translated to higher surgery- and anesthesia-related charges in the transumbilical group ($1574 ± $433 and $731 ± $190). The charges in the laparoscopic group were $1299 ± $311 for surgery and $ 586 ± $137 for anesthesia. Charges in the open group were $1237 ± $411 and $578 ± $167. In conclusion, the laparoscopic approach was cost effective, efficient, and safe. **Figs. 7** and **8** are postoperative films of healed incisions after an open and laparoscopic pyloromyotomy, respectively.

A note here about comfort level with this procedure might be appropriate. This is not an emergency procedure. If a community general surgeon has not done this procedure for some time, or if a community anesthesiologist is not comfortable with providing the anesthesia to a small infant, it is completely appropriate to begin resuscitation and refer the patient to a center where this case is considered routine and is done commonly.

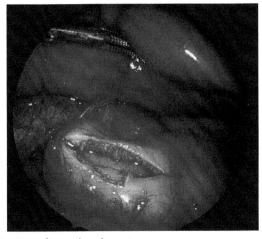

**Fig. 6.** Laparoscopic view of completed myotomy.

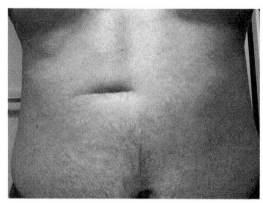

**Fig. 7.** Healed right upper quadrant scar in a 22-year-old man who had an open pyloromyotomy as an infant.

## POSTOPERATIVE CONSIDERATIONS
### Feedings

Historically, patient feedings were held for a time in an attempt to decrease postoperative vomiting. More contemporary thoughts suggest that early feedings within a few hours after recovery are safe and effective at starting the patient's progress to discharge. Beginning ad libitum feeds 3 hours after the patient returns from the recovery room is tolerated well. Withholding feeds for a day or a nursing shift may decrease vomiting overall, but will delay the infant who is ready to progress. Starting

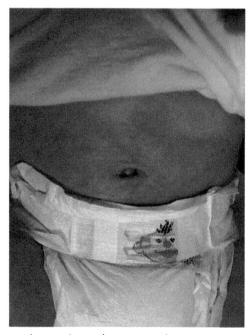

**Fig. 8.** Healed laparoscopic scars 1 month postoperative.

feeds shortly after recovery allows most infants to advance to full feedings and be ready for discharge by the time their apnea monitoring is completed.[34]

## IV Fluids

Maintenance fluids of D5.45 NS with 2 mEq of KCl per 100 mL can be continued postoperatively at 4 mL/kg/h until the patient is tolerating a diet. Once the infant has started feeding, decreasing the fluids to keep-open rate, or heparin locking the IV may be useful to encourage the infant to eat by decreasing total fluid intake.

## Monitoring

A large number of patients with PS are in the 2- to 8-week age range, and are susceptible to postoperative apnea risks because of their immaturity. This may occur even when properly resuscitated and is related to the influence of anesthetic agents on the immature central nervous system, not on the adequacy of the resuscitation. A child who was born prematurely (ie, <37 week's gestational age) may have postoperative apnea problems, even when properly resuscitated. This susceptibility for postoperative apnea persists until the child is approximately 52 weeks corrected age.

For this reason, after recovery in the postanesthesia care unit, the patient should be monitored using a cardiac and apnea monitor for the first 24 hours. Most apneas in this period only require minimal stimulation of the patient to resume normal breathing. Monitoring the patient for that time period allows apneas to be noticed and treated. The risk decreases to normal level after the first 24 hours following the general anesthesia.

## Dealing with Vomiting and Pain

Parents must be informed during the consent process that the patient is expected to vomit postoperatively. The stomach is irritated and if over distended, will likely result in vomiting. Continuing to feed the child will result in more food being tolerated as the postoperative period continues. An inadequate myotomy will cause persistent vomiting, but in most cases, when the myotomy is adequate during intraoperative testing, any vomiting that occurs postoperatively will be because of pyloric and antral spasm and will resolve with continued feedings.

Most patients can be easily managed with acetaminophen as the only postoperative pain medication. A dosage of 10 mg/kg/dose is adequate for most infants.

## Hygiene

The baby can be sponge bathed on the first day after the operation. Sponge bathing for the first week is probably sufficient with a more liberal bath after the first week.

## DISCHARGE CRITERIA

When the child is afebrile, able to tolerate maintenance feeds, has acceptable pain control, and does not have other problems, such as apnea, the child can be safely discharged home. Appropriate follow up with the pediatrician in a few days and the surgeon within a month is a reasonable approach. Most postoperative questions can be dealt with by phone.

## SUMMARY

PS is a common pediatric surgical problem that is easily diagnosed by US. When resuscitated properly with adequate electrolyte replacement and volume resuscitation, the perioperative care is usually quite smooth. Appropriate postoperative monitoring and early feeding allow consistent and timely discharge within 24 to 48 hours. Intraoperative surgical care focused on the avoidance of perforation and adequate myotomy provides a consistent and satisfying result. Although the driving principle of a sutureless extramucosal myotomy has remained the same over the last century, a variety of approaches have been used to achieve this goal. Minimally invasive surgery is safe and effective with improved cosmetic results but requires subspecialty expertise.

## ACKNOWLEDGMENTS

The authors would like to acknowledge Dr Linda Dultz for her valuable input in this article.

## REFERENCES

1. Potts W. Pyloric stenosis. In: The surgeon and the child. Philadelphia: WB Saunders; 1959. p. 153–8.
2. Garcia VF, Randolph JG. Pyloric stenosis: diagnosis and management. Pediatr Rev 1990;11(10):292–6.
3. Huang IF, Tiao MM, Chiou CC, et al. Infantile hypertrophic pyloric stenosis before 3 weeks of age in infants and preterm babies. Pediatr Int 2011;53:18–23.
4. MacMahon B. The continuing enigma of pyloric stenosis of infancy: a review. Epidemiology 2006;17(2):195–201.
5. Ramstedt WC, Clinic R, Spicer D. Proffered review infantile hypertrophic pyloric stenosis: a review. Br J Surg 1982;69:128–35.
6. Panteli C. New insights into the pathogenesis of infantile pyloric stenosis. Pediatr Surg Int 2009;25(12):1043–52.
7. Carter CO, Evans KA. Inheritance of congenital pyloric stenosis. J Med Genet 1969;6:233–54.
8. SanFilippo J. Infantile hypertrophic pyloric stenosis related to ingestion of erythromycine estolate: a report of five cases. J Pediatr Surg 1976;11:177–80.
9. Mahon BE, Rosenman MB, Kleiman MB. Maternal and infant use of erythromycin and other macrolide antibiotics as risk factors for infantile hypertrophic pyloric stenosis. J Pediatr 2001;139:380–4.
10. Rogers IM. The true cause of pyloric stenosis is hyperacidity. Acta Paediatr 2006; 95(2):132–6.
11. Dodge JA. Production of duodenal ulcers and hypertrophic pyloric stenosis by administration of pentagastrin to pregnant and newborn dogs. Nature 1970; 225(5229):284–5.
12. Spicer RD. Infantile hypertrophic pyloric stenosis: a review. Br J Surg 1982;69(3): 128–35.
13. La Ferla G, Watson J. The role of prostaglandins E2 and F2 alpha in infantile hypertrophic pyloric stenosis. J Pediatr Surg 1986;21(5):410–2.
14. Shinohara K, Shimizu T. Correlation of prostaglandin E2 production and gastric acid secretion in infants with hypertrophic pyloric stenosis. J Pediatr Surg 1998;33(10):1483–5.
15. Ricketts RR. Workup of neonatal intestinal obstruction. Am Surg 1984;50(10): 517–21.
16. Zenn MR, Redo SF. Hypertrophic pyloric stenosis in the newborn. J Pediatr Surg 1993;28(12):1577–8.
17. Senquiz AL. Use of decubitus position for finding the "olive" of pyloric stenosis. Pediatrics 1991;87(2):266.

18. Hernanz-Schulman M. Pyloric stenosis: role of imaging. Pediatr Radiol 2009; 39(Suppl 2):S134–9.
19. Malcom GE 3rd, Raio CC, Del Rios M, et al. Feasibility of emergency physician diagnosis of hypertrophic pyloric stenosis using point-of-care ultrasound: a multi-center case series. J Emerg Med 2009;37(3):283–6.
20. Macdessi J, Oates RK. Clinical diagnosis of pyloric stenosis: a declining art. BMJ 1993;306(6877):553–5.
21. Alain JL, Grousseau D, Terrier G. Extramucosal pyloromyotomy by laparoscopy. Surg Endosc 1991;5(4):174–5.
22. Dozier K, Kim S. Vascular clamp stabilization of pylorus during laparoscopic pyloromyotomy. Pediatr Surg Int 2007;23(12):1237–9.
23. Turial S, Enders J, Schier F. Microlaparoscopic pyloromyotomy in children: initial experiences with a new technique. Surg Endosc 2011;25(1):266–70.
24. Muensterer O, Adibe O, Harmon C, et al. Single-incision laparoscopic pyloromyotomy: initial experience. Surg Endosc 2010;24(7):1589–93.
25. Ostlie D, Woodall C, Wade K, et al. An effective pyloromyotomy length in infants undergoing laparoscopic pyloromyotomy. Surgery 2004;136(4):827–32.
26. Eltayeb AA, Othman MH. Supraumbilical pyloromyotomy: a comparative study between intracavitary and extracavitary techniques. J Surg Educ 2011;68(2): 134–7.
27. Fischer JD. Smaller scars–what is the big deal: a survey of the perceived value of laparoscopic pyloromyotomy. J Pediatr Surg 2008;43(8):1580 [author reply: 1580–1].
28. Hall NJ, Van Der Zee J, Tan HL, et al. Meta-analysis of laparoscopic versus open pyloromyotomy. Ann Surg 2004;240(5):774–8.
29. Leclair MD, Plattner V, Mirallie E, et al. Laparoscopic pyloromyotomy for hypertrophic pyloric stenosis: a prospective, randomized controlled trial. J Pediatr Surg 2007;42(4):692–8.
30. Sola JE, Neville HL. Laparoscopic vs open pyloromyotomy: a systematic review and meta-analysis. J Pediatr Surg 2009;44(8):1631–7.
31. St Peter SD, Holcomb GW 3rd, Calkins CM, et al. Open versus laparoscopic pyloromyotomy for pyloric stenosis: a prospective, randomized trial. Ann Surg 2006; 244(3):363–70.
32. St Peter SD, Ostlie DJ. Pyloric stenosis: from a retrospective analysis to a prospective clinical trial - the impact on surgical outcomes. Curr Opin Pediatr 2008;20(3):311–4.
33. Kim SS, Lau ST, Lee SL, et al. Pyloromyotomy: a comparison of laparoscopic, circumumbilical, and right upper quadrant operative techniques. J Am Coll Surg 2005;201:66–70.
34. Puapong D, Kahng D, Ko A, et al. Ad libitum feeding: safely improving the cost-effectiveness of pyloromyotomy. J Pediatr Surg 2002;37(12):1667–8.

# Pediatric Gastroesophageal Reflux Disease

Felix C. Blanco, MD[a], Katherine P. Davenport, MD[a],
Timothy D. Kane, MD[b,c],*

## KEYWORDS

- Gastroesophageal reflux disease • Laparoscopy • Nissen fundoplication
- Hiatal hernia

## KEY POINTS

- Gastroesophageal reflux is extremely common in infants and children.
- Pathologic reflux or gastroesophageal reflux disease (GERD) causes symptoms secondary to esophageal damage or respiratory disease but remains a clinical diagnosis.
- The diagnostic confirmation of GERD is challenging and often requires multiple diagnostic studies.
- Surgical management of GERD is reserved for infants and children who fail maximal medical therapy or develop complications from severe GERD.
- Minimally invasive surgery is considered the standard of care for the treatment of infants and children with severe GERD.

Gastroesophageal reflux (GER) is a condition in which the protective barrier mechanisms of the esophagus are ineffective in preventing the reflux of gastric contents. Gastroesophageal reflux disease (GERD) refers to a clinical complex that develops as a result of persistent gastric reflux causing bothersome symptoms as well as secondary respiratory disease and esophageal damage. In large part, GER in young children is physiologic and self-limiting and responds effectively to nonoperative treatment. Surgery is indicated when the maximal medical management of GERD fails or when there is evidence of ongoing esophageal injury.

The authors have nothing to disclose.
[a] Sheikh Zayed Institute for Pediatric Surgical Innovation, Children's National Medical Center, 111 Michigan Avenue NW, Washington, DC 20010, USA; [b] The George Washington University School of Medicine & Health Sciences, Washington, DC, USA; [c] Department of Surgery, Sheikh Zayed Institute for Pediatric Surgical Innovation, Children's National Medical Center, 111 Michigan Avenue NW, Washington, DC 20010, USA
* Department of Surgery, Sheikh Zayed Institute for Pediatric Surgical Innovation, Children's National Medical Center, 111 Michigan Avenue NW, Washington, DC 20010.
E-mail address: TKane@cnmc.org

In recent years, increasing knowledge on the pathogenesis of GERD has led to the implementation of new diagnostic techniques and the discovery of highly effective pharmacologic agents. Without a doubt, these medications have considerably altered the management of the disease. When required, the surgical correction of GERD plays a role in the multidisciplinary management of these patients, which is especially challenging in children with neurologic impairment.

This article reviews the mechanisms responsible for GERD, available techniques for diagnosis, and current medical management. In addition, it extensively discusses the surgical treatment of GERD, emphasizing the use of minimally invasive techniques.

## ANATOMY AND PHYSIOLOGY OF THE LOWER ESOPHAGEAL SPHINCTER COMPLEX

The lower esophageal sphincter (LES) complex is formed by a set of specialized anatomic structures tightly regulated by multiple physiologic forces. It is formed by a thickening of the circular muscle layer of the lower esophagus and the oblique muscle fibers of the gastric cardia or collar of Helvetius. In this area, the acute angle formed by the distal esophagus and the gastric fundus or angle of His acts as a valve to prevent reflux. The LES is strategically located in the esophageal hiatus between the fibers of the right crus, where it is exposed to a pressure gradient across the diaphragm. During each breath, as the thoracic pressure changes, the hiatus squeezes the distal esophagus, reducing its diameter and preventing reflux.[1] To maintain an intact antireflux mechanism, the abdominal portion of the esophagus must measure at least 1 cm in length. As expected, neonates and infants have a proportionally shorter intra-abdominal esophagus.[2]

Neural and humoral influxes are the main regulators of the LES tone, which remains closed most of the time. The sphincter relaxes in response to esophageal peristaltic waves originated by swallowing and occasionally to transient relaxations.[3] During the initial stages of digestion, the release of numerous gastrointestinal (GI) hormones triggers signals of positive and negative feedback to either close or relax the LES. Positive feedback signals mediated by gastrin, motilin, and substance P keep the sphincter closed. Negative feedback signals relax the LES, allowing the passage of the esophageal contents into the stomach. These are mediated by cholecystokinin, secretin, glucagon, vasoactive intestinal peptide, and nitric oxide.[4]

Swallowing initiates propulsive and coordinated esophageal contractions that travel through the esophageal wall as peristaltic waves (type 1). Type 2 contractions occur in response to residual swallowed material or gastric refluxate in the esophagus and are therefore considered clearance contractions. Finally, type 3 contractions are independent of swallowing or clearance, are poorly coordinated, and occur sporadically.

Between periods of swallowing and esophageal clearance, the parasympathetic nervous system (vagus nerve) maintains the LES closed with a resting tone of 6 to 26 mm Hg.[5] The LES primarily relaxes in response to the esophageal peristalsis initiated by swallowing (types 2 and 3 LES relaxation). Type 1 relaxation or transient LES relaxation (TLESR) is independent of swallowing and has been implicated in the pathogenesis of GER in neurologically normal children.[6] Reflux in neurologically impaired children appears to be unrelated to TLESR.[6,7]

## CLASSIFICATION
### Physiologic GER

Most healthy infants have occasional regurgitation known as physiologic reflux. Nelson reported an incidence of GER in up to 60% of infants aged 6 months, which declined to 5% at the end of the first year of life.[8] GER at this age is mainly due to the immaturity of the LES (obtuse angle of His and a short intra-abdominal esophagus) and a predominantly liquid diet. As solids are introduced in the diet and the anatomic maturity of the LES is reached, reflux disappears by 12 months of age.[9]

## Pathologic GER or GERD

Persistent and bothersome GER in children may be the cause of secondary respiratory symptoms, apnea, and failure to thrive; therefore it is considered pathologic (GERD). The mechanisms responsible for GERD can be divided into anatomic or physiologic.

### Anatomic abnormalities causing GERD

These include hiatal hernia, short esophagus, esophageal atresia, and esophageal strictures. Similarly, the surgical correction of congenital defects of the abdominal wall such as omphalocele or gastroschisis indirectly predisposes to GERD by increasing the intra-abdominal pressure,[10,11] as does the presence of ascites or occasionally peritoneal dialysis.

### Functional causes of GERD

Pharmacologic agents such as caffeine, calcium channel blockers, or xanthines predispose to GERD by relaxing the LES as well as poor dietary habits, smoking, and alcohol intake, which are common among adolescents.

Increases in intragastric pressure secondary to delayed emptying or abnormal gastric motility result in reflux especially in neurologically impaired patients who also have decreased parasympathetic tone of the LES, increased gagging reflex, esophageal dysmotility, and muscle spasticity with resultant increased intra-abdominal pressure.[7]

GERD has been commonly described in children with congenital diaphragmatic hernia (CDH), although no intrinsic anatomic or physiologic abnormality of the esophagus or LES has been found.[12] It is possible that the return of the herniated viscera into a constricted and poorly developed peritoneal cavity at the time of surgical correction of CDH could increase abdominal pressure, resulting in GER. This may explain in part why reflux in CDH survivors resolves with time as the abdominal domain is regained.[13] Limited evidence has demonstrated that large CDH defects requiring patch repair and the requirement for extracorporeal life support (ECMO) are risk factors for long-term GERD; therefore these children may be candidates for early antireflux surgery.[13]

## CLINICAL PRESENTATION

Most children with GERD have one or more of the following symptoms:

- Regurgitation and vomiting (70%)
- Chronic cough (50%)[14]
- Epigastric pain (36%) and irritability—which has been described in up to 17% of infants with GERD[15]
- Feeding difficulties and feeding refusal (29%)
- Failure to thrive (28%)[16]
- Apnea or apparent life-threatening event (ALTE)—An ALTE episode is defined as the occurrence of apnea in association with choking, gagging, cyanosis, hypotonia, lethargy, or unresponsiveness.[17] It is postulated to occur during a GERD episode as a result of laryngospasm. Although commonly present, reflux is not suspected

to be the cause of apnea in the majority of children with ALTE. Similarly, ALTE was identified only in 5% of children suffering from GERD.[18,19]

- Bronchospasm and asthma—Asthma secondary to GERD is caused by micro-aspiration of acid and and/or digestive enzymes and reflex bronchospasm.[20–22] GERD should be suspected in children with steroid-dependent asthma who have failed to respond to standard treatments, especially when asthma attacks are nocturnal and are associated with concurrent symptoms of reflux and/or recurrent pneumonitis.[23] It is typical for these children to have completed a course of empiric therapy with acid-suppressive medications before GERD was investigated.[24]
- Sandifer syndrome or spasmodic torsional dystonia—This condition is a postural expression of GERD manifested by arching of the back and neck (Sandifer posturing) and abdominal wall contractions.[25] This posturing can be mistaken for a seizure with subsequent referral to neurology.

## DIAGNOSIS

A thorough medical history and physical examination should always precede the use of any diagnostic test to investigate GERD. Patient age, neurologic development, and history regarding length of nonoperative management, medications and previous anti-reflux surgeries should be carefully reviewed. Before a test is ordered, the clinician should keep in mind that GERD is a dynamic process with notorious variability and often unrelated to food intake.

Despite advances in technology, there is not a single study to accurately diagnose GERD in children, and a combination of tests is generally required.

### Radiography of the Chest

Chest radiography is frequently obtained as part of the work-up of a child with recurrent respiratory symptoms but is not necessarily indicated in the investigation of GERD. Incidental findings on chest radiography include hiatal hernia or a dilated esophagus.

### Esophagram

Esophagram is a static and purely anatomic study in which a swallowed contrast agent delineates the esophagus and proximal stomach. This study identifies esophageal lesions as well as abnormal esophageal configurations, strictures, and hiatal hernia. Unfortunately, esophagram is neither sensitive nor specific.

### Upper GI Series

Similar to esophagram, upper GI series help identify anatomic abnormalities of the esophagus, stomach, and duodenum which are found in approximately 4% of children with GERD.[26] Due to its poor sensitivity and the low incidence of anatomic abnormalities in children with reflux, this test should not be used alone to diagnose GERD.[26,27]

Despite these limitations, surgeons routinely obtain preoperative upper GI series to rule out anatomic abnormalities and delayed gastric emptying. Upper GI series may expose the child to prolonged radiation times, as provocative maneuvers are often performed to elicit reflux.[28]

### Esophagogastroduodenoscopy

Esophagogastroduodenoscopy (EGD) allows direct visualization of the upper GI tract, helping identify strictures, infections, or inflammatory changes of the esophagus and stomach. EGD enables biopsy of suspicious lesions of the esophagus such as Barrett metaplasia and eosinophilic esophagitis.[29]

When interpreting the results of endoscopy, the clinician should remember that children with GERD rarely have pathologic changes; hence, the absence of esophageal abnormalities does not rule out GERD.[18,28] In fact, nonerosive esophageal disease (NERD) is a well known clinical entity described in children with GERD. The treatment of NERD is mainly guided by the resolution of symptoms.[18]

### Twenty-Four Hour pH Monitoring

Twenty-four hour pH monitoring is the gold standard test for the diagnosis of GERD. It identifies with precision the presence of acid reflux in the esophagus while the patient performs routine age-related activities and receives a normal diet. Thus, a pH-metry study will accurately demonstrate the relationship between the symptoms and reflux episodes.[30] The data obtained from pH-metry will also allow the clinician to monitor the response to medical management.

Monitoring is performed by placing a probe in the distal esophagus. The pH level and the duration and frequency of acid reflux episodes are determined for 24 hours. A result with a pH less than 4 in at least 5% of the measured time is considered positive.[7] Due to a higher number of physiologic reflux episodes in infants, a total reflux time of up to 9.7% is considered normal for this age.[31] The buffering effect of milk and formula should also be taken into consideration when interpreting a pH-metry study.[23,32]

The introduction of wireless pH probes has obviated the need for trans-nasal catheters. Unfortunately, besides needing sedation for placement, these probes were tested only in patients older than 6 years of age.[33]

The main limitation of 24-hour pH-metry is the inability to detect alkaline and weak acid reflux, which are present in 2% and 70% of children with GERD, respectively.[34,35] False-negative results may be due to daily variations of reflux in children.

### Gastroesophageal Scintigraphy

Gastroesophageal scintigraphy or milk scan has been frequently used to determine GERD in children. Upper GI tract images are obtained after formula labeled with [99]Technetium is ingested by the patient. Normally, radiotracer material is found in the stomach and proximal intestine. In addition to reflux, scintigraphy often detects delays in gastric emptying, nonacid reflux, and aspiration.

Scintigraphy has fallen out of favor due to its low sensitivity and specificity. Current guidelines do not recommend its routine use in the evaluation of children with GERD.[28]

### Esophageal Manometry

Manometry provides useful information on esophageal peristalsis and the presence of esophageal motility disorders. It helps locate the LES in relation to the diaphragmatic hiatus and to determine the length as well as the ability of the LES to relax. Due to the rarity of esophageal motility abnormalities in children with GERD, manometry is of limited use. A subset of children with severe reflux esophagitis occasionally have transient impairment of esophageal motility, which usually resolves after the esophagitis is treated.[36]

### Multiple-channel Intraluminal Esophageal Impedance

Esophageal impedance (EI) is one of the most commonly used tests to diagnose GERD in children today. During the test, a catheter with multiple electrodes monitors distension of the esophagus during the passage of food as well as during reflux episodes.[34] The addition of a pH probe helps distinguish acid and nonacid reflux.[32] The additional information provided by the pH probe during impedance testing is particularly useful for identifying infants with GERD due to weak acid reflux.[35] Similar to pH monitoring, symptoms such as cough, cry, pain, or vomiting are recorded by the parent and can then be correlated with the findings of the EI and pH probe.[37]

Since EI has mainly been tested in children with GERD, normal parameters have not been identified for comparison.

### Bronchoalveolar Lavage

Bronchoalveolar lavage (BAL) was designed to detect silent aspiration of gastric contents in children with respiratory disease believed to be secondary to GERD. The test relies on the detection of lipid-laden alveolar macrophages in BAL fluid. Although initially used to complement the diagnosis of GERD, BAL has fallen out of favor due to its poor sensitivity and specificity.[38] Recent studies with multichannel impedance could not find a significant correlation between the presence of lipid-laden alveolar macrophages in BAL and reflux in children with GERD.[39]

Similar to lipid-laden macrophages, the detection of pepsin in the BAL fluid has been found to correlate with GERD-related respiratory aspiration.[40]

## MEDICAL MANAGEMENT

The management of children with GERD involves a sequence of steps that are usually nonoperative and often result in resolution of symptoms. The goals of medical management include change of the gastric pH with acid-suppressive medications, improvement in the transit of gastric contents with prokinetic agents, and, lifestyle modifications.

Physiologic reflux is common in healthy infants with postprandial regurgitation or non-bilious vomiting. As mentioned before, symptoms of reflux in small children frequently resolve in the first year of life without surgery.[41,42] The introduction of thickened foods (antiregurgitation formula, rice cereal) is often sufficient to resolve GER. In the past, advocates for the prone or lateral positions believed these would alleviate GER. Currently, they are not considered safe in children less than 1 year of age due to the association with sudden infant death syndrome (SIDS).[28]

If an infant with continuous regurgitation or vomiting has poor weight gain, cow's milk allergy should be ruled out first. According to current guidelines, a 2-week trial of thickened hydrolyzed formula or amino acid-based formula with increased caloric intake should be offered before GERD is investigated.[28]

Symptoms such as heartburn, dyspepsia, or postprandial substernal discomfort in older children and adolescents should be initially managed with lifestyle modifications, avoidance of known substances in the diet, and a trial of proton pump inhibitors (PPIs). The persistence or recurrence of symptoms after the medications have been discontinued should prompt investigation of GERD.

When esophagitis is detected at EGD, a 3-month trial of acid-suppressive medication should be started, followed by repeat endoscopy. Failure of treatment or recurrence of esophagitis are indications for antireflux surgery.

### Histamine-2 Receptor Antagonists

Histamine-2 receptor antagonists are the most commonly used acid-suppressive agents in children. These medications are effective in reducing the gastric pH, relieving symptoms of GERD, and resolving esophagitis. Prolonged use may cause tachyphylaxis or tolerance.[43]

### Proton Pump Inhibitors

PPIs are safe and effective in children with GERD. Long-term PPIs are commonly indicated for the treatment of esophagitis and are routinely used as adjuvants after surgery. Twenty-four hour pH studies demonstrate that children require greater than standard doses of PPIs. To achieve the desired effect, incremental doses may be required.[9,44–46]

### Prokinetics

Cisapride, a 5HT-4 antagonist, has been shown to improve esophageal motility and gastric emptying when used in children with severe and chronic reflux. The main reported side effects of cisapride are cardiac conduction abnormalities (prolongation of QT interval), leading to fatal arrhythmias and occasionally death.[47–49] Arrhythmias were particularly reported when cisapride was used in combination with other medications competing for enzymatic pathways involving cytochrome P450 in the liver. Despite attempts to establish safe dosing in children, the US Food and Drug Administration (FDA) has regulated its use to limited access programs.

Metoclopramide, another prokinetic agent commonly used in children, promotes esophageal motility, increases the tone of the LES, and has antiemetic properties. Long-term use of metoclopramide has been associated with significant adverse effects in children, including gynecomastia and extrapyramidal symptoms,[50] therefore, its use is no longer widespread.

Baclofen, a $\gamma$–aminobutyric acid (GABA) receptor antagonist, appears to decrease the frequency of transient LES relaxation, thereby reducing the episodes of GERD. Baclofen may also accelerate the gastric emptying.[51]

### SURGICAL MANAGEMENT

Current guidelines favor the surgical management of children with GERD when the diagnosis has been unquestionably ascertained.

### Indications

The main indications for surgery are:

1. Poor response or refractive to medical management
2. Failure to thrive
3. ALTE[52]
4. Severe pulmonary disease with associated GERD
5. GERD in neurologically impaired children
6. Complicated GERD (recurrent esophagitis, esophageal stricture, Barrett esophagus)
7. Severe, steroid-dependent asthma associated with GERD.[28]

### Surgical Principles

The main goal of surgery for GERD is to eradicate the reflux of gastric contents into the esophagus, whether acid or nonacid. This is achieved by creating a valve mechanism at the gastroesophageal junction (fundoplication) and promoting gastric emptying.

Commonly, as part of the initial operation, many children require a concomitant feeding gastrostomy, especially those who have not been able to feed orally and those who depend on tube feeding.

### Types of fundoplication

The type of fundoplication depends on whether the wrap around the esophagus is partial or total (circumferential). Nissen, Toupet, Thal, and Dor fundoplications are techniques with variable success and specific indications. The following sections describe the two most common techniques.

**Nissen fundoplication** Since the initial description of the technique in 1959, Nissen fundoplication has evolved to become the standard surgical treatment of GERD in both children and adults. While minimally invasive techniques have been introduced in surgery, laparoscopic Nissen fundoplication has become one of the most commonly performed procedures in children with GERD. The procedure involves several steps.

**Patient positioning** After general anesthesia and preoperative antibiotics, the patient is placed in a supine position in slight reverse Trendelenburg. This position allows gravity to move the visceral contents of the upper abdomen away from the operative area. For older children and adolescents, a modified Lloyd-Davies or lithotomy position is preferred; this permits the surgeon to stand between the patient's legs and have better handling of the laparoscopic instruments. Infants and small children (under 20 kg) are positioned at the end of the operating table in a frog-legged position.

**Trocar placement** The first trocar is inserted at the umbilicus (#1 in **Fig. 1**) to gain access to the peritoneal cavity. Through this port, a 5 mm 30° or 45° angled scope is introduced in the abdomen. Four additional 3 to 5 mm ports are then placed in the subcostal area under direct vision, 2 in each side of the midline. The ports located on the patient's right side are used for liver retraction (see #2 in **Fig. 1**) and the surgeon's left hand (see #3 in **Fig. 1**). The left-sided ports are dedicated to the surgeon's right hand (see #5 in **Fig. 1**) and assistant surgeon's hand for retraction (see #4 in **Fig. 1**). It is important to note that position #4 in **Fig. 1** will also become the eventual gastrostomy tube site in some patients. Therefore, this site should be

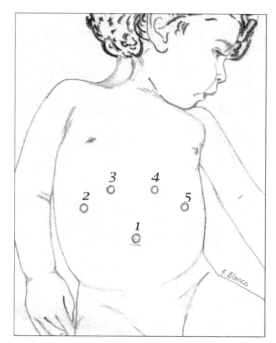

**Fig. 1.** Port placement for laparoscopic fundoplication. 1. Port for laparoscope, 2. Port for liver retraction, 3 and 5. Ports for surgeon's left and right hands, and 4. Port for assistant.

selected before insufflation of pneumoperitoneum to place it sufficiently away from the costal margin but not too far inferiorly so as to make the stomach difficult to reach.

**Gastroesophageal mobilization** The mobilization of the GE junction is initiated by dividing the gastrohepatic ligament parallel to the lesser curvature of the stomach. This is extended to the level of the esophageal hiatus. (**Fig. 2**A) During this maneuver, the main vagi trunks are identified and preserved. Occasionally, an aberrant left hepatic artery runs in the ligament; its presence should be anticipated and the artery preserved.

**Hiatal dissection** A combination of blunt and sharp dissection is done in this area. The use of hook cautery or harmonic scalpel facilitates the division of the phrenoeso-phageal and phrenogastric ligaments to release the gastroesophageal junction and mobilize the distal esophagus (see **Fig. 2**B). This step is intended to gain esophageal length; however, recent evidence has shown that extensive mobilization of the gastro-esophageal junction at the hiatus is unnecessary and that limited dissection with pres-ervation of the phrenoesophageal ligament effectively prevents the migration of the wrap and preserves the intrinsic pressure of the LES.[53]

When a hiatal hernia is encountered, traction of the fundus brings the herniated stomach back into the abdomen. If adhesions between the hernia and the diaphragm are encountered, these may be divided and the hernia sac removed.

A wrap around the intra-abdominal esophagus provides a valve mechanism against gastric reflux. To achieve this, the gastric fundus is mobilized from its attachments to the spleen by dividing the gastrosplenic ligament. Care should be taken to avoid tearing the ligament as it incorporates the short gastric vessels (see **Fig. 2**C). After the greater curvature of the stomach is mobilized, the retro-esophageal space is entered above the left gastric vessels and carefully dissected to create a window. While doing this, the surgeon should avoid injury to the posterior vagus nerve, which lies in close contact to the esophageal and gastric walls.

**Crural approximation** The mobilization of the gastroesophageal junction will expose the fibers of the right crus, which split and hug the distal esophagus, forming the diaphragmatic hiatus. Once exposed, the hiatus is approximated with interrupted nonabsorbable sutures with a Maloney bougie in the esophagus and across the hiatus. This helps estimate the desired esophageal diameter and tightness of the crura (see **Fig. 2**D). While others place sutures to secure the esophagus to the hiatus to prevent the migration of the wrap, the authors do not routinely perform this step.

**Creation of a 360° wrap** A grasper is passed through the retro-esophageal window to grasp the mobilized fundus, which is then pulled behind the esophagus from left to right; a second grasper is used to hold the fundus on the opposite side. The mobilized fundus is rocked back and forth behind the esophagus (see **Fig. 2**E). This maneuver, known as the shoe shine maneuver, will ensure the mobility of the wrap.

As a last step, the edges of the wrap are approximated at the 10 o'clock or 11 o'clock position in front of the esophagus with nonabsorbable suture. Three separate stitches secure the wrap in a distance of no more than 2 cm (see **Fig. 2**F). The authors prefer to incorporate part the esophageal wall with each stitch to prevent telescoping of the wrap around the esophagus.

Under most circumstances, the authors insert an appropriate-sized Maloney bougie in the esophagus as the wrap is constructed. This will ensure that the wrap is not too tight.

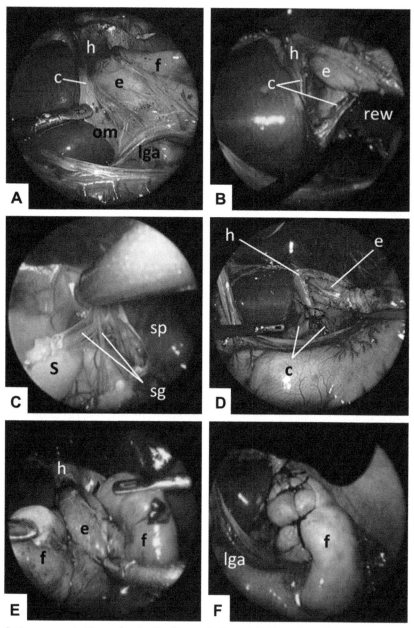

**Fig. 2.** Laparoscopic Nissen fundoplication technique. (*A*) Dissection of the lesser omentum (om) and exposure of the esophageal hiatus (h), crura (c), esophagus (e), and left gastric artery (lga). (*B*) Hiatal dissection, esophageal mobilization and creation of retroesophageal window (rew). (*C*) Division of short gastric vessels (sg) after traction of stomach (S) away from spleen (sp). (*D*) Crural approximation with nonabsorbable sutures. (*E*) Shoe shine maneuver after gastric fundus (f) is mobilized and passed behind esophagus. (*F*) 360° wrap creation.

**Gastrostomy placement** While most patients undergoing fundoplication receive a gastrostomy, children with intact swallowing and those who were not dependent on gastrostomy or tube feeding before fundoplication are candidates for fundoplication alone.

When gastrostomy is performed in addition to Nissen fundoplication, the authors use the U-stitch technique described by Georgeson.[54] In children with a pre-existing gastrostomy, the authors prefer to take down the old site, suture this closed, and replace it at the end of the procedure if the tube is in the way for the dissection of the hiatus and wrap or there is too much tension on the fundus from the gastrostomy to create an appropriate Nissen fundoplication.

**Toupet fundoplication** Toupet or partial fundoplication involves the creation of a 270° degree wrap around the esophagus. The operation is often performed in patients with impaired esophageal motility in whom a complete wrap would cause postoperative dysphagia.

The surgical steps are similar to that of Nissen fundoplication with the exception that, after the fundus is mobilized, the edges of the wrap are secured anteriorly on either side of the distal esophagus. The wrap encircles only three-quarters of the circumference of the esophagus. Pediatric surgeons experienced with the Toupet report similar outcomes compared with the Nissen fundoplication in neurologically normal children and may prefer this technique.[55] Others have shown that children who undergo Nissen fundoplication have a lower recurrence rate than for partial wraps.[56] It is clear from the adult literature that partial wraps are inferior as an antireflux barrier compared with the Nissen wrap.[57]

### Gastrostomy

The difficult management of failed fundoplication has led to the implementation of alternative antireflux procedures. Gastrostomy without fundoplication appears to be an effective technique to treat children with GERD. According to one study, symptoms of GERD were alleviated in 76% of children with gastrostomy alone; from these, only 7% eventually required an antireflux procedure. The group of children with partial response to gastrostomy had improved symptoms when doses of antireflux medications were increased. Interestingly, 75% of children in this series were neurologically impaired.[58]

The mechanisms for which gastrostomy resolves GERD are not clear. The authors believe that for many patients, gastrostomy alone may not be sufficient to treat GERD, since a valve mechanism is essential to prevent reflux.

### Gastrojejunal feeding

There is controversy about the use of gastrojejunal (GJ) tubes as a single treatment of children with GERD. Reports indicate that GJ tubes are a good alternative to fundoplication, especially in children with neurological impairment who are at greater risk for operative complications. In one study, the complication rates for GJ tubes were similar to that of fundoplication.[59] However, tube dislodgement and enteral intussusceptions were common with this form of therapy (16%) and appeared to be related to the pigtail-shaped tip of some jejunostomy tubes.[60] There are reported cases of jejunal perforation and intestinal volvulus around jejunal tubes. Similar to gastrostomy, patients treated with GJ tubes alone will require lifelong antireflux medications.

Frequently, GJ or transpyloric tubes are used as adjuvants in children with neurological impairment who have undergone fundoplication but have delayed gastric emptying.

## Total esophagogastric dissociation

Originally described by Bianchi, total esophagogastric dissociation (TEGD) is considered the procedure of choice after repeatedly failed fundoplication, because it permanently eradicates GERD.

As its name implies, in TEGD the esophagus is transected from the stomach and anastomosed to a divided loop of proximal jejunum brought in a retrocolic fashion. The biliopancreatic limb draining the gastric contents is then anastomosed to the jejunal loop 30 cm distal to the esophagojejunal anastomosis. If not already present, a gastrostomy is placed in the gastric remnant to allow drainage until return of bowel function; then oral and tube feedings can be initiated.

TEGD is usually offered to children with severe neurological impairment and to those with repeated fundoplication failure. Some justify primary use of this procedure, since each reoperation places the patient at an even greater risk for complications.[61]

Recently, as with other antireflux procedures, laparoscopic TEGD has been shown to be a feasible technique in children.[62]

## Roux-en-Y gastrojejunal diversion

With this technique, a Roux-en-Y gastrojejunostomy is constructed to facilitate gastric emptying. A divided jejunal limb is anastomosed to the stomach distal to a pre-existent or newly created fundoplication wrap. Laparoscopic Roux-en-Y gastrojejunal diversion was succesful in a group of neurologically impaired children with delayed gastric emptying. The procedure improved gastric emptying and decreased GERD recurrence.[63]

## Endoluminal endoscopic gastroplication

Endoluminal gastroplication involves the endoscopic creation of multiple folds or plicae in the stomach below the LES. Although reported recurrence rates are as high as 25%, more than half of patients treated with gastroplication had excellent outcomes with improvement of symptoms and no need for antireflux medications at a 3-year follow-up.[64] The experience for endoluminal plication techniques (Endocinch and Esophyx) for adult patients has been less satisfactory compared with those undergoing fundoplication. However, the less invasive nature of this approach may be benefitial.[65] There are no data regarding the long-term outcomes of gastroplication in children.

## OUTCOMES

Recent reviews comparing laparoscopic versus open fundoplication established the superiority of the laparoscopic technique. Shorter length of stay, reduced need for postoperative analgesia, and lower surgical complication rates were reported with laparoscopic fundoplication.[66–69] Although initially questioned, the safety, effectiveness, and outcomes of laparoscopic Nissen fundoplication in small children weighting less than 5 kg were similar to that of older children.[70] The absence of a large incision in the upper abdomen worked in favor of the lung mechanics of many of these patients who have variable degrees of pulmonary compromise.

In one comparative prospective study, total fundoplication (Nissen) and partial fundoplication (Thal) had similar operative times, intraoperative complications, time to full feeds, and length of stay.[71] Even though Nissen fundoplication seemed to be particularly associated with postoperative dysphagia, other studies have reported that partial fundoplication had a higher incidence of persistent or recurrent reflux.[72]

Due to the high failure rates of conventional antireflux procedures in children with neurological impairment (75%), some believe that TGED should be used as a primary procedure in these patients.[73]

## SURGICAL COMPLICATIONS
### Short-Term Complications

#### Intraoperative complications
Bleeding, gastric and esophageal perforation, pneumothorax, and vagus nerve injury have been reported in up to 0.7% of patients after laparoscopic fundoplication.[67,74]

#### Postoperative complications
Delayed gastric emptying is frequently reported after fundoplication, especially in children with neurological impairment.[74] It is believed that this is not a complication of fundoplication but a pre-existing condition in both neurologically normal and neurologically impaired children. Therefore, the need for pyloroplasty during fundoplication procedures has been long debated, especially in children with associated delayed gastric emptying. Evidence has shown that the outcome of children who have undergone Nissen fundoplication with pyloroplasty was similar to those who have been treated without pyloroplasty. Postoperative complications have been reported to be higher when pyloroplasty was added to the antireflux procedure.[75] In addition, studies have demonstrated improved gastric emptying following fundoplication as documented by preoperative and postoperative gastric emptying scans in both adults and children.[76,77]

As mentioned previously, 360° wraps had a higher incidence of postoperative dysphagia, but seemed to subside within 24 months after the procedure.[71,72] The ability to create a loose wrap that also prevents reflux is a skill acquired from a large experience with antireflux operations. It is especially important in non-neurologically impaired children to avoid an overly tight wrap, since the resultant dysphagia is often considered worse than reflux in these children.

Gastrostomy tube complications occurred in up to 9% of patients undergoing fundoplication in one series with the majority of these related to tube dislodgement and entry site infections.[71,74]

### Long-Term Complications

Failure of fundoplication occurs in 2% of neurologically normal and in up to 12% of neurologically impaired children.[78] Failure of fundoplication typically occurs 16 months after surgery and is recognized by recurrent GERD symptoms.[74] In neurologically impaired children the presence of uncoordinated swallowing, frequent supine position, seizures, spasticity, aerophagia, delayed gastric emptying, chronic constipation, and scoliosis contribute to fundoplication failure.[59]

Fundoplication failure is classified as follows

Type 1. Disruption of the wrap
Type 2. Sliding hernia with intact wrap
Type 3. Slippage of stomach above the wrap (slipped Nissen)
Type 4. Intrathoracic herniation of the wrap.

Multiple reports have indicated that "redo" fundoplication is a reasonable option and that, in experienced hands, laparoscopic Nissen fundoplication is a feasible technique with a failure rate of 6% at 2 years.[67]

## POSTOPERATIVE MANAGEMENT OF NISSEN FUNDOPLICATION

Liquids are allowed the morning after surgery. For those patients with gastrostomy, tube feedings are resumed on the first postoperative day. Once oral intake is tolerated, the patients are kept on a pureed diet for at least 3 weeks. Follow-up visits should document the improvement in symptoms as well as appropriate weight gain. Upper GI studies are not routinely needed and should be ordered only when the patient has recurrent symptoms or when there is evidence of recurrent GERD.

## GERD IN THE NEUROLOGICALLY IMPAIRED CHILD

Neurologically impaired (NI) children with GERD pose a particular challenge for the surgeon. As described previously, functional abnormalities such as poor esophageal coordination, impaired swallowing, delayed gastric emptying, altered parasympathetic tone, and increased retching contribute to surgical failure, recurrence, and increased risk of complications.[79–82] Therefore, the selection of an antireflux procedure for NI children must be carefully planned and individualized for each patient.

While fundoplication with gastrostomy appears to be the best strategy for a NI child with poor swallowing and dependence on tube feedings, the operative risks should be considered. Gastrostomy alone, GJ tubes, and TGED are valid alternatives for selected patients with neurological impairment, but each procedure carries inherent risks/benefits. Although delayed gastric emptying seems to play an important role in the failure of fundoplication and may be recognized before surgery, there has been no consensus as to how this should be managed surgically. In deciding which procedure to perform for enteral access or GERD, the surgeon must keep in mind the general and nutritional status of the patient, the risk factors for fundoplication failure, and the patient's expected survival and quality of life.

## REFERENCES

1. Goldani HA, Fernandes MI, Vicente YA, et al. Lower esophageal sphincter reacts against intraabdominal pressure in children with symptoms of gastroesophageal reflux. Dig Dis Sci 2002;47:2544.
2. Boix-Ochoa J, Canals J. Maturation of the lower esophagus. J Pediatr Surg 1976; 11:749.
3. Hoffman I, De Greef T, Haesendonck N, et al. Esophageal motility in children with suspected gastroesophageal reflux disease. J Pediatr Gastroenterol Nutr 2010; 50(6):601–8.
4. Chang DH, Evers BM. The digestive system. In: O'leary P, editor. The physiologic basis of surgery. Philadelphia: Lippincot Williams & Wilkins; 2007. p. 485.
5. Maish M. Esophagus. In: Townsend CM, editor. Sabiston textbook of surgery. 18th edition. Philadelphia: Elsevier; 2007. p. 1057–60.
6. Omari TI, Barnett CP, Benninga MA, et al. Mechanisms of gastro-oesophageal reflux in preterm and term infants with reflux disease. Gut 2002;51:475.
7. Pensabene L, Miele E, Del Giudice E, et al. Mechanisms of gastroesophageal reflux in children with sequelae of birth asphyxia. Brain Dev 2008;30(9):563–71.
8. Nelson SP, Chen EH, Syniar GM, et al. Prevalence of symptoms of gastroesophageal reflux during infancy. A pediatric practice-based survey. Pediatric Practice Research Group. Arch Pediatr Adolesc Med 1997;151(6):569–72.
9. Barron JJ, Tan H, Spalding J, et al. Proton pump inhibitor utilization patterns in infants. J Pediatr Gastroenterol Nutr 2007;45(4):421–7.

10. Beaudoin S, Kieffer G, Sapin E, et al. Gastroesophageal reflux in neonates with congenital abdominal wall defect. Eur J Pediatr Surg 1995;5(6):323–6.
11. Koivusalo A, Rintala R, Lindahl H. Gastroesophageal reflux in children with a congenital abdominal wall defect. J Pediatr Surg 1999;34(7):1127–9.
12. Kawahara H, Okuyama H, Nose K, et al. Physiological and clinical characteristics of gastroesophageal reflux after congenital diaphragmatic hernia repair. J Pediatr Surg 2010;45(12):2346–50.
13. Qi B, Soto C, ez-Pardo JA, et al. An experimental study on the pathogenesis of gastroesophageal reflux after repair of diaphragmatic hernia. J Pediatr Surg 1997;32:1310–3.
14. Borrelli O, Marabotto C, Mancini V, et al. Role of gastroesophageal reflux in children with unexplained chronic cough. J Pediatr Gastroenterol Nutr 2011;53(3):287–92.
15. Feranchak AP, Orenstein SR, Cohn JF. Behaviors associated with onset of gastro-esophageal reflux episodes in infants: prospective study using split-screen video and pH probe. Clin Pediatr 1994;33:654–61.
16. Lee WS, Beattie RM, Meadows N, et al. Gastro-oesophageal reflux: clinical profiles and outcome. J Paediatr Child Health 1999;35(6):568–71.
17. Brand DA, Altman RL, Purtill K, et al. Yield of diagnostic testing in infants who have had an apparent life-threatening event. Pediatrics 2005;115(4):885–93.
18. Vandenplas Y, Rudolph CD, Di Lorenzo C, et al. North American Society for Pediatric Gastroenterology Hepatology and Nutrition, European Society for Pediatric Gastroenterology Hepatology and Nutrition. Pediatric gastroesophageal reflux clinical practice guidelines: joint recommendations of the North American Society for Pediatric Gastroenterology, Hepatology, and Nutrition (NASPGHAN) and the European Society for Pediatric Gastroenterology, Hepatology, and Nutrition (ESPGHAN). J Pediatr Gastroenterol Nutr 2009;49(4):498–547.
19. Semeniuk J, Kaczmarski M, Wasilewska J, et al. Is acid gastroesophageal reflux in children with ALTE etiopathogenetic factor of life threatening symptoms? Adv Med Sci 2007;52:213–21.
20. Field SK. Underlying mechanisms of respiratory symptoms with esophageal acid when there is no evidence of airway response. Am J Med 2001;111(Suppl 8): 37S–40S.
21. Moser G, Vacariu-Granser GV, Schneider C, et al. High incidence of esophageal motor disorders in consecutive patients with globus sensation. Gastroenterology 1991;101:1512–21.
22. Canning BJ, Mazzone SB. Reflex mechanisms in gastroesophageal reflux disease and asthma. Am J Med 2003;115(Suppl 3A):45S–8S.
23. Rudolph CD, Mazur LJ, Liptak GS, et al. Guidelines for evaluation and treatment of gastroesophageal reflux in infants and children: recommendations of the North American Society for Pediatric Gastroenterology and Nutrition. J Pediatr Gastroenterol Nutr 2001;32:S1–31.
24. Gold BD. Asthma and gastroesophageal reflux disease in children: exploring the relationship. J Pediatr 2005;146(Suppl 3):S13–20.
25. Frankel EA, Shalaby TM, Orenstein SR. Sandifer syndrome posturing: relation to abdominal wall contractions, gastroesophageal reflux, and fundoplication. Dig Dis Sci 2006;51(4):635–40.
26. Valusek PA, St Peter SD, Keckler SJ, et al. Does an upper gastrointestinal study change operative management for gastroesophageal reflux? J Pediatr Surg 2010;45(6):1169–72.
27. Simanovsky N, Buonomo C, Nurko S. The infant with chronic vomiting: the value of the upper GI series. Pediatr Radiol 2002;32(8):549–50.

28. Boyle JT. Gastroesophageal reflux disease in 2006. The imperfect diagnosis. Pediatr Radiol 2006;36(Suppl 2):192–5.
29. Heine RG, Nethercote M, Rosenbaum J, et al. Emerging management concepts for eosinophilic esophagitis in children. J Gastroenterol Hepatol 2011;26(7): 1106–13.
30. Colletti RB, Christie DL, Orenstein SR. Indications for pediatric esophageal pH monitoring. J Pediatr Gastroenterol Nutr 1995;21:253–62.
31. Gold BD. Review article: epidemiology and management of gastro-oesophageal reflux in children. Aliment Pharmacol Ther 2004;19:22–7.
32. Van Wijk MP, Benninga MA, Omari T. Role of the multichannel intraluminal impedance technique in infants and children. J Pediatr Gastroenterol Nutr 2009;48(1): 2–12.
33. Hochman JA, Favaloro-Sabatier J. Tolerance and reliability of wireless pH monitoring in children. J Pediatr Gastroenterol Nutr 2005;41(4):411–5.
34. Salvatore S, Hauser B, Devreker T, et al. Esophageal impedance and esophagitis in children: any correlation? J Pediatr Gastroenterol Nutr 2009;49(5): 566–70.
35. López-Alonso M, Moya MJ, Cabo JA, et al. Twenty-four-hour esophageal impedance-pH monitoring in healthy preterm neonates: rate and characteristics of acid, weakly acidic, and weakly alkaline gastroesophageal reflux. Pediatrics 2006;118(2):e299–308.
36. Cucchiara S, Staiano A, Di Lorenzo C. Esophageal motor abnormalities in children with gastroesophageal reflux and peptic esophagitis. J Pediatr 1986; 108(6):907–10.
37. Salvatore S, Arrigo S, Luini C, et al. Esophageal impedance in children: symptom-based results. J Pediatr 2010;157(6):949–54, e1–2.
38. Krishnan U, Mitchell JD, Tobias V, et al. Fat laden macrophages in tracheal aspirates as a marker of reflux aspiration: a negative report. J Pediatr Gastroenterol Nutr 2002;35(3):309–13.
39. Rosen R, Fritz J, Nurko A, et al. Lipid-laden macrophage index is not an indicator of gastroesophageal reflux-related respiratory disease in children. Pediatrics 2008;121(4):e879–84.
40. Farrell S, McMaster C, Gibson D, et al. Pepsin in bronchoalveolar lavage fluid: a specific and sensitive method of diagnosing gastro-oesophageal reflux-related pulmonary aspiration. J Pediatr Surg 2006;41(2):289–93.
41. Hegar B, Dewanti NR, Kadim M, et al. Natural evolution of regurgitation in healthy infants. Acta Paediatr 2009;98(7):1189–93.
42. Khoshoo V, Ross G, Brown S, et al. Smaller volume, thickened formulas in the management of gastroesophageal reflux in thriving infants. J Pediatr Gastroenterol Nutr 2000;31(5):554–6.
43. Vandenplas Y. Gastroesophageal reflux: medical treatment. J Pediatr Gastroenterol Nutr 2005;41(Suppl 1):S41–2.
44. Bishop J, Furman M, Thomson M. Omeprazole for gastroesophageal reflux disease in the first 2 years of life: a dose-finding study with dual-channel pH monitoring. J Pediatr Gastroenterol Nutr 2007;45:50–5.
45. Tolia V, Ferry G, Gunasekaran T, et al. Efficacy of lansoprazole in the treatment of gastroesophageal reflux disease in children. J Pediatr Gastroenterol Nutr 2002; 35:S308–18.
46. Hassall E, Israel D, Shepherd R, et al. Omeprazole for treatment of chronic erosive esophagitis in children: a multi center study of efficacy, safety, tolerability and dose requirements. J Pediatr 2000;137:800–7.

47. Dalby-payne J, Morris AM, Craig JC. Meta-analysis of randomized controlled trials on the benefits and risks of using cisapride for the treatment of gastroesophageal reflux in children. J Gastroenterol Hepatol 2003;18:196–202.

48. Shulman RJ, Boyle JT, Colletti RB, et al. The use of cisapride in children. The North American Society for Pediatric Gastroenterology and Nutrition. J Pediatr Gastroenterol Nutr 1999;28:529–33.

49. Hill SL, Evangelista JK, Pizzi AM, et al. Proarrhythmia associated with cisapride in children. Pediatrics 1998;101:1053–6.

50. Chicella MF, Batres LA, Heesters MS, et al. Prokinetic drug therapy in children: a review of current options. Ann Pharmacother 2005;39(4):706–11.

51. Omari TI, Benninga MA, Sansom L, et al. Effect of baclofen on esophagogastric motility and gastroesophageal reflux in children with gastroesophageal reflux disease: a randomized controlled trial. J Pediatr 2006;149(4):468–74.

52. Valusek PA, St Peter SD, Tsao K, et al. The use of fundoplication for prevention of apparent life-threatening events. J Pediatr Surg 2007;42(6):1022–4.

53. St Peter SD, Barnhart DC, Ostlie DJ, et al. Minimal vs extensive esophageal mobilization during laparoscopic fundoplication: a prospective randomized trial. J Pediatr Surg 2011;46(1):163–8.

54. Aprahamian CJ, Morgan TL, Harmon CM, et al. U-stitch laparoscopic gastrostomy technique has a low rate of complications and allows primary button placement: experience with 461 pediatric procedures. J Laparoendosc Adv Surg Tech A 2006;16(6):643–9.

55. Esposito C, Montupet P, van Der Zee D, et al. Long-term outcome of laparoscopic Nissen, Toupet, and Thal antireflux procedures for neurologically normal children with gastroesophageal reflux disease. Surg Endosc 2006;20(6):855–8.

56. Kubiak R, Andrews J, Grant HW. Long-term outcome of laparoscopic nissen fundoplication compared with laparoscopic thal fundoplication in children: a prospective, randomized study. Ann Surg 2011;253(1):44–9.

57. Nijjar RS, Watson DI, Jamieson GG, et al. International Society for the Diseases of the Esophagus-Australasian Section. Five-year follow-up of a multicenter, double-blind randomized clinical trial of laparoscopic Nissen vs anterior 90 degrees partial fundoplication. Arch Surg 2010;145(6):552–7.

58. Wilson GJ, van der Zee DC, Bax NM. Endoscopic gastrostomy placement in the child with gastroesophageal reflux: is concomitant antireflux surgery indicated? J Pediatr Surg 2006;41(8):1441–5.

59. Wales PW, Diamond IR, Dutta S, et al. Fundoplication and gastrostomy versus image-guided gastrojejunal tube for enteral feeding in neurologically impaired children with gastroesophageal reflux. J Pediatr Surg 2002;37(3):407–12.

60. Hughes UM, Connolly BL, Chait PG, et al. Further report of small-bowel intussusceptions related to gastrojejunostomy tubes. Pediatr Radiol 2000;30(9): 614–7.

61. Morabito A, Lall A, Lo Piccolo R, et al. Total esophagogastric dissociation: 10 years' review. J Pediatr Surg 2006;41(5):919–22.

62. Boubnova J, Hery G, Ughetto F, et al. Laparoscopic total esophagogastric dissociation. J Pediatr Surg 2009;44(10):e1–3.

63. Mattioli G, Buffa P, Gandullia P, et al. Laparoscopic proximal Roux-en-Y gastrojejunal diversion in children: preliminary experience from a single center. J Laparoendosc Adv Surg Tech A 2009;19(6):807–13.

64. Thomson M, Antao B, Hall S, et al. Medium-term outcome of endoluminal gastroplication with the EndoCinch device in children. J Pediatr Gastroenterol Nutr 2008;46(2):172–7.

65. Zagol B, Mikami D. Advances in transoral fundoplication for oesophageal reflux. Dig Liver Dis 2011;43(5):361–4.
66. Rhee D, Zhang Y, Chang DC, et al. Population-based comparison of open vs laparoscopic esophagogastric fundoplication in children: application of the Agency for Healthcare Research and Quality pediatric quality indicators. J Pediatr Surg 2011;46(4):648–54.
67. Kane TD, Brown MF, Chen MK. Members of the APSA New Technology Committee. Position paper on laparoscopic antireflux operations in infants and children for gastroesophageal reflux disease. American Pediatric Surgery Association. J Pediatr Surg 2009;44(5):1034–40.
68. Rothenberg SS. Experience with 220 consecutive laparoscopic Nissen fundoplications in infants and children. J Pediatr Surg 1998;33:274–8.
69. Mauritz FA, van Herwaarden-Lindeboom MY, Stomp W, et al. The effects and efficacy of antireflux surgery in children with gastroesophageal reflux disease: a systematic review. J Gastrointest Surg 2011;15(10):1872–8.
70. Shah SR, Jegapragasan M, Fox MD, et al. A review of laparoscopic Nissen fundoplication in children weighing less than 5 kg. J Pediatr Surg 2010;45(6):1165–8.
71. Kubiak R, Andrews J, Grant HW. Laparoscopic Nissen fundoplication versus Thal fundoplication in children: comparison of short-term outcomes. J Laparoendosc Adv Surg Tech A 2010;20(7):665–9.
72. Davis CS, Baldea A, Johns JR, et al. The evolution and long-term results of laparoscopic antireflux surgery for the treatment of gastroesophageal reflux disease. JSLS 2010;14(3):332–41.
73. Goyal A, Khalil B, Choo K, et al. Esophagogastric dissociation in the neurologically impaired: an alternative to fundoplication? J Pediatr Surg 2005;40(6):915–8.
74. Rothenberg SS. The first decade's experience with laparoscopic Nissen fundoplication in infants and children. J Pediatr Surg 2005;40(1):142–6.
75. Maxson RT, Harp S, Jackson RJ, et al. Delayed gastric emptying in neurologically impaired children with gastroesophageal reflux: the role of pyloroplasty. J Pediatr Surg 1994;29(6):726–9.
76. Pacilli M, Pierro A, Lindley KJ, et al. Gastric emptying is accelerated following laparoscopic Nissen fundoplication. Eur J Pediatr Surg 2008;18(6):395–7.
77. Bais JE, Samsom M, Boudesteijn EA, et al. Impact of delayed gastric emptying on the outcome of antireflux surgery. Ann Surg 2001;234(2):139–46.
78. Capito C, Leclair MD, Piloquet H, et al. Long-term outcome of laparoscopic Nissen-Rossetti fundoplication for neurologically impaired and normal children. Surg Endosc 2008;22:876–80.
79. Gibbon TE, Stockwell JA, Kreh RP, et al. The status of gastroesophageal reflux disease in hospitalized US children, 1995-2000. J Pediatr Gastroenterol Nutr 2001;33(4):197.
80. Fonkalsrud EW, Ashcraft KW, Coran AG, et al. Surgical treatment of gastroesophageal reflux in children: a combined hospital study of 7467 patients. Pediatrics 1998;101:419–22.
81. Weir KA, McMahon S, Taylor S, et al. Oropharyngeal aspiration and silent aspiration in children. Chest 2011;140(3):589–97.
82. Danielson PD, Emmens RW. Esophagogastric disconnection for gastroesophageal reflux in children with severe neurological impairment. J Pediatr Surg 1999;34(1):84–6.

# Pediatric Obesity

Mark J. Holterman, MD, PhD*, Ai-Xuan Le Holterman, MD,
Allen F. Browne, MD

## KEYWORDS

- Pediatric • Obesity • Diabetes • Weight management • Adolescent

## KEY POINTS

- Obesity is the most common chronic disease among children.
- The cause of the increase in the incidence of obesity in children is multifactorial.
- Obesity is the root cause for many comorbidities.
- Obese children become obese adults.
- Bariatric procedures are necessary, safe, and effective components of a comprehensive weight management program for adolescents.
- Guidelines for the best bariatric surgical procedure for adolescents and preteens depends on the age and degree of obesity.
- Multi-institutional cooperative studies are necessary to develop better evidence-based guidelines.

*Obesity represents the most common chronic illness of children and adolescents.*
—*Sandra Gibson Hassink*[1]

*Until we know how to prevent it, treating obesity is our only choice.*
—*Barbara Moore & Louis Martin*[2]

Obesity is a serious life-threatening disease that affects an increasing number of children in the developed world. Obese children suffer in many physical and psychosocial ways and their burden has important consequences to our society. Although obesity prevention is the ultimate goal, currently and into the foreseeable future, there will be a significant subset of our children suffering from significant life-altering weight comorbidities. Currently, nonsurgical weight loss strategies have met with limited success,

Disclosure: The authors are involved in 2 separate Food and Drug Administration safety and efficacy trials testing the use of the Laparoscopic Adjustable Band System. One of these trials is sponsored by Allergan, Inc, makers of this device.
Division of Pediatric Surgery, Children's Hospital of Illinois, Order of St. Francis Medical Center, University of Illinois College of Medicine-Peoria, 420 Northeast Glen Oak Avenue, Suite 201, Peoria, IL 61603, USA
* Corresponding author.
*E-mail address:* Mark.J.Holterman@osfhealthcare.org

but weight management clinics that offer a surgical treatment option have been effective at achieving sustained weight loss and resolution of weight-related comorbidities. A collaborative multidisciplinary approach to the management and care of obese children is essential for success. Choosing a weight loss surgical strategy for children and adolescents should be patient specific and based on their age, severity of comorbidities, and their body mass index (BMI). The authors have developed a treatment algorithm for the care of obese adolescents and a plan for the development of aggressive treatment options for obese preteen-aged children based on the limited existing literature and their experience treating adolescents and children at The New Hope Pediatric and Adolescent Weight Management Clinic between 2005 and 2011 at the University of Illinois College of Medicine.[3] As surgeons, we must continually test our treatments, evaluate our results, and improve the care we offer our patients.

## THE DISEASE OF OBESITY

It is not surprising that modern society is faced with an obesity epidemic. Our energy intake and storage mechanisms are uniquely adapted to our previously primitive diets, which often included irregularly spaced, low-caloric density foods encased in slow-to-digest cellulose. This diet required the ability to quickly ingest a large quantity of food into the stomach and upper gastrointestinal (GI) tract. A long length of small intestine was necessary to allow for digestion and nutrient absorption. Only when the food reached the distal gastrointestinal tract and there was a risk of caloric wasting via dumping and diarrhea did the brain receive signals to stop consumption. The storage of surplus energy was crucial for survival during famine. Now in modern times, our primitive GI tracts and energy homeostasis mechanisms have not been able to adapt to the improved economic infrastructure that enables and encourages a sedentary lifestyle with little energy expended on food hunting and gathering; where large quantities of high-caloric-density and easy-to-digest food are readily available; and where enhanced public sanitation and infectious disease control decreases the burden of chronic health problems. The net result is the creeping epidemic of obesity.

### Obesity Throughout History

Ancient figurines from 20,000 to 25,000 years ago depicted obvious obesity, and in more recent times, obesity was seen as a sign of affluence and success. In the past 200 years, obesity has become a negative physical attribute linked to an increasing number of medical and psychosocial problems. Common-sense approaches to the treatment of obesity were aimed at limiting food intake and increasing physical activity. Such measures clearly can work for the slightly overweight to minimally obese motivated individual who has the discipline to undergo significant lifestyle change. For most seriously overweight people, diet modification and exercise have minimal success and a high recidivism rate.[4,5]

In the second half of the twentieth century, the increasing prevalence of patients with life-altering obesity prompted the development of surgical procedures for the treatment of obesity. Initial bariatric procedures, such as the jejunoileal bypass, were designed with limited understanding of the underlying physiologic mechanisms controlling hunger, satiety, caloric absorption, malnutrition, and the bystander effects on the liver and the body as a whole.[6] In the past quarter century, weight loss surgery has become more refined with combinations of intestinal bypass to interfere with caloric absorption and a variety of restrictive procedures and devices to restrict caloric ingestion. Research has been slow to unravel the puzzle of obesity and has discovered an increasingly complex array of signals that control energy homeostasis.[7] Significant work remains to be done to understand how these mechanisms increasingly fail when interacting with the social, economic, and environmental changes of our modern society. The long-term goal is to prevent and treat obesity with nonsurgical means. This goal is currently well out of reach.

## Definition

Obesity is defined as a long-term positive imbalance between energy intake and expenditure, with increased adipose tissue lipid storage and number of fat cells.[8] The Centers for Disease Control and Prevention[9] (CDC) recommend using the percentile BMI-for-age and gender (BMI-for-age) charts to screen children who are overweight or obese. Children with BMI at greater than the 85th percentile are considered overweight and those with BMI greater than the 95th percentile are considered obese.[10] Those with BMI greater than the 99th percentile are considered severely obese.

## Incidence

In the past 30 years, the incidence of obesity in children has increased from less than 5% to approximately 20% in the United States.[10] Childhood obesity in most developing countries is a problem of urban children of a higher socioeconomic class. In the United States, the largest increase of obesity in children is seen in the urban poor.[11]

A closer analysis of these trends reveals that between 1976 to 1980 and 2007 to 2008, obesity increased from 5.0% to 10.4% in children aged 2 to 5 years, from 6.5% to 19.6% in children aged 6 to 11 years, and from 5% to 18% in adolescents aged 12 to 19 years.[10,12] Despite these numbers, pediatric research in surgical procedures, surgical devices, and drugs has been almost exclusively performed in adolescents and not in the preteen years. Preventive dietary counseling, activity recommendations, and behavioral support for younger children have been mostly unsuccessful but may be somewhat responsible for the recent leveling off in the rate of increase of obesity among our youngsters. At present, 15% to 20% of our children are still faced with the medical, social, and economic challenges of obesity.[12]

## Cause

The metabolic constitution of patients who are morbidly obese seems to disrupt the normal balance of energy inflow and energy outflow in violation of the basic law of physics and thermodynamics. How can children from the same parents in the same household with similar consumption of calories vastly differ in body compositions? There are aspects of energy homeostasis underlying the body's energy balance set-point accounting for these differences, which we do not fully understand in morbidly obese children, and which may be difficult to modify after a certain stage of postnatal development. The most visible and obvious indicator of this aberrant set-point is increased body fat mass. Intensive research is ongoing to better understand how the metabolically active fat "organ" interacts with and dynamically responds to signals from its environment, the central and peripheral nervous system, and other key organ systems in the body.[13]

### Calories: Supply and Demand

When combined with increased sedentary activities (accompanied by the opportunity and expectation of snacking outside mealtime), our high caloric-density diet is a major contributor to obesity. Historically, our caloric expenditure was part of the physical activities of daily living, such as food and water procurement, manual labor, or walking. In modern society, fewer engage in heavy manual labor. Physical activity has instead become something we voluntarily perform to maintain our health in our leisure time. In addition, rather than eating because of hunger and satiety, we eat out of habit and expectation. Our current diet frequently consists of meals, fluids, and snacks that have a high-caloric density and a high glycemic index (a measure of how rapidly glucose appears in the blood after carbohydrates are ingested).

The biologic controls of caloric intake are hunger and satiety. The physiology of these sensations involves hormones, neural transmitters, and their receptors.[13,14] One such signal is mediated by leptin, which is produced by fat tissue and suppresses hunger; its level is proportional to fat mass. Patients with the rare syndrome of congenital leptin deficiency suffer from severe obesity. With leptin replacement, they stop eating and lose fat mass and weight. Obese patients are not leptin deficient but are considered to be leptin insensitive because the administration of leptin does not reverse their obesity.[13]

Ghrelin, a hormone produced in the stomach and duodenum, stimulates hunger and enhances visceral fat deposition. Ghrelin is a potent stimulator of growth hormone production.[13] Surgical procedures that bypass a large portion of the stomach (Roux-en-Y gastric bypass [RYGB]) or that excise a large portion of the stomach (sleeve gastrectomy [SG]) are associated with reduced ghrelin levels. Research scientists have developed a vaccine targeting ghrelin that interferes with ghrelin signaling in the central nervous system and that reduces weight gain in rodents and pigs.[13]

PYY and GLP-1 hormones are produced in the ileum and the colon; they suppress hunger in response to intraluminal food. Obese people have significantly longer small intestines than nonobese people and this may delay the release of these important satiety signals.[13] Procedures that increase the speed of arrival of food in the ileum may suppress hunger.

External factors, such as obesogens (eg, Tributyltin and tetrabromobisphenol A), may affect our caloric use. Obesogens, or endocrine disruptors, are functionally defined as chemicals that inappropriately alter lipid homeostasis and fat storage, change metabolic set-points, disrupt energy balance, or modify the regulation of appetite and satiety to promote fat accumulation and obesity.[15] Their increased presence in our environment parallels the increase in obesity in our society. The effects of exposure to these chemicals in childhood and the development of obesity are currently being investigated.[16,17]

Another potential obesity modulator is GI tract flora.[18] The guts of obese mice and obese people harbor an array of microbes (microbiota) that are different from that of their lean counterparts.[19] The gut microbiota and its microbiome (gene content) change with obesity and during weight loss.[20] Although intriguing, these observations may simply be associative and require further study to establish the cause-or-effect relationship and its mechanisms.

### Effects of Medications

Medications are a part of our modern environment. Many medications have effects on salt and water retention and on hunger. Others may have effects on calorie utilization. Medications, such as glucocorticoids, antidiabetic drugs, antidepressants, antiepileptics, and antihistamines, are known to be associated with weight gain.[21,22] Children with a tendency toward obesity may be susceptible to weight gain with the use of these drugs. The interaction of drugs and obesity is an important consideration for all pediatric providers caring for an obese child.

### Genetics

Obesity can be thought of as maladaptation of a child's physiology to genetic or epigenetic factors in our modern environment. Although the children of obese parents are much more likely to be obese themselves and identical twins raised separately are more likely to be obese if their biologic parents were obese,[23] the mother and father from the same household with similar diet and opportunities for physical activity can also have both lean and obese children.

In fact, the causes of childhood obesity may be polygenic.[24] Specific genetic mutations are involved in the rare cases of Prader-Willi syndrome and leptin deficiency. Genome-wide association studies revealed that common variants in the first intron of a gene called *FTO* and variants near the melanocortin-4 receptor gene (*MC4R*) are strongly associated with obesity and seem to be involved in energy homeostasis signals in the central nervous system. These genetic findings have identified important pathways in energy homeostasis for certain obese children and may become useful genetic markers to identify at-risk children who might benefit from earlier or more aggressive interventions.[25,26]

### Comorbidities: Physical and Psychosocial

Obesity is a significant health risk. As the incidence of childhood obesity grows, pediatric clinicians now detect in childhood and adolescence many of the same chronic illnesses and risk factors that are seen in adults. Comorbidities of pediatric obesity include insulin resistance and Type 2 diabetes,[27] polycystic ovary syndrome (PCOS),[28] hypertension,[29] hypercholesterolemia,[30] dyslipidemia and cardiovascular disease,[31,32] sleep apnea,[33] asthma,[34] nonalcoholic fatty liver disease and nonalcoholic steatohepatitis (NASH),[35] orthopedic disease conditions,[36,37] and pseudotumor cerebri.[38]

Obesity is causing a rapid increase in the incidence of Type II diabetes, which historically is a disease of obese, middle-aged patients. Now a significant number of new patients with Type II diabetes are children, some presenting in the preteen years.[27] In its early stages, Type II diabetes is a problem of insulin insensitivity that can be treated with weight loss. The prolonged demand on the pancreatic beta cells to produce supraphysiologic amounts of insulin eventually results in pancreatic insufficiency, at which point significant weight loss will not reverse the need for exogenous insulin.[39] The course and development of complications of Type II diabetes in children has a similar timeline to that seen in adults. It is logical to expect that diabetes-associated comorbidities (cardiac, renal, peripheral vascular, and ocular problems) will prematurely occur in these obese children as they grow into adulthood.[40,41]

Briefly, common obesity-related medical comorbidities in children[42] include the following:

(1) Sleep apnea has a negative effect on school and work performance and is associated with premature death in young adults who developed obesity as children. (2) NASH is the second most common reason for pediatric liver transplantation. (3) PCOS is a major source of social difficulties for obese teenage girls and is associated with anemia and infertility in obese young women, many of whom became obese as children. (4) Slipped capital femoral epiphysis and Blount disease are becoming more common in obese children and frequently result in multiple orthopedic interventions with the risks for permanent disabilities. (5) Metabolic syndrome is associated with obesity and defined in adults as a combination of 3 or more of the following: elevated blood pressure, elevated fasting glucose, increased waist circumference, low high-density lipoprotein cholesterol, and elevated triglycerides. In children, there is little agreement on the parameters of metabolic syndrome mostly because of the wide range of normal values for these metabolic measurements in childhood and adolescence. These comorbidities are preventable and, to a large extent, treatable with weight loss.

Obesity also has a major impact on an individual's mental, psychosocial, and economic health.[43] Emotional comorbidities include low self-esteem, negative body image, and depression. These comorbidities can be directly related to a child's obesity as demonstrated when his or her quality-of-life evaluation improves after successful weight loss.[44] Social comorbidities include isolation, stigmatization, negative stereo-typing, discrimination, teasing, and bullying.[45] Social science analysis clearly demonstrates the prejudice against obese children by their nonobese peers, teachers, and general society. In obese children, these social comorbidities often result in poor school performance and incorrect diagnosis of learning disabilities. Frequently, these children end up in home-schooling situations.[45] Economic comorbidities take the form of wage penalties, fewer promotions, and wrongful termination.[46] As the children become wage earners, their poor school performance, their lack of advanced training, the physical limitations of their size and weight, and their absenteeism caused by their obesity-related clinical comorbidities lead to a reduction in their wage-earning potential.[46]

## OBESITY: A PROBLEM FOR PATIENTS, PARENTS, HEALTH CARE SYSTEMS, AND SOCIETY

All children want to be able to fit in with their peer group and to do the things the other children do. Quality-of-life questionnaires and personal interviews with obese adolescents consistently demonstrate a sense of desperation from their inability to keep up with their peers in all physical and social activities.[44] Obese adolescents often present to the weight management clinic with a sense of resignation and helplessness brought on by years of emotional scarring and failed attempts at weight loss.

The obese child's parents in turn experience significant blame and guilt for their child's obesity. These parents are often told by others, not the least by health care professionals, that they are the cause of their child's problem for having the wrong genes, for their parenting style, and for their personal ignorance, laziness, thoughtlessness, lack of love, or selfishness.[47]

Hospitals and the health care system have a responsibility to treat the disease of obesity in children. They need to be aware of obesity-specific issues of the obese child presenting with standard medical problems,[48] including the need for specialized furniture and equipment, such as sphygmomanometers and commodes; different transfer techniques; the variability in how their body composition and physiology change the pharmacodynamics of different drugs; and the direct correlation of obesity with the increased length of hospitalization and complication rates.[49] Furthermore, hospitals and health care personnel need specific training to overcome their bias and lack of knowledge about obesity and obese children. To address these issues, obesity should be a diagnostic item in patients' problem lists to identify them at the time of admission as a special patient population and alert the personnel and health care providers to their particular needs.

From the point of view of an economist, the long-term societal effect of childhood obesity is sobering. Health care costs associated with obesity-related illnesses for children and adults are estimated at $147 billion per year.[50] The costs of caring for obese children with typical pediatric diseases, such as asthma and appendicitis, are increased by their longer hospitalizations and their higher incidence of complications.[51] Obesity comorbidities are chronic, progressive, and pediatric obesity health care costs are likely to be carried over into adulthood. On an individual basis, some progress is seen on payers' reimbursement of obesity-related services, but for the most part, coverage of recommended treatments for pediatric obesity through Medicaid or private insurance is available in only a few states.[52,53] Furthermore, it has been well established that obese people have fewer educational opportunities and, therefore, fewer and lower-paying job opportunities.[46] Their economic productivity is also compromised because of the work time lost from the high rate of associated comorbidities and disabilities.[54] National security may be adversely affected because greater than 20% of young men and 40% of young women do not qualify for the United States armed forces because of their obesity.[55] The gloomy economic outlook for obese children growing into adulthood boils down to less economic productivity and more cost to society.

## OBESITY TREATMENT
### Why Treat Obesity?

Society demands that health care providers aggressively treat children suffering from an illness that has serious clinical life-threatening consequences. Therefore, it is puzzling why leaders in pediatric health care, government, and third-party payers have been loath to embrace aggressive treatment of morbid obesity in children. This reluctance denies the fact that the child suffers from serious clinical, psychological, and social comorbidities directly related to obesity and that the best treatment of any of these comorbidities is for the child to achieve a healthy weight. Reluctance to effectively treat childhood obesity ignores the serious economic burden of the comorbidities of obese children, which will be carried into adulthood. Although there might be opinions that children do not need treatment of obesity because they will grow out of it, the data clearly demonstrate that adult obesity usually starts in childhood and is correlated with the duration and degree of childhood obesity.[56,57] Aggressive management strategies for children are, therefore, needed.

For obesity and bariatric interventions, many treatment recommendations are currently restricted to adolescents (aged 14 through 18 years). The inclusion of bariatric procedures in weight management protocols for children should be *need* related not *age* related.[58] The surgical and device options must be carefully considered and developed to minimize risks and anatomic rearrangements and maximize control of the comorbidities associated with obesity. The risks need to be balanced against the larger benefits of weight reduction on comorbidities.

From a philosophic standpoint, the idea of exposing a child to a bariatric surgical procedure has traditionally met with significant opposition from pediatric primary care physicians and society at large. This philosophic resistance is inconsistent with our current management approaches for other pediatric diseases. Sick children receive treatment when they have a problem, regardless of their age. A problem is first recognized and the best treatment of their problem is devised. Treatment regimens are frequently multidisciplinary and involve risks (eg, radiotherapy and chemotherapy for cancer, immunotherapy for inflammatory bowel disease, surgical reconstruction for GI tract anomalies, and cardiac surgery for cardiac anomalies). These risks are accepted because the benefits of treatment outweigh the disease. Similarly, obesity shares many of the life-threatening aspects of cancer or coronary artery disease albeit on a longer time scale because obesity currently remains a chronic and incurable disease.[59] The same issues of obesity treatment pertaining to how to work with children in different developmental stages, how to facilitate treatment adherence, how to deal with families of different capabilities, and how to provide chronic, multidisciplinary care are questions pediatric health care providers have already addressed for many other diseases.

Prevention measures may one day lead to a significant decrease in obesity. A more complete understanding of the multiple factors involved in obesity and how they interact with each other will someday lead to effective and individualized nonsurgical treatment protocols or new pharmacologic agents that curb appetite, decrease calorie absorption, or increase metabolic rates without significant side effects. Additionally, endoscopic techniques will be developed that allow for the deployment of devices that interfere with absorption or appetite without significant surgical risk. In the meantime, without bariatric treatment, a generation of obese youngsters is at risk of prolonged morbidity and early death without some form of effective intervention.

### Core Treatment Program for Weight Management

There are 3 essential core elements to any adult, adolescent, or pediatric weight management program: nutrition education, activity guidance, and behavioral modification/support. Ideally, the pediatric/adolescent multidisciplinary weight management team should include pediatric specialists in the following disciplines: medicine, surgery, nursing, nutrition, activity, and mental health. Pediatric subspecialists need to be available to manage obesity-related comorbidities.

Nutritional guidance and training is a basic tool of weight management. With an increasing number of families not eating at home and not preparing their own food, families come under the influence of advertising and convenience rather than healthy nutrition. Certainly larger portions, additives in foods to improve shelf life, and sweeteners in liquids are correlated with the increase in obesity statistics, but direct physiologic pathways remain to be worked out. Instruction in portion size, reading labels for additives, and noting calories in liquids is basic education to improve everyone's nutritional health.[60] The dietician considers economic and cultural issues when developing educational materials.

Activity prescription is designed to achieve basic cardiorespiratory fitness, matching activity to the physical capabilities of each person. Obese people cannot successfully participate in activities designed for lean people. They need unique equipment, unique intensity goals, and unique duration goals. In a sense, obese people are physically handicapped and can be best served by physical therapists. Raising awareness about the economic, cultural, geographic, and seasonal obesity-potentiating aspects of our modern society, such as where to park the car, who walks the dog, the safety of the neighborhood, the availability of indoor facilities in inclement weather, and how long to walk at the mall before shopping, can be part of the activity education.[61]

Ongoing psychological/behavioral support remains the third basic component of weight management in obese children. Using the same quality-of-life assessment tool, it has been shown that obese children's rating of their quality of life was lower than that of a group of children with cancer.[62] No child wants to be obese; almost all have failed previous attempts at achieving a healthy weight. Childhood obesity is associated with emotional and behavioral problems from as young as 3 years of age, with boys being especially at risk.[63] Although obese children and their families respond when using the tools of nutrition, activity, and behavioral support,[64] the 10% loss of excess body weight[65] and the high rate of recidivism are disappointing and speak to the need for further research and efforts into the treatment of obese children.

### Adjunct Therapies to the Core Treatment Program

#### Pharmacologic treatment

There is no pharmacologic cure for obesity. In general, drug investigations have been conducted as a single treatment but should only be considered within the context of a long-term, multidisciplinary weight management program. Specific drugs used in obesity therapy are discussed in this section.

Orlistat (Xenical) is approved for use in obese children 12 years of age and older. Orlistat inhibits pancreatic lipase production to reduce fat absorption. Its long-term applicability for a chronic disease like obesity is limited by the major side effects of liquid, fatty stools, and abdominal pain. Orlistat may be useful during the initiation phase of a multidisciplinary weight management program or for intermittent use to help maintain weight loss/control.[5]

Other drugs are related to amphetamines and suppress appetite. Sibutramine (Meridia) was recently removed from the market because of the risk of myocardial infarction and stroke. Rimonabant is a cannabinoid CB1 receptor antagonist that failed to gain Food and Drug Administration (FDA) approval because of its psychiatric side effects.[5]

Hormone analogues, such as a GLP-1 analogue and an Amylin analogue, suppress appetite and are being studied as antiobesity drugs.[66] GLP-1 is produced in the ileum and colon in the presence of food, whereas Amylin is produced in the pancreas in response to the presence of food in the proximal small bowel. Lorcaserin (a serotonergic receptor agonist-appetite suppressant) and the combination drugs Qnexa (appetite suppressant/stimulant and anticonvulsive) and Contrave (antidepressant and antiaddiction) are currently being studied.[66]

### Bariatric surgical procedures in adolescents

As previously mentioned, the nonsurgical options for weight loss in morbidly obese adolescents have limited effectiveness. Surgical interventions for obesity were initially developed for morbidly obese adults and later applied to adolescents.[67] In response to concerns for the unique aspects of adolescent children, several pediatric surgeons rose to the challenge of adolescent bariatric surgery by beginning in-depth studies of the various surgical options and developing adolescent weight management programs.[68–74] Overall, there is no one perfect bariatric procedure for all obese adolescents. The ability to test these procedures in cooperative multi-institutional prospective trials should allow this field to advance rapidly. Historically, weight loss procedures were developed to minimize caloric intake (restrictive procedures), control caloric digestion (malabsorptive procedures), or to combine both effects. **Table 1** offers a detailed comparison of the more commonly performed procedures, including the laparoscopic adjustable gastric band (LAGB), SG, and RYGB.

### Surgical Approaches to Weight Loss in Adolescents

The ideal bariatric procedure would result in durable and substantial weight loss, with minimal risk from short-term procedural complications and long term malnutrition, growth limitation, liver problems, malignancy or mechanical complications. These issues are crucial in the process of choosing a suitable weight loss procedure for adolescents. However, significant disagreement on the best bariatric surgical procedure for adults, much less for children, remains. Each of the procedures has advantages and disadvantages (see **Table 1**). There is no randomized clinical trial comparing the effectiveness among bariatric procedures in adolescents. Definitive comparative studies are rare and sometimes yield contradictory results.[75,76] It is, however, encouraging that individual adolescent weight management programs are increasingly reporting on their own adolescent experience.[77–85] Overall, very good weight loss response and rapid improvements in all comorbidities, including enhanced physical and psychosocial quality of life along with low morbidity, have been reported.

## FACTORS IN EVALUATING WEIGHT LOSS PROCEDURES IN ADOLESCENTS

As previously mentioned, the current literature does not provide easy answers to the ideal operation for morbidly obese adolescents. There are no available parallel

**Table 1**
Bariatric surgery comparison chart

| Modality of Weight Loss | Restrictive and Malabsorptive (Stomach and Intestines) | Restrictive (Stomach Only) | |
|---|---|---|---|
| **Type of Operation** | **RYGB** | **SG** | **Laparoscopic Adjustable Gastric Band** |
| Anatomy | Small 30 cc gastric pouch<br>Pouch connected to the small intestine<br>Food excluded from digestive juices for 100–150 cm | Long narrow gastric sleeve (100 cc)<br>No intestinal bypass performed<br>Majority stomach removed | An adjustable silicone band is placed around the top part of the stomach creating a small 30–60 cc pouch |
| Mechanism | Food volume is restricted<br>Mild malabsorption<br>Negative feedback in the form of dumping syndrome when sugar or fats are consumed<br>Faster release of GLP-1 and PYY increases early satiety | Food volume is restricted<br>NO malabsorption<br>NO dumping<br>Good physiologic sense of fullness from restriction in reduced stomach<br>Increased GLP-1 and PYY<br>Decreased ghrelin levels curb appetite | Food volume is restricted<br>Adjustable tightness of band delay pouch emptying and prolong sense of fullness |
| Weight Loss<br>United States average statistical loss at 10 y | Excess weight loss 60%–70%<br>Lost within 12–18 mo<br>Initially greater weight loss, which levels off | Excess weight loss 50%–60%<br>Lost within 12–24 mo<br>Initially greater weight loss, which levels off | Excess weight loss 50%–60%<br>Lost over 36 mo<br>Weight loss gradual over first year but similar to other procedures by 2–3 y postop<br>Requires the most effort of all bariatric procedures to be successful |

| | RYGB | Sleeve Gastrectomy | Adjustable Gastric Band |
|---|---|---|---|
| Long-term Dietary Modification (Excessive carbohydrate/high calorie intake will defeat all procedures) | 3 small high-protein meals per d; Must avoid sugar and fats to prevent dumping syndrome; Vitamin deficiency/protein deficiency usually preventable with supplements | No dumping, no diarrhea; Weight regain may be more likely than in other procedures if dietary modifications not adopted for life | Certain dense foods can get stuck if not chewed well (causing pain and vomiting); No liquids with meals |
| Nutritional Supplements Needed (Lifetime) | Multivitamin; Vitamin B12; Calcium; Iron (menstruating women) | Multivitamin; Calcium | Multivitamin; Calcium |
| Potential Problems | Dumping syndrome; Stricture; Ulcers; Bowel obstruction; Anemia; Vitamin/mineral deficiencies (iron, vitamin B12, folate); Anastomotic leak; Weight regain; Technically challenging | Nausea and vomiting; Heartburn; Inadequate weight loss; Weight regain; Staple line leak; Additional procedure may be needed to obtain adequate weight loss; Technically easy | Slow weight loss; Slippage; Erosion; Infection; Port problems/device malfunction; Additional procedure may be needed to obtain adequate weight loss; Technically easy |
| Hospital Stay | 2–3 d | 1–2 d | Overnight (<1 d) |
| Time out of School | 2–3 wk | 1–2 wk | 1 wk |
| Operating Time | 2 h | 1.5 h | 1 h |
| Insurance coverage | Most payers will cover the RYGB even in adolescents | Third-party payers have been reluctant to cover the SG, especially in children because it is considered an experimental procedure | The adjustable gastric band is not FDA approved for use in patients aged 18 years or younger. Many payers will NOT authorize this procedure. Medicaid will pay in some states |

comparisons of the RYGB and LAGB in teens; limited data are now available describing the use of the SG in adolescents. Current clinical guidelines for adolescent weight loss surgical procedures are primarily based on the pros and cons analyses of the various procedures for both adults and adolescents.[86–90] To address this lack of definitive data, the Longitudinal Assessment of Bariatric Surgery (LABS) consortium was established and supported by the National Institutes of Health (NIH) in 2003 to promote collaborations between surgeons working with obesity. The adolescent version of this consortium, Teen-LABS, was started in 2007 to collect available data with the hope to develop guidelines for the optimal adolescent weight loss management strategy.[71]

At this juncture, the authors' recommendations are based on their evaluation of the more extensive adult data combined with the limited adolescent series and their own experience. A brief review of the existing bariatric procedures in use in children follows to help frame the discussion and offer standardized treatment protocols.

The LAGB is an effective procedure for 60% to 80% of patients and is especially effective for patients with a BMI of 50 or less, with an expected loss of 50% to 60% of their excess weight over a 2- to 3-year period.[91] The LAGB procedure has a short learning curve. Most complications, with incidence as high as 15%, are related to mechanical issues, such as the band's position, pouch enlargement, or mechanical port and catheter problems. In the authors' experience, these problems were primarily experienced by patients with poor weight loss who aggregate into a higher BMI (>50) group. (Holterman and colleagues, *Journal of Pediatric Surgery*. Article submitted for publication.) The authors have elected to subsequently offer SG in most of these patients or have referred them for RYGB to adult bariatric surgeons.

In comparison, the RYGB is an effective procedure that provides excellent rapid weight loss in most adolescent patients but with a slightly higher mortality rate.[92] The positive weight loss response needs to be balanced against the more serious short- and long-term surgical complications, including micronutrient and vitamin deficiencies from the aggressive anatomic rearrangement. Short- and longer-term safety concerns associated with the RYGB may limit the referral of morbidly obese patients to centers that only offer this procedure.

The SG is a technically simple procedure that has become a stand-alone, first-line weight loss procedure for many adult surgeons. After SG, patients have minimal risk of micronutrient and vitamin deficiencies and complications are infrequent and manageable. In support of the encouraging midterm data from adult patients, the American Society for Metabolic and Bariatric Surgery (ASMBS) "has accepted the SG as an approved bariatric surgical procedure primarily because of it potential value as a first-stage operation for high risk patients, with the full realization that successful long-term weight reduction in an individual patient after SG would obviate the need for a second-stage procedure."[93] The SG has also been successfully performed as a salvage operation for adolescent patients who do not respond sufficiently to or have mechanical issues with the LAGB (Dr Robert Kanard, personal communication, 2011). Short-term data of the SG as an initial operation in adolescents are encouraging.[94] Concerns for the use of SG in adolescent patients center on decreased ghrelin production and on its adverse effects on growth hormone production and growth.[95] This concern may be less relevant because adolescents should respond to supplemental growth hormone injections and most adolescents treated for weight loss surgery have already achieved growth plate fusion.

The biliopancreatic diversion/duodenal switch (BPD/DS) is an effective weight loss procedure that is technically challenging with significant short-term risks and long-term nutritional concerns.[96] This procedure is best understood as a combination of a sleeve gastrectomy and a bypass procedure in which the food that enters the duodenal bulb from the tubularized stomach is diverted into a roux limb (the new duodenum). This limb of intestine carrying the ingested food mixes with digestive enzymes carried by the native duodenum and jejunum at a downstream enteroenterostomy and limits the available time for digestion and nutrient absorption. The profound anatomic rearrangements and risk of long-term nutrient absorption problems associated with BPD/DS is unsettling to most physicians caring for adolescents and, therefore, precludes its use as a first-line bariatric procedure in this age group. The role of the BPD/DS may be as a salvage procedure after insufficient weight loss with the RYGB or SG.

## DEVICES AND NEW PROCEDURES

In addition to the previously described bariatric procedures, several new devices and one new procedure are under development. Currently, the adjustable gastric band is the only weight loss device in general use. Other devices under consideration have been designed to interfere with normal gastrointestinal physiology in a reversible and adjustable fashion and may be attractive alternatives but require extensive clinical testing before they will be available for use in children.

In this section, the authors first discuss the process of FDA approval for device use in the United States and give a brief overview of the new weight loss devices under development, including various intragastric balloons, the vagal stimulator, the gastric stimulator, and the duodenojejunal bypass device, new minimally invasive procedures, including gastric imbrications, and a procedure that combines the gastric sleeve, omentectomy, and a mid–small bowel resection.

## THE FDA AND BARIATRIC DEVICES

Devices for the treatment of obesity in children may be an ideal alternative to weight loss surgery because they are seen as a less-invasive treatment, may have lower morbidity, and are adjustable, reversible, and removable. These factors may make weight loss devices more acceptable as part of a multidisciplinary weight management strategy in children. It is important to appreciate that the FDA has jurisdiction over the use of medical devices (but not surgical procedures) in the United States. Medical devices for use in obesity, therefore, require extensive testing in FDA-monitored trials. These FDA-approved trials have been performed almost exclusively in adult patients.

The FDA-approved clinical indication of a device or medication frequently excludes or ignores the product's use in children, citing the lack of data or inadequate theoretical grounds. Therefore, by necessity, many pediatric health care professionals frequently resort to the use of devices and drugs that will never undergo the required clinical testing to attain FDA-approved-use-in-children status, thus exposing themselves to a potentially vulnerable medicolegal position. Indeed, the pediatric providers have traditionally used clinical judgment in their decision making to use off-label medications and devices/equipment and frequently make necessary modifications. Unfortunately, many third-party payers will not reimburse for off-label usage of a device, and hospital risk management often prevents practitioners from the use of off-label items. Furthermore, device manufacturers frequently make a business-based decision to avoid the expense of clinical trials in children for a market that is small and more prone to liability. These factors deter the development of weight loss devices for preadults and limit the available treatment options to surgical procedures that are outside the jurisdiction of the FDA. It can be argued that this lack of attention to device development and evaluation is a form of discrimination against children.

## Temporary Procedures

The intragastric balloon (IB) and the Endosleeve are intraluminal devices that can be considered to be temporary because they are removed or changed on a regular basis. These procedures would be attractive in children whose bodies would revert to a more normal physiology when they achieve a healthy body fat mass. These devices could help children attain a healthy percentage body fat at which time their use might be able to be discontinued.

### Intragastric balloon

The IB is designed to be inflated in the stomach and causes a continual sensation of gastric fullness and satiety. Early versions of this concept were not tolerated well because they were not adjustable and caused significant discomfort and vomiting when inflated; they also slowly deflated over time and moved into the lower GI tract, sometimes causing obstruction. Newer versions are expected to address some of these problems.[97,98]

Current IBs under development include 2 nonadjustable free-floating balloons filled either with saline (BioEnterics intragastric balloon [BIB] [Allergan Corp, Irvine, CA, USA])[98] or with air (Heliosphere [Helioscopie SA, Vienne, France])[99] and 2 adjustable systems (Endogast [Districlass Médical SA, Saint-Etienne, France][100] and Spatz, Adjustable Balloon System [Spatz FGIA, Inc, Jericho, NY, USA][101]). The Endogast is fixed in position in the proximal stomach via a transgastric catheter system that connects to a subcutaneous port and is adjusted with air insertion or removal. The Spatz is a free-floating system with a tube attached that is retrieved endoscopically for adjustments with saline. This adjustability may allow patients to adapt without vomiting and to better tolerate the presence of the device. Adjustability will also allow the balloon size to be titrated to the size of the patient and to the desired effect. The intragastric balloon systems have been used in adults and a small number of children outside the United States. Based on reports from this limited clinical experience, these devices seem to be safe and effective for temporary use.[102,103]

### Endosleeve

The EndoBarrier Gastrointestinal Liner (GI Dyamics, Lexington, MA, USA) involves a sleeve of impermeable material placed inside the intestine from the proximal duodenum distally into the jejunum. Current versions extend distally for about 60 cm. The sleeve is placed and removed endoscopically. The gastrointestinal liner creates a mechanical bypass situation (as opposed to surgical) by having the food go through the inner lumen of the sleeve where it is excluded from the digestive juices outside the sleeve.[104] This separation interferes with absorption and the usual neuro-hormonal cascade of the bypassed intestine (CCK and Amylin) is not stimulated by contact with chyme. The mixing of food and digestive enzymes at a point further down the GI tract limits time for calorie absorption and prematurely initiates the satiety-inducing neuro-hormonal feedback loop when PYY and GLP-1 are released from the distal ileum. The length of sleeve necessary for an effective device has been determined in adults but a pediatric version would need to vary in diameter and length based on age. Current design and early studies on adults anticipate that the individual GI liners will have a lifespan of about 6 months, at which time they require endoscopic retrieval and possible deployment of a new EndoBarrier. A FDA-monitored trial of the Endobarrier is ongoing in adults in the United States, South America, and Europe. It is currently not FDA approved for use in the United States.

### Semipermanent Procedures

The vagal-blocking devices, the gastric-stimulating devices, and the endoscopic gastroplasty techniques are designed for long-term usage without permanent anatomic change and can be removed or reversed.

#### Vagal-blocking devices

The vagal-blocking devices are based on the observation of the lack of appetite and weight loss frequently seen in post-vagotomy patients. Subsequent analysis has identified the existence of vagal afferent pathways to the central nervous system that control appetite. This knowledge prompted the development of electronic vagal-blocking devices that place leads around the vagus nerves in the abdomen or in the thorax with minimally invasive techniques. These leads are then connected to a subcutaneous power source/control device similar to a cardiac pacemaker or a phrenic-nerve-stimulating diaphragmatic pacing device. Of note, stimulation of the cervical portion of the vagus nerve has been used for years to control seizure activity. These devices seem to be well tolerated in the long term. The frequency, amplitude, and wave form of the stimulation can then be customized to gain maximal effect on satiety in a given individual. The current subcutaneous boxes are bulky but will decrease in size and become easier for children to tolerate. Early studies of the Maestro System (EnteroMedics Inc, St Paul, MN, USA) in adults show modest weight loss.[105] Trials are now underway in the United States.

#### Gastric stimulators

The use of gastric stimulation to induce weight loss is based on several possible mechanisms. The stimulation may interfere with ghrelin production or simulate the sensation of a full stomach, sending afferent messages via the vagus nerve. Trials in adults to date have been disappointing but an effect was realized in some patients.[106] Patient selection or a comprehensive weight management approach may improve its effectiveness in children. One gastric stimulation system (Tantalus, MedaCure, Orangeburg, NY, USA), has been used in Europe and is undergoing FDA trial in the United States in patients aged more than 17 years.[107]

### New Procedures

#### Gastric imbrication

Gastric imbrication involves plicating the greater curve, fundus, and body of the stomach to leave a tube along the lesser curvature from the gastroesophageal junction to the pylorus. It mimics the SG without excision of the stomach. The mechanism is presumed to be restrictive with reduction of ghrelin production. In this procedure, gastric ghrelin production is not stimulated because the food stream is excluded from the stomach. The procedure can be performed open, laparoscopically, or endoluminally. The endoluminal approach is restricted by the size of the endoscopes necessary to do the suturing. This factor may be limiting in children. Whether the lack of stimulation on ghrelin changes the effect on growth hormone in children remains to be determined. The safety of this procedure probably lies somewhere between the devices and the other surgical procedures, and its effectiveness and durability need to be studied. Similarly to the SG, the gastric imbrication procedure should have minimal effect on micronutrient absorption.[108,109]

#### Combined gastric sleeve resection and mid–small bowel resection

This procedure combines a gastric sleeve resection and omentectomy with a mid–small bowel resection. The mechanism of effect for this approach is fivefold: (1) mechanical restriction; (2) reduced stimulation of appetite (lower ghrelin levels);

(3) increased suppression of appetite (higher GLP-1 and PYY levels); (4) diminished surface area for caloric absorption; and (5) the inflammatory cytokines released from the omental fat are removed helping to spare the liver.[110] Theoretically, malabsorption is avoided by leaving the proximal small bowel intact and in line with the remaining GI tract to maintain fat-soluble vitamin absorption and the enterohepatic circulation of bile salts in the terminal ileum. Small series of this procedure in adults and adolescents have been reported with encouraging results but a longer follow-up will be required.[110,111] It is also not clear as to the optimal resection amount of the mid–small intestine. The sequential addition of a mid–small bowel resection to patients who do not lose adequate weight after an SG or RYGB may be a logical and safer next step rather than the BPD/DS.

## SUGGESTED CLINICAL MANAGEMENT PROTOCOL FOR WEIGHT LOSS IN ADOLESCENTS AND CHILDREN

It is becoming increasingly clear to the medical community, and society at large, that better treatment strategies need to be developed for the care of morbidly obese children. Nonoperative treatments have mostly failed or have met with minimal and temporary success. Primary care physicians are frustrated with the current ineffectiveness of nonmedical weight loss for morbid obesity but remain unwilling to condone aggressive bariatric surgical procedures. In the absence of clear-cut class I evidence for the relative effectiveness of the various bariatric surgical protocols, it is challenging to set exact guidelines for the management of morbid obesity in adolescents and children. The pediatric committee for the ASMBS published their recommended guidelines in 2012, which built on earlier NIH consensus guidelines.[86] According to these guidelines, children aged 13 to 18 years with a BMI of greater than or equal to 40 or greater than or equal to 35 with significant comorbidities qualify for surgery. In addition, the children must have failed 6 months of monitored weight loss attempts and be competent to assent to their procedure. In light of the complex causes and variable extent of morbid obesity, a rational approach customizes protocols to patients' individual needs by taking into account their age, BMI, type and severity of comorbidities, and psychosocial factors. These treatment protocols would provide the structure for clinical trials to evaluate and refine treatment strategies. The authors recommend multi-institutional cooperative treatment protocols with critical long-term safety and efficacy analysis, in the same manner the Children's Oncology Group has approached childhood cancer.

It seems most prudent to offer a common-sense practical and step-wise intensification of the management options. Resolution of the medical and psychosocial comorbidities must be the primary and overarching goal, secondary to the achievement of normal or near-normal weight. Choosing a bariatric procedure based on the morbidity (frequency and severity) and the risk of mortality prioritizes these goals.

### ADOLESCENTS: SUGGESTED CLINICAL MANAGEMENT PROTOCOL FOR WEIGHT LOSS

*Group I:* Patients aged 13 to 19 years with BMI less than or equal to 50 (**Fig. 1**)
Because of their simplicity and low morbidity, the LAGB or SG can be a good first choice for these patients. Morbidly obese adolescents with a lower BMI respond well to the gentle progressive pattern of LAGB weight loss.
*Group II:* Patients aged 13 to 15 years with BMI greater than 50
From the authors' experience, adolescents with BMI greater than 50 experienced difficulties with LAGB. They lose the same net weight as their lower-BMI adolescent counterparts (Holterman A, and colleagues, *Journal of Pediatric Surgery*, article submitted for publication.), but the large amount

**Surgical Approach to the Obese Teenagers**

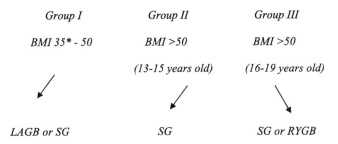

| Group I | Group II | Group III |
|---------|----------|-----------|
| BMI 35* - 50 | BMI >50 | BMI >50 |
| | (13-15 years old) | (16-19 years old) |
| LAGB or SG | SG | SG or RYGB |

Insufficient responders to the LAGB can undergo SG or RYGB

Insufficient responders to SG can undergo RYGB, BPD/DS, or mid-small bowel resection

*= BMI 35-39 with obesity related comorbidities

BMI >35 represents a BMI that is >97 percentile for age and gender (CDC Website)

LAGB = Laparoscopic Adjustable Gastric Band

SG = Sleeve Gastrectomy

RYGB = Roux-en-Y Gastric Bypass

BPD/DS = Biliopancreatic Diversion with Duodenal Switch

Insufficient responder = insufficient weight loss or resolution of comorbidities

with LAGB or SG and/or persistent mechanical problems with the LAGB

**Fig. 1.** Surgical decision protocol for bariatric surgery in adolescents.

of excess weight that remains and the slower pace of the LAGB leads to frustration and unmet expectations. Further tightening of the band to help accelerate weight loss often results in pouch enlargement, necessitating subsequent loosening of the band at the risk of regaining weight. The authors, therefore, recommend a more aggressive initial procedure, such as the SG, which would provide additional appetite suppression without the risk of micronutrient deficiencies along with an earlier and faster weight loss response.

*Group III*: Patients aged 16 to 19 years with BMI greater than 50

In addition to the same factors that limit the effectiveness of LAGB in group II, the age-related maturational independence of this group often leads to less-than-ideal adherence to treatment. In addition, insurance coverage changes for these adolescents can create a financial barrier to their ongoing care. The authors, therefore, recommend a more aggressive initial procedure, such as the SG or RYGB, which would provide an earlier and faster weight loss response. The shallow learning curve for laparoscopic SG compared with the more technically challenging RYGB and its lower risk of micronutrient deficiencies may make the SG particularly attractive for this mobile population.

For the subset of patients who require salvage operations for a recalcitrant response to the LAGB, the SG and RYGB may be appropriate. A failed SG is probably best salvaged by an RYGB or BPD/DS procedure or with the addition of a mid–small bowel resection. It is the authors' hope that these patient selection criteria will enhance the success rate of the LAGB and reduce the frustration of patients and parents from unmet expectations and wasted multiple operations.

## CHILDREN: GUIDELINES FOR DEVELOPING WEIGHT LOSS STRATEGIES

Although obesity can start in infancy and its comorbidities can occur in the very young, treatment outside behavior modification, activity programs, and diet training for obese children younger than 13 years is nearly nonexistent. One needs to be cognizant of many age-specific physiologic and psychological issues in the treatment of these obese children. For instance, obese children younger than 13 years old frequently have not completed their linear growth. Their BMI can improve when their weight gain is arrested while their linear growth remains. It is not clear whether this process reduces the body fat mass and resolves obesity related comorbidities. As obese children advance through the developmental stages of infancy, toddler, school age, preteen, and early teenage years (before reaching 13 years of age), the dynamics of food consumption, food choices, and activity decisions are much different from that of the adolescent. Their behavior may be more malleable and parents or health care providers may have a better chance at influencing their compliance. Any treatment program should have a multidisciplinary approach that recognizes the previously described basic tools of weight management, especially when surgical procedures and pharmacologic use are part of the therapy. Large study groups with shared protocols and databases are strongly recommended.

Of note, it has been the authors' experience that under physician and parents' guidance, younger adolescents are more accepting of the LAGB lifestyle modifications. Because of the excellent safety profile, reversibility, and adjustability of the LAGB, which allow controlled caloric ingestion and nutrition without malabsorption, the use of LAGB may be appropriate to the treatment of younger patients in their prepubertal and early puberty years (10–13 years of age with advanced obesity with or without comorbidities). Control of food ingestion in this group may allow them to undergo the longitudinal growth that leads to a normalization of their BMI without malnutrition. The adjustable gastric band can then be emptied, and if weight remains within an acceptable range, it could be easily removed.

The FDA can play a larger role in the development of drugs and devices for obesity treatment in children by supporting parallel studies in children, adolescents, and adults, taking into account their physical, physiologic, and psychological differences, and their differential responses. The traditional approach to wait for the completion of adult trials before proceeding with studies in children neglects the fact that 20% to 30% of children aged less than 13 years affected by obesity are still waiting for treatment. A new paradigm of cooperation is needed between industry, the FDA, the CDC, the NIH, and professional health care associations (American Academy of Pediatrics, National Association of Children's Hospitals and Related Institutions, American Academy of Family Physicians, American Pediatric Surgical Association, American Society for Metabolic and Bariatric Surgery, and so forth) to assist pediatric health care providers with tools and techniques to care for obese children. Rather than placing blame on parents for the lack of effective therapy and taking these children away from their families, the health care system needs to come to terms with the challenge of developing effective pediatric obesity treatment schemes.

## SUMMARY

Childhood obesity is a tremendous burden for children, their families, and society. Obesity prevention remains the ultimate goal, but rapid development and deployment of effective nonsurgical treatment options is not currently achievable given the complexity of this disease. In the meantime, hundreds of thousands of our world's youth are facing discrimination, a poor quality of life, and a shortened lifespan from the burdens of this illness. Surgical options for adolescent obesity have been proven to be safe and effective and should be offered. The development of stratified protocols of increasing intensity (ie, surgical aggressiveness) should be individualized for each patient based on their disease severity and risk factors. These protocols should be offered in the context of multidisciplinary, cooperative clinical trials to critically evaluate and develop optimal treatment strategies for morbid obesity. Long-term cooperation between families, schools, communities, government, health care professionals, media, insurers, and industry is essential in addressing the prevention and treatment of childhood obesity.

## REFERENCES

1. Hassink SG. A clinical guide to pediatric weight management and obesity. Philadelphia: Lippencott; 2007. p. vii.
2. Moore BJ, Martin LF. Why should obesity be treated? In: Martin LF, editor. Obesity surgery. New York: McGraw-Hill; 2004. p. 1–15.
3. Browne AF, Browne NT. Lap-Band® in adolescents. In: Rosenthal RJ, Jones DB, editors. Weight loss surgery: a multidisciplinary approach. Edgemont (PA): Matrix Medical Communications; 2008. p. 477–88.
4. Franz MH, VanWormer JJ, Crain AL, et al. Weight-loss outcomes: a systematic review and meta-analysis of weight-loss clinical trials with a minimum 1-year follow-up. J Am Diet Assoc 2007;107:1755–67.
5. Freemark M. Pharmacotherapy of childhood obesity and pre-diabetes. In: Freemark M, editor. Pediatric obesity. New York: Springer; 2010. p. 339–56.
6. Martin LF. The evolution of surgery for morbid obesity. In: Martin LF, editor. Obesity surgery. New York: McGraw-Hill; 2004. p. 15–48.
7. Ikramudden S, Leslie D, Whitson B, et al. Energy metabolism & biochemistry of obesity. In: Rosenthal RJ, Jones DB, editors. Weight loss surgery: a multidisciplinary approach. Edgemont (PA): Matrix Medical Communications; 2008. p. 17–26.
8. Lakka HM, Bouchard C. Etiology of obesity. In: Buchwald H, Cowan G, Pories W, editors. Surgical management of obesity. Philadelphia: Saunders; 2007. p. 18–28.
9. Clinical growth charts. Centers for Disease Control and Prevention, National Center for Health Statistics; 2009. Available at: www.cdc.gov/growthcharts/clinical_charts.htm. Accessed April 10, 2012.
10. Ogden CL, Carroll MD, Curtin LR, et al. Prevalence of high body mass index in US children and adolescents, 2007–2008. JAMA 2010;303(3):242–9.
11. Popkin B. Global dynamics in childhood obesity: reflections on a life of work in the field. In: Freemark M, editor. Pediatric obesity. New York: Springer; 2010. p. 3–12.
12. National Center for Health Statistics. Health, United States, 2010: with special features on death and dying. Hyattsville (MD): U.S. Department of Health and Human Services; 2011.
13. Lustig RH. The neuroendocrine control of energy balance. In: Freemark M, editor. Pediatric obesity. New York: Springer; 2010. p. 15–32.
14. Vincent RP, Le Roux CW. Changes in gut hormones after bariatric surgery. Clin Endocrinol 2008;69(2):173–9.

15. Grün F, Blumberg B. Endocrine disrupters as obesogens. Mol Cell Endocrinol 2009;304(1–2):19–29.
16. Decherf S, Demeneix BA. The obesogen hypothesis: a shift of focus from the periphery to the hypothalamus. J Toxicol Environ Health B Crit Rev 2011; 14(5–7):423–48.
17. Grün F. Obesogens. Curr Opin Endocrinol Diabetes Obes 2010;17(5):453–9.
18. Tsai F, Coyle WJ. The microbiome and obesity: is obesity linked to our gut flora? Curr Gastroenterol Rep 2009;11(4):307–13.
19. DiBaise JK, Zhang H, Crowell MD, et al. Gut microbiota and its possible relation-ship with obesity. Mayo Clin Proc 2008;83(4):460–9.
20. Ley RE. Obesity and the human microbiome. Curr Opin Gastroenterol 2010; 26(1):5–11.
21. Malone M. Medications associated with weight gain. Ann Pharmacother 2005; 39(12):2046–55.
22. Leslie WS, Hankey CR, Lean ME. Weight gain as an adverse effect of some commonly prescribed drugs: a systematic review. QJM 2007;100(7):395–404.
23. Stunkard AJ, Harris JR, Pedersen NL, et al. The body-mass index of twins who have been reared apart. N Engl J Med 1990;322(21):1483–7.
24. Hinney A, Hebebrand J. Polygenic obesity. In: Freemark M, editor. Pediatric obesity. New York: Springer; 2010. p. 75–90.
25. Dina C, Meyre D, Gallina S, et al. Variation in FTO contributes to childhood obesity and severe adult obesity. Nat Genet 2007;39:724–6.
26. Loos R, Lindgren C, Li S, et al. Common variants near MC4R are associated with fat mass, weight and risk of obesity. Nat Genet 2008;40(6):1–8.
27. Weiss R, Cali A, Caprio S. Pathogenesis of insulin resistance and glucose intol-erance in childhood obesity. In: Freemark M, editor. Pediatric obesity. New York: Springer; 2010. p. 163–74.
28. Glueck CJ, Morrison JA, Umar M, et al. The long-term metabolic complications of childhood obesity. In: Freemark M, editor. Pediatric obesity. New York: Springer; 2010. p. 253–64.
29. Hunley RE, Kon V. Pathogenesis of hypertension and renal disease in obesity. In: Freemark M, editor. Pediatric obesity. New York: Springer; 2010. p. 223–40.
30. McGill HC Jr, McMahan CA, Gidding SS. Childhood obesity, atherogenesis, and adult cardiovascular disease. In: Freemark M, editor. Pediatric obesity. New York: Springer; 2010. p. 265–78.
31. McCrindle BW. Pathogenesis and management of dyslipidemia in obese children. In: Freemark M, editor. Pediatric obesity. New York: Springer; 2010. p. 175–200.
32. Shah AS, Khoury PR, Dolan LM, et al. The effects of obesity and type 2 diabetes mellitus on cardiac structure and function in adolescents and young adults. Di-abetologia 2011;54(4):722–30.
33. Erler T, Paditz E. Obstructive sleep apnea syndrome in children: a state-of-the-art review. Treat Respir Med 2004;3(2):107–22.
34. Verhulst S. Sleep-disordered breathing and sleep duration in childhood obesity. In: Freemark M, editor. Pediatric obesity. New York: Springer; 2010. p. 241–52.
35. Lindback SM, Gabbert C, Johnson BL, et al. Pediatric nonalcoholic fatty liver disease: a comprehensive review. Adv Pediatr 2010;57(1):85–140.
36. Montgomery CO, Young KL, Austen M, et al. Increased risk of Blount disease in obese children and adolescents with vitamin D deficiency. J Pediatr Orthop 2010;30(8):879–82.
37. Peck D. Slipped capital femoral epiphysis: diagnosis and management. Am Fam Physician 2010;82(3):258–62.

38. Wall M. Idiopathic intracranial hypertension (pseudotumor cerebri). Curr Neurol Neurosci Rep 2008;8(2):87–93.

39. Elder DA, Woo JG, D'Alessio DA. Impaired beta-cell sensitivity to glucose and maximal insulin secretory capacity in adolescents with type 2 diabetes. Pediatr Diabetes 2010;11(5):314–21.

40. Pinhas-Hamiel O, Zeitler P. Acute and chronic complications of type 2 diabetes mellitus in children and adolescents. Lancet 2007;369(9575):1823–31.

41. Shiga K, Kikuchi N. Children with type 2 diabetes mellitus are at greater risk of macrovascular complications. Pediatr Int 2009;51(4):563–7.

42. Daniels SR. Complications of obesity in children and adolescents. Int J Obes (Lond) 2009;33(Suppl 1):S60–5.

43. Washington RL. Childhood obesity: issues of weight bias. Prev Chronic Dis 2011;8(5):A94.

44. Holterman AX, Browne A, Dillard BE 3rd, et al. Short-term outcome in the first 10 morbidly obese adolescent patients in the FDA-approved trial for laparoscopic adjustable gastric banding. J Pediatr Gastroenterol Nutr 2007;45(4):465–73.

45. Puhl RM, Latner JD. Stigma, obesity, and the health of the nation's children. Psychol Bull 2007;133(4):557–80.

46. Puhl RM, Heuer CA. The stigma of obesity: a review and update. Obesity 2009; 17:941–64.

47. Edmunds LD. Parents; perceptions of health professionals' responses when seeking help for their overweight children. Fam Pract 2005;22(3):287–92.

48. Young KL, Demeule M, Stuhlsatz K, et al. Identification and treatment of obesity as a standard of care for all patients in children's hospitals. Pediatrics 2011; 128(Suppl 2):S47–50.

49. Ghobadi C, Johnson TN, Aarabi M, et al. Application of a systems approach to the bottom-up assessment of pharmacokinetics in obese patients: expected variations in clearance. Clin Pharmacokinet 2011;50(12):809–22.

50. Finkelstein EA, Trogdon JG, Cohen JW, et al. Annual medical spending attributable to obesity: payer-and service-specific estimates. Health Aff 2009;28(5):w822–31.

51. Woolford SJ, Gebremariam A, Clark SJ, et al. Incremental hospital charges associated with obesity as a secondary diagnosis in children. Obesity 2007; 15(7):1895–901.

52. Simpson LA, Cooper J. Paying for obesity: a changing landscape. Pediatrics 2009;123(Suppl 5):S301–7.

53. Lee JS, Sheer JL, Lopez N, et al. Coverage of obesity treatment: a state-by-state analysis of Medicaid and state insurance laws. Public Health Rep 2010;125(4): 596–604.

54. Finkelstein EA, DiBonaventura M, Burgess SM, et al. The costs of obesity in the workplace. J Occup Environ Med 2010;52(10):971–6.

55. Cawley J, Maclean JC. Unfit for service: the implications of rising obesity for US military recruitment. Health Econ 2011. DOI: 10.1002/hec.1794. [Epub ahead of print].

56. Lee JM, Lim S, Zoellner, et al. Don't children grow out of their obesity? Weight transitions in early childhood. Clin Pediatr (Phila) 2010;49(5):466–9.

57. Whitaker RC, Wright JA, Pepe MS, et al. Predicting obesity in young adulthood from childhood and parental obesity. N Engl J Med 1997;337:869–73.

58. Browne AF, Inge T. How young for bariatric surgery in children? Semin Pediatr Surg 2009;18(3):176–85.

59. Bray FA, Ryan DH. Medical approaches to the treatment of the obese patient. In: Mantzoros CS, editor. Obesity and diabetes. Totowa (MJ): Humana Press; 2006. p. 457–69.

60. American Dietetic Association (ADA). Position of the American Dietetic Association: individual-, family-, school-, and community-based interventions for pediatric overweight. J Am Diet Assoc 2006;106(6):925–45.
61. Bennett B, Sothern MS. Diet, exercise, behavior: the promise and limits of lifestyle change. Semin Pediatr Surg 2009;18(3):152–8.
62. Schwimmer JB, Burwinkle TM, Varni JW. Health-related quality of life of severely obese children and adolescents. JAMA 2003;289(14):1813–9.
63. Griffiths LJ, Dezateux C, Hill A. Is obesity associated with emotional and behavioural problems in children? Findings from the Millennium Cohort Study. Int J Pediatr Obes 2011;6(2–2):e423–32.
64. Epstein LF, Paluch RA, Roemmich JN, et al. Family-based obesity treatment, then and now: twenty-five years of pediatric obesity treatment. Health Psychol 2007;26(4):381–91.
65. Whitlock E, Williams S, Gold R, et al. Screening and interventions for childhood overweight: a summary of evidence for the US Preventive Services Task Force. Pediatrics 2005;116(1):e125–44.
66. Klonoff DC, Greenway F. Drugs in the pipeline for the obesity market. J Diabetes Sci Technol 2008;2(5):913–8.
67. Sugerman JH, Sugerman EL, DeMaria EJ, et al. Bariatric surgery for severely obese adolescents. J Gastrointest Surg 2003;7(1):102–7.
68. Garcia VF, Langlord L, Inge TH. Application of laparoscopy for bariatric surgery in adolescents. Curr Opin Pediatr 2003;15(3):248–55.
69. Inge TH, Garcia V, Daniels S, et al. A multidisciplinary approach to the adolescent bariatric surgical patient. J Pediatr Surg 2004;39(3):442–7.
70. Inge TH, Krebs NF, Garcia VF, et al. Bariatric surgery for severely overweight adolescents: concerns and recommendations. Pediatrics 2004;114(1):217–23.
71. Inge TH, Zeller M, Harmon C, et al. Teen-longitudinal assessment of bariatric surgery: methodological features of the first prospective multicenter study of adolescent bariatric surgery. J Pediatr Surg 2007;42(11):1969–71.
72. Nadler EP, Youn HA, Ginsburg HB, et al. Short-term results in 53 US obese pediatric patients treated with laparoscopic adjustable gastric banding. J Pediatr Surg 2007;42(1):137–41.
73. Warman J. The application of laparoscopic bariatric surgery for treatment of severe obesity in adolescents using a multidisciplinary adolescent bariatric program. Crit Care Nurs Q 2005;28(3):276–87.
74. Zitsman JL, Fennoy I, Witt MA, et al. Laparoscopic adjustable gastric banding in adolescents: short-term results. J Pediatr Surg 2011;46(1):157–62.
75. Buchwald H, Avidor Y, Braunwald E, et al. Bariatric surgery: a systematic review and met-analysis. JAMA 2004;292(14):1724–37.
76. Franco JV, Ruiz PA, Palermo M, et al. A review of studies comparing three laparoscopic procedures in bariatric surgery: sleeve gastrectomy, Roux-en-Y gastric bypass and adjustable gastric banding. Obes Surg 2011;21(9):1458–68.
77. Conroy R, Lee EJ, Jean A, et al. Effect of laparoscopic adjustable gastric banding on metabolic syndrome and its risk factors in morbidly obese adolescents. J Obes 2011;2011:906384.
78. Dillard BE 3rd, Gorodner V, Galvani C, et al. Initial experience with the adjustable gastric band in morbidly obese US adolescents and recommendations for further investigation. J Pediatr Gastroenterol Nutr 2007;45(2):240–6.
79. Holterman AX, Browne A, Tussing L, et al. A prospective trial for laparoscopic adjustable gastric banding in morbidly obese adolescents: an interim report of weight loss, metabolic and quality of life outcomes. J Pediatr Surg 2010;45(1):74–8.

80. Lawson ML, Kirk S, Mitchell T, et al. One-year outcomes of Roux-en-Y gastric bypass for morbidly obese adolescents: a multicenter study from the Pediatric Bariatric Study Group. J Pediatr Surg 2006;41(1):137–43.

81. Loux TJ, Haricharan RN, Clements RH, et al. Health-related quality of life before and after bariatric surgery in adolescents. J Pediatr Surg 2008;43(7):1275–9.

82. Nadler EP, Youn HA, Ren CJ, et al. An update on 73 US obese pediatric patients treated with laparoscopic adjustable gastric banding: comorbidity resolution and compliance data. J Pediatr Surg 2008;43(1):141–6.

83. Nadler EP, Reddy S, Isenalumhe A, et al. Laparoscopic adjustable gastric banding for morbidly obese adolescents affects android fat loss, resolution of comorbidities, and improved metabolic status. J Am Coll Surg 2009;209(5):638–44.

84. O'Brien PE, Sawyer SM, Laurie C, et al. Laparoscopic adjustable gastric banding in severely obese adolescents: a randomized trial. JAMA 2010;303(6):519–26.

85. Zitsman JL, Digiorgi MF, Marr JR, et al. Comparative outcomes of laparoscopic adjustable gastric banding in adolescents and adults. Surg Obes Relat Dis 2011;7(6):720–6.

86. Michalsky M, Reichard K, Inge T, et al. ASMBS pediatric committee best practice guidelines. Surg Obes Relat Dis 2012;8(1):1–7.

87. Michalsky M, Kramer RE, Fullmer MA, et al. Developing criteria for pediatric/adolescent bariatric surgery programs. Pediatrics 2011;128(Suppl 2):S65–70.

88. Fullmer MA, Abrams SH, Hrovat K, et al. Nutritional strategy for the adolescent patient undergoing bariatric surgery: report of a Working Group of the Nutrition Committee for the North American Society of Pediatric Gastroenterology, Hepatology and Nutrition and National Association of Children's Hospital and Related Institutions. J Pediatr Gastroenterol Nutr 2012;54(1):125–35.

89. Barnett SJ. Contemporary surgical management of the obese adolescent. Curr Opin Pediatr 2011;23(3):351–5.

90. Baur LA, Fitzgerald DA. Recommendations for bariatric surgery in adolescents in Australia and New Zealand. J Paediatr Child Health 2010;46(12):704–7.

91. Cunneen SA. Review of meta-analytic comparisons of bariatric surgery with a focus on laparoscopic adjustable gastric banding. Surg Obes Relat Dis 2008;4(Suppl 3):S47–55.

92. Xanthakos SA. Bariatric surgery for extreme adolescent obesity: indications, outcomes, and physiologic effects on the gut-brain axis. Pathophysiology 2008;15(2):135–46.

93. American Society for Metabolic and Bariatric Surgery. Updated position statement on sleeve gastrectomy as a bariatric procedure. Surg Obes Relat Dis 2010;6(1):1–5.

94. Nadler EP, Barefoot LC, Qureshi FG. Early results after laparoscopic sleeve gastrectomy in adolescents with morbid obesity. Oral presentation at the 7th Annual Academic Surgical Congress, Las Vegas (NV), February, 2012.

95. Inge RH, Xanthakos S. Sleeve gastrectomy for childhood morbid obesity: why not? Obes Surg 2010;20(1):118–20.

96. Scopinaro N, Adami FG, Marinari GM, et al. Biliopancreatic diversion. World J Surg 1998;22(9):936–46.

97. Stimac D, Majanović SK, Turk T, et al. Intragastric balloon treatment for obesity: results of a large single center prospective study. Obes Surg 2011;21(5):551–5.

98. Dumonceau JM. Evidence-based review of the Bioenterics intragastric balloon for weight loss. Obes Surg 2008;18(12):1611–7.

99. Lecumberri E, Krekshi W, Matía P, et al. Effectiveness and safety of air-filled balloon Heliosphere BAG® in 82 consecutive obese patients. Obes Surg 2011;21(10):1508–12.

100. Gaggiotti F, Tack J, Garrido AB Jr, et al. Adjustable totally implantable intragastric prosthesis (ATIIP)-Endogast for treatment of morbid obesity: one-year follow-up of a multicenter prospective clinical survey. Obes Surg 2007;17(7):949–56.

101. Machytka E, Klvana P, Kombluth A, et al. Adjustable intragastric balloons: a 12-month pilot trial in endoscopic weight loss management. Obes Surg 2011; 21(10):1499–507.

102. Swidnicka-Siergiejko A, Wróblewski E, Andrezej D, et al. Endoscopic treatment of obesity. Can J Gastroenterol 2011;25(11):627–33.

103. Genco A, Bruni T, Doldi SB, et al. BioEnterics Intragastric Balloon: the Italian experience with 2,515 patients. Obes Surg 2005;15(8):1161–4.

104. Gersin KS, Torhstein RI, Tosenthal RJ, et al. Open-label, sham-controlled trial of an endoscopic duodenojejunal bypass liner for preoperative weight loss in bariatric surgery candidates. Gastrointest Endosc 2010;71(6):976–82.

105. Camilleri M, Toouli J, Herrera MF, et al. Selection of electrical algorithms to treat obesity with intermittent vagal block using an implantable medical device. Surg Obes Relat Dis 2009;5(2):224–9.

106. Shikora SA, Bergenstal R, Bessler M, et al. Implantable gastric stimulation for the treatment of clinically severe obesity: results of the SHAPE trial. Surg Obes Relat Dis 2009;5(1):31–7.

107. Sanmiguel CP, Conklin JL, Cunneen SA, et al. Gastric electrical stimulation with the TANTALUS system in obese type 2 diabetes patients: effect on weight and glycemic control. J Diabetes Sci Technol 2009;3(4):964–70.

108. Skrekas G, Antiochos K, Stafyla VK. Laparoscopic gastric greater curvature placation: results and complications in a series of 135 patients. Obes Surg 2011;21(11):1657–63.

109. Brethauer SA, Harris JL, Kroh M, et al. Laparoscopic gastric plication for treatment of severe obesity. Surg Obes Relat Dis 2011;7(1):15–22.

110. Velhote MC, Damiani D. Bariatric surgery in adolescents: preliminary 1-year results with a novel technique (Santoro III). Obes Surg 2010;20(12):1710–5.

111. Heap AJ, Cummings DE. A novel weight-reducing operation: lateral subtotal gastrectomy with Silastic ring plus small bowel reduction with omentectomy. Obes Surg 2008;18(7):819–28.

# Congenital Cervical Cysts, Sinuses, and Fistulae in Pediatric Surgery

Cabrini A. LaRiviere, MD, MPH, John H.T. Waldhausen, MD*

## KEYWORDS

- Branchial anomalies • Cervical cysts • Cervical sinuses • Cervical fistulae
- Thyroglossal duct cysts • Congenital

## KEY POINTS

- Thyroglossal duct cysts are the most common congenital anomaly of the neck in children. Resection must include resection of the mid portion of the hyoid bone along with the tract to the base of the tongue.
- Branchial cleft anomalies are the second most common congenital anomaly of the neck in children. Second branchial cleft cysts and sinuses are the most common type. Whereas thyroglossal duct cysts are midline structures, second branchial cleft cysts and sinuses are lateral along the anterior border of the sternocleidomastoid muscle in the mid neck, and third and fourth sinuses are found lower in the neck.
- Branchial cleft cysts and sinuses as well as thyroglossal duct cysts are best dealt with by surgical resection. Dissection must carefully include the entire tract that is associated with these lesions. Detailed knowledge of the vascular anatomy and surrounding nerves is necessary for safe and complete resection, especially for branchial cleft anomalies.

Congenital cervical cysts, sinuses, and fistulae are lesions that a surgeon must include in the differential diagnosis of head and neck masses in children and adults. The most common congenital neck masses encountered in practice are thyroglossal duct cysts, followed by branchial cleft anomalies and dermoid cysts. It is essential for the surgeon to fully comprehend the embryology and anatomy of each lesion to attain the correct preoperative diagnosis and plan for an appropriate surgical management in order to prevent the most common complication in these lesions, recurrence. The following sections discuss the embryology, anatomy, common presentation, evaluation, and the current principles of surgical treatment for each of the congenital lesions.

The authors have nothing to disclose.
Department of Surgery, Seattle Children's Hospital, University of Washington School of Medicine, 4800 Sand Point Way, NE, Seattle, WA 98105, USA
* Corresponding author.
E-mail address: john.waldhausen@seattlechildrens.org

## THYROGLOSSAL DUCT ANOMALIES

Thyroglossal duct anomalies are the most common congenital anomaly of the neck and the second most common neck mass found in children after inflammatory masses.[1,2] Thyroglossal duct remnants occur in approximately 7% of the population, and although the majority will remain asymptomatic, the index of suspicion should remain high until a final diagnosis of any neck mass is complete.[1]

### Embryology

The thyroid gland develops during the third week of gestation and forms out of the ventral diverticulum (median thyroid anlage) comprising endoderm of the first and second pharyngeal pouches.[2] The diverticulum migrates caudally as the embryo develops and descends anteriorly or through the hyoid bone and laryngeal cartilage.[3,4] As the median thyroid anlage descends caudally, a tract forms the thyroglossal duct (**Fig. 1**).[4] The thyroglossal duct originates at the base of the tongue and during the fifth to eighth week of gestation, the thyroglossal duct obliterates to leave the proximal remnant, the foramen cecum, at the base of the tongue.[3] The distal remnant of the tract forms the pyramidal lobe of the thyroid.[3] If the tract persists and fails to obliterate along any portion of the thyroid's descent to the pretracheal position in the neck, a midline cystic remnant persists as the thyroglossal duct cyst.[1,3]

### Clinical Presentation and Diagnosis

The majority (two-thirds) of patients with thyroglossal duct anomalies are diagnosed before 30 years of age, and greater than half of these are identified before age 10 years.[1] Patients present commonly with an asymptomatic, cystic neck mass in the midline near the hyoid bone (**Figs. 2 and 3**).[2,3] The most common location for the cystic mass is adjacent to the hyoid bone (66%), but they are also located between the tongue and hyoid bone, between the hyoid and pyramidal lobe, within the tongue,

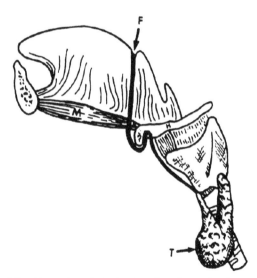

**Fig. 1.** The course of the thyroglossal duct extending from the foramen cecum (F) to the thyroid (T). (*Reprinted from* Som PM, Smoker WRK, Curtin HD, et al. Congenital lesions in head and neck imaging. In: Som PM, Curtin HD, editors. Head and Neck Imaging. St Louis (MO): Mosby; 2003. p. 121–5; with permission.)

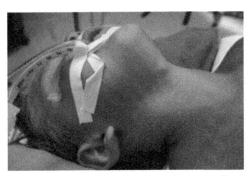

**Fig. 2.** Thyroglossal duct cyst, uncomplicated. (*From* Foley DS, Fallat ME. Thyroglossal duct and other congenital midline cervical anomalies. Semin Pediatr Surg 2006;15(2):70–5; with permission.)

or within the thyroid gland.[3] The neck mass will typically move with swallowing or protrusion of the tongue on examination. Approximately one-third of thyroglossal duct cysts present with an active infection or clinical history consistent with prior infection of the neck mass, and infection of the mass is the typical presentation of thyroglossal duct cysts in the adult population.[3,5] One-fourth of patients present with a draining sinus that either has ruptured spontaneously or is the result of surgical drainage of a thyroglossal duct cyst abscess.[3] The material draining from the sinus can result in a foul taste in the mouth if the drainage occurs at the foramen cecum. Thyroglossal duct cyst remnants may rarely present with severe respiratory distress or sudden infant death syndrome related to lesions at the base of the tongue. These lesions may also present as lateral cystic neck masses, anterior tongue fistulae, or be coexistent with branchial anomalies.[3]

The preoperative evaluation for a patient with a suspected thyroglossal duct cyst includes a complete history and physical examination with a preoperative ultrasonogram, and a screening thyroid-stimulating hormone (TSH) level to enhance the history and physical when necessary. For patients with history, examination findings, or elevated TSH levels suggesting hypothyroidism or a solid mass, scinti-scanning to rule out a median ectopic thyroid is helpful.[3] When median ectopic thyroid is present it may contain the only functioning thyroid tissue, and removal of the structure would render the patient permanently dependent on thyroid replacement.[2] The management of median ectopic thyroid is controversial.[6] Some investigators believe patients can be treated with exogenous thyroid hormone to suppress the gland, whereas others

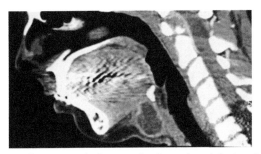

**Fig. 3.** Sagittal computed tomography image of a thyroglossal duct cyst demonstrating the close relationship to the hyoid bone. (*Courtesy of* Glenn Isaacson, MD, Philadelphia, PA.)

advocate for resection, for reasons that are discussed below.[3] Although median ectopic thyroid only occurs in 1% to 2% of thyroglossal duct cysts, some investigators advocate for scinti-scans in all patients.[7]

## Treatment

Elective surgical excision is the treatment of choice for uncomplicated thyroglossal duct cysts, so that cyst infection is prevented. The Sistrunk procedure, which includes removal of the central portion of the hyoid bone, is performed rather than simple excision to reduce recurrence risk.[3] With the patient in the supine position and the neck extended, a transverse incision is made over the mass. The dissection is carried down to the cyst, then caudally to determine if there is a tract to the pyramidal lobe. If present, it is excised en bloc with the cyst. The surgeon then dissects cranially toward the hyoid bone and a block of tissue around the proximal tract is also excised. The central portion of the hyoid bone must be excised, and the tract is further dissected with a core of tissue from the muscle at the base of the tongue to the foramen cecum (**Fig. 4**).[3] After confirming adequate proximal dissection by pressure on the base of the tongue from the mouth, the tract is ligated and transected. Intrathyroidal thyroglossal duct cysts should also undergo a Sistrunk procedure if there is a transhyoidal fistulous tract, but can be treated with thyroidectomy if no tract can be identified.[8]

Infected cysts or sinuses are first managed by relieving the infection. The cysts are usually infected via the mouth, thus the most common organisms are *Haemophilus influenzae*, *Staphylococcus aureus*, and *Staphylococcus epidermidis*.[3] Antibiotic coverage targeting these organisms should be initiated, and needle aspiration may be indicated to allow for decompression and identification of the causal organism. Formal incision and drainage should be avoided, if possible, to prevent seeding of ductal cells outside the cyst, which may increase the risk of recurrence.[2] If incision and drainage is necessary, the incision should be placed so it can be completely excised with an ellipse at the time of definitive resection. Once the infection clears and the incision heals, the patient may undergo an elective Sistrunk procedure.[3]

If a solid mass is encountered during excision of a suspected thyroglossal duct cyst, it should be sent for frozen section to rule out a median ectopic thyroid. If the biopsy returns as normal thyroid tissue and the patient has functional thyroid tissue in the correct location, the mass should be excised by the Sistrunk procedure.[3] If the

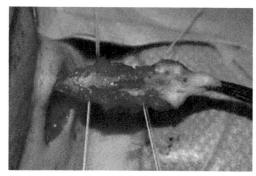

**Fig. 4.** Sistrunk procedure resection of a thyroglossal duct cyst. Note that the specimen includes the cyst, hyoid bone, and proximal tract en bloc. (*From* Foley DS, Fallat ME. Thyroglossal duct and other congenital midline cervical anomalies. Semin Pediatr Surg 2006;15(2):70–5; with permission.)

mass is possibly the patient's only functional thyroid tissue, the management becomes controversial. One option involves leaving the ectopic thyroid, either in situ or repositioning it laterally below the strap muscles or into the rectus or quadriceps muscles. This option is intended to prevent the patient from becoming permanently hypothyroid; however, many patients still require long-term thyroid hormone replacement for the treatment of hypothyroidism or to control the size of the ectopic thyroid tissue for cosmetic or functional reasons.[2] The need for long-term therapy and the possibility of malignant degeneration have led some to recommend excision of the median ectopic thyroid regardless of the presence of additional thyroid tissue.[3]

Thyroglossal duct cysts are lined with ductal epithelium, or contain solid thyroid tissue. Fewer than 1% will have malignant tissue, usually well-differentiated thyroid carcinoma.[9] This carcinoma occurs more often in adults, but has been reported in children as young as 6 years old.[10] It is usually identified incidentally at the time of surgery for a suspected thyroglossal duct cyst. Papillary carcinoma is seen most often, although all types of thyroid carcinoma except medullary carcinoma have been reported.[3,5] If there is no evidence of capsular invasion, or distant or regional metastasis, the Sistrunk procedure has been associated with a 95% cure rate, although careful follow-up is necessary.[3] Other investigators recommend completion thyroidectomy regardless of capsular invasion, citing the benefits of full pathologic examination of the gland, facilitation of radioactive iodine ablation, and increased sensitivity of radioisotope screening for recurrence.[1] If capsular invasion is present, completion thyroidectomy, nodal dissection, and radioiodine ablation should be pursued as indicated by type and stage of disease.[3]

Recurrence of thyroglossal duct cyst after complete excision using the Sistrunk procedure is reported to be 2.6% to 5%.[1,5] Several factors have been identified predisposing patients to increased risk of recurrence. Failure to completely excise the cyst (especially simple excision alone) can result in recurrence rates of 38% to 70%.[1,5] In children younger than 2 years, intraoperative cyst rupture and presence of a cutaneous component increases the risk of recurrence. Preoperative or concurrent infections of the cyst has been historically reported as a risk factor because of the increased difficulty of complete resection, although some have found that postoperative rather than preoperative infections were associated with increased recurrence.[3,11] Recurrent thyroglossal cyst excision has a higher risk of recurrence (20%–35%) and requires a wider en bloc resection.[3]

## BRANCHIAL CLEFT ANOMALIES

Branchial anomalies are the second most common congenital neck masses in children, and comprise approximately 30% of all head and neck lesions after thyroglossal ducts cysts and sinuses.[1,12] Branchial lesions affect males and females equally, and most abnormalities are diagnosed in infancy or childhood, although some lesions may not be recognized until adulthood.[12,13]

### Embryology

The fourth week of gestation marks the development of the 4 pairs of well-defined branchial arches and 2 rudimentary arches not visible on the surface of the embryo.[12] The branchial arches are covered with ectoderm on the surface, the inside branchial pouches consist of foregut endoderm, and mesodermal tissue lies between the 2 layers.[14] The mesodermal tissue contains the dominant artery, nerve, cartilage rod, and muscle for each branchial arch.[12,14] Six arches in fish and amphibians form into gills, but in humans only 5 arches (1, 2, 3, 4, and 6) become the head and neck structures after gradual obliteration of the clefts (grooves) and pouches by mesenchymal tissue (**Fig. 5**).[12,14] The incomplete obliteration of the clefts and pouches results in branchial anomalies.[12]

Throughout gestation each arch transforms into a defined anatomic pattern. Understanding the pattern of transformation and the relationship to normal structures in the neck are essential in the diagnosis and treatment of these anomalies. Branchial anomalies are classified by the cleft or pouch of origin, and this is determined by the internal opening of the sinus and its relationship to nerves, arteries, and muscles. It is important to understand these anatomic relationships to prevent injury to surrounding structures and ensure complete resection.[12] The essential embryology and anatomy is described here for each arch.

## Pathology

Branchial anomalies may be lined with respiratory epithelium or squamous epithelium, or may contain both tissue types. Cysts are often lined with squamous epithelium, whereas sinuses and fistulae are more likely to be lined with ciliated, columnar epithelium.[12] Lymphoid tissue, sebaceous glands, salivary tissue, or cholesterol crystals in mucoid fluid within the cysts can be seen. Squamous cell cancer can be found within branchial lesions in adults, although it is extremely rare, and it is difficult to distinguish between a primary lesion arising from within an anomaly and a metastasis lesion from an occult primary lesion.[15]

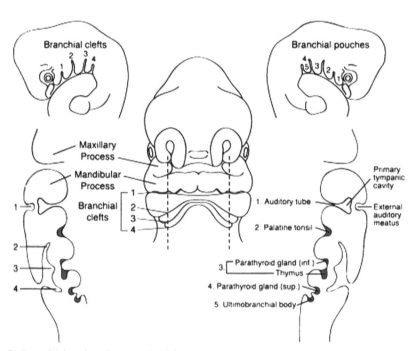

**Fig. 5.** Branchial embryology at the fifth week of gestation. Sagittal sections demonstrate the anatomic relationship of the external clefts and internal pouches as well as the derivation of important head and neck structures. (*From* Waldhausen JH. Branchial cleft and arch anomalies in children. Semin Pediatr Surg 2006;15(2):64–9; with permission.)

## Diagnosis

Branchial anomalies present as cysts, sinuses, or fistulae. The clinical terms used to describe the branchial remnants are often inconsistent, and it is important to distinguish the manifestations of each type of anomaly.[1,2] Cysts do not communicate with any body surface; sinuses have an opening to a single body surface, often skin or the pharynx; and fistulae abnormally connect 2 body surfaces.[1] Cysts are remnants of the cervical sinus without an external opening. A persistent cervical sinus with an external opening is diagnosed as a sinus, and a fistula contains remnants of the branchial groove with breakdown of the branchial membrane that results in a pharyngocutaneous fistula.[16] The presentation for branchial anomalies varies according to the arch of origin, and the details of specific arch types are described below.[1]

The evaluation for branchial lesions begins with a complete history and physical examination. In classic cases, no additional evaluation may be necessary. Evaluation may include upper airway endoscopy to determine the presence of a pharyngeal opening.[1] A careful examination of the pyriform sinus and the tonsillar fossa will help identify fistulae present. In adults, a fine-needle aspiration (FNA) should be performed to rule out metastatic carcinoma or to clarify the diagnosis.[12,13] FNA does not need to be performed in children and an incisional biopsy should be avoided, because this will make the branchial lesion resection technically more difficult.[12] Ultrasonography, computed tomography (CT), and magnetic resonance imaging (MRI) can be helpful in defining the lesion and its anatomic course.[12] CT with thin slices is the current study of choice, when necessary, in providing 3-dimensional relationships and evaluation of the surrounding soft tissue and bone structures, and may demonstrate a fistula in up to 64% of cases.[17] Barium esophagography may play a role in the diagnosis of branchial lesions with a 50% to 80% sensitivity for third-arch and fourth-arch fistulae; however, the modality is not required and should not replace pharyngoscopy or CT in the workup for branchial lesions.[18,19]

## Treatment

The definitive treatment for branchial anomalies is complete surgical excision. Cysts and sinuses that remain unresected have a high risk of infection, and the incomplete resection of lesions may result in higher rates of recurrence.[12] The timing of resection is debated; some advocate early resection to prevent infection, whereas others support waiting until age 2 to 3 years.[12,15,20] One-fifth of lesions that present for operative resection have already become infected at least once before surgery.[15] As in the case of thyroglossal duct cysts, acute infections should be first treated with antibiotics, needle aspiration and, if necessary, incision and drainage, followed by complete resection after resolution of the infection.[6] Considerations for each of the arch anomalies are discussed here.

## First-Cleft Anomalies

First branchial anomalies comprise 1% of branchial cleft malformations.[12] The mandible and a portion of the maxillary process are derivatives of the paired first branchial arches.[12] The first arch also contributes to the development of the inner ear, while the external auditory canal, eustachian tube, middle ear cavity, and mastoid air cells are derivatives of the first branchial clefts and pouches. First branchial cleft anomalies course through the external auditory canal and, less commonly, through the middle ear.[12] First branchial cleft anomalies are found in close proximity to the parotid gland, with a potential for the superficial lobe of the parotid to overlie the anomaly and even course superiorly, inferiorly, or through the branches of the facial nerve.[2,12] The 2 classifications of first cleft anomalies describe their anatomic position: type I lesions are found lateral to the facial nerve, and type II lesions pass medial to the facial nerve (**Figs. 6** and **7**).[12] Type I lesions are duplications of the membranous external auditory canal, contain only ectoderm, and can have attachments to the skin of the external auditory canal or the tympanic membrane.[2] Type II cleft lesions may contain cartilage components and are made up of both ectoderm and mesoderm.[12] Type II first-cleft anomalies can be found as preauricular, infra-auricular, or postauricular swellings inferior to the angle of the mandible or anterior to the sternocleidomastoid muscle.[1,6,12]

First branchial cleft anomalies can be a challenge to the provider, because of their anatomic position and proximity to the facial nerve.[2] First-cleft lesions can present as cysts, sinuses, or fistulae located between the external auditory canal and the angle of the mandible.[2,12] The lesions may be asymptomatic, but patients may present with cervical, parotid, or auricular pain or discomfort.[6] Cervical symptoms may consist of drainage from a pitlike depression at the angle of the mandible, and if infected can become purulent.[12] Parotid symptoms result from a mass effect of the lesion, which becomes more prominent with rapidly increased size resulting from inflammation of the anomaly. Auricular symptoms include otorrhea with mucus or purulent discharge from the ear. Ten percent of first-cleft anomalies will have an asymptomatic membranous attachment from the floor of the external auditory canal to the tympanic membrane.[6,21]

The appropriate surgical treatment of first branchial arch anomalies will generally require careful avoidance of the facial nerve and parotid gland. The surgical resection should include complete removal of the lesion as well as excision of involved skin or

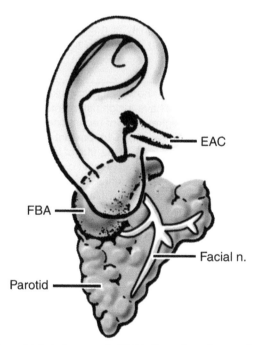

**Fig. 6.** Type I first branchial cleft anomaly (FBA). Note that the cyst is located within the parotid gland and does not connect to the external auditory canal (EAC). (*From* Mukherji SK, Fatterpekar G, Castillo M, et al. Imaging of congenital anomalies of the branchial apparatus. Neuroimaging Clin N Am 2000;10:75–93; with permission.)

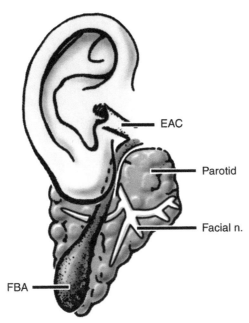

**Fig. 7.** Type II first branchial cleft anomaly. Note that the cyst (FBA) communicates with the external auditory canal (EAC) and extends into the deep lobe of the parotid gland. (*From* Mukherji SK, Fatterpekar G, Castillo M, et al. Imaging of congenital anomalies of the branchial apparatus. Neuroimaging Clin N Am 2000;10:75–93; with permission.)

cartilage components of the external auditory canal.[2,6] The lesion may have a tract that extends medial to the tympanic membrane, and the complete excision may necessitate transection of the tract with removal of the medial portion at a later, second procedure.[1] If the tract courses to the middle ear, it will typically lie deep to the facial nerve in contrast to a tract that enters the external auditory canal.[17] The position of the tracts can be variable, however, and a course that divides around the facial nerve can be observed.[21] The average number of procedures to completely excise first-cleft lesions is reported to be 2.4 per patient, as it is uncommon to successfully excise the entire lesion at the first procedure.[22] Repeated drainage procedures or failed attempts to remove the lesions carry an increased risk of injury to the facial nerve from scarring, which emphasizes the importance of a complete resection at the first attempt when possible.[12]

### Second-Cleft Anomalies

The most common type of branchial cleft malformations is second-cleft anomalies, accounting for 95% of all lesions. The second arch, or hyoid arch, forms the hyoid bone and adjacent areas of the neck. The second-pouch endodermal layer forms the epithelium of the palatine tonsil and the supratonsillar fossae.[2,14] Second-pouch anomalies can form a fistulous tract and connect the palatine tonsil to the lateral neck, at the anterior border of the sternocleidomastoid muscle.[2,14] A second-cleft anomaly enters the supratonsillar fossa and passes adjacent to the glossopharyngeal and hypoglossal nerves as the fistula courses to the fossa.[12] Second-arch anomalies are classified into 4 types as demonstrated in **Fig. 8**. Type I lesions lie anterior to the sternocleidomastoid muscle (SCM) and do not contact the carotid sheath. Type II

**A**   **C**

**B**   **D**

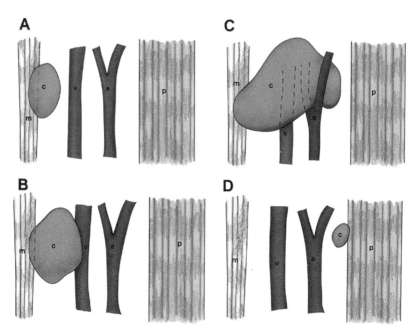

**Fig. 8.** Types I–IV second branchial cleft anomalies. (*A*) Type I: the cyst (c) is superficial to the anterior border of the sternocleidomastoid muscle (m). (*B*) Type II: the cyst is adjacent to the carotid sheath. (*C*) Type III: the cyst passes between the internal and external carotid arteries and extends to the lateral wall of the pharynx (p). (*D*) Type IV: the cyst is deep to the carotid sheath abutting the pharynx. a, artery; v, vein. (*From* Mukherji SK, Fatterpekar G, Castillo M, et al. Imaging of congenital anomalies of the branchial apparatus. Neuroimaging Clin N Am 2000;10:75–93; with permission.)

lesions are the most common and pass deep to the SCM, and pass either anterior or posterior to the carotid sheath. Type III lesions pass between the internal and external carotid arteries and are adjacent to the pharynx. Type IV lesions lie medial to the carotid sheath close to the pharynx, adjacent to the tonsillar fossa.

Second branchial cleft anomalies may present as cysts, sinuses, or fistulae in the lower anteriolateral neck. Most second-cleft cysts are diagnosed in the third to fifth decades, and present as a nontender, soft mass deep to the anterior border of the SCM.[1] Patients may present with acute increase in the size of cystic lesions and/or abscess formation, most likely during an upper respiratory tract infection.[1] Depending on the size, the acute transformation of the lesion may lead to respiratory compromise, torticollis, or dysphagia.[1,6] Fistulae are typically diagnosed in infancy or childhood, and manifest as chronic drainage from an opening along the anterior border of the SCM in the lower third of the neck.[12]

Resection of a second-cleft anomaly can be approached using a transverse cervical incision within a natural skin fold. A cyst may be found superficial or deep to the cervical fascia, so a local exploration should leave the surgeon confident there is no associated fistulous tract.[12] If a fistula is encountered, care must be taken to completely excise the tract to decrease the risk of recurrence.[12] Fistula excision may be aided with cannulation of the tract with a 2-0 or 3-0 monofilament suture or a lacrimal probe.[6] The tract may be injected with methylene blue; however, this can stain surrounding tissue and make the rest of the dissection more challenging.[12]

Once a fistulous tract is identified, the skin incision may need extension superiorly to completely expose the course of the tract. Alternatively, a step-ladder incision may be used to provide optimal visualization of the superior portion of the tract as it enters the pharynx.[1,6] The spinal accessory, hypoglossal, and vagus nerves must be protected from injury during the dissection.[6] Digital palpation or a bougie in the oropharynx may help identify the opening in the tonsillar fossa. The thin tract must be carefully ligated and divided at the proximal opening. A drain is not necessary if the fistulous tract is completely excised.[12]

### Third-Cleft and Fourth-Cleft Anomalies

Third and fourth branchial anomalies are rare, although their presentation is similar to second branchial anomalies.[6] The third branchial pouch divides superiorly to become the inferior parathyroid tissue and inferiorly to differentiate into thymic tissue.[2] Third and fourth pouches form the pharynx below the hyoid bone, and lesions usually arise from the pyriform sinus of the hypopharynx.[19] Third and fourth branchial anomalies contain thymic tissue as well as cysts and sinuses that result from thymic or parathyroid rests; however, only the branchial anomalies connect to the pyriform sinus. Third-arch lesions present as cystic structures located at the lower, anterior border of the SCM, and pass deep to the internal carotid artery and glossopharyngeal nerve, entering the thyrohyoid membrane above the superior laryngeal nerve and piercing the pyriform sinus (**Fig. 9**).[1] A third-arch cyst may present with hypoglossal nerve palsy if infected. The course of the fourth-arch anomalies depends on the side of the lesion (**Fig. 10**). Lesions on the right side of the body loop around the subclavian artery and pass deep to the internal carotid artery, ascend to the level of the hypoglossal nerve, and descend along the anterior border of the SCM to finally enter the pharynx at the pyriform apex or cervical esophagus. A fourth-arch lesion on the left tracts into the mediastinum, loops around the aortic arch medial to the ligamentum arteriosus, remaining superficial to the recurrent laryngeal nerve, and ascends in a similar course to the right side to enter the pharynx at the pyriform apex or cervical esophagus.[1,12] Third or fourth branchial lesions may present at any age, from in utero to adulthood.[6] Either lesion may present with tracheal compression or airway compromise in the neonate, owing to the rapid enlargement of the lesion with infection. Other presentations may include upper respiratory tract infections, neck or thyroid pain, or thyroid abscess.

As with second-arch anomalies, complete surgical excision of third- and fourth-arch anomalies is necessary to prevent recurrence. Fiberoptic endoscopy may be necessary to identify the entry point of third and fourth lesions to the pyriform sinus. Identification of the entry point allows for cannulation or injection of the tract to aid the dissection. There are reports of successful chemical cauterization of the tracts; however, there are no long-term results regarding this approach.[23] Fourth-arch anomalies require ipsilateral hemithyroidectomy for complete excision of the tract and may require partial resection of the thyroid cartilage to provide adequate exposure of the pyriform sinus.[24]

## DERMOID CYSTS AND TERATOMAS

Dermoid cysts are germ cell tumors that result from the inclusion of embryonic epithelial elements with embryonal median and paramedian fusion planes, and contain ectodermal and endodermal components.[1,2] Dermoids are lined with apparently normal epithelium on histology but also contain epithelial appendages such as hair, follicles, or sebaceous glands.[3] Dermoid cysts are commonly found on the face and head, but

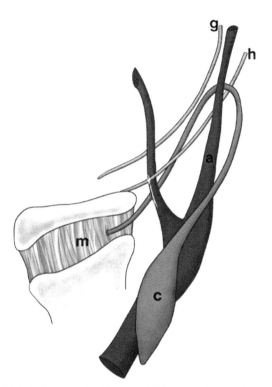

**Fig. 9.** Third branchial cleft anomaly. The cyst (c) is posterior to the sternocleidomastoid muscle (m), and the tract ascends posterior to the internal carotid artery (a). It then passes medially to pass between the hypoglossal (h) and glossopharyngeal (g) nerves. It pierces the thyroid membrane to enter the pyriform sinus. (*From* Mukherji SK, Fatterpekar G, Castillo M, et al. Imaging of congenital anomalies of the branchial apparatus. Neuroimaging Clin N Am 2000;10:75–93; with permission.)

also frequently present in the midline of the neck in the submental region, and although attached to overlying skin are painless unless infected.[2] Cervical dermoid cysts represent 20% of head and neck dermoids and are typically diagnosed before age 3 years.[1] Dermoid cysts in the neck can be close to the hyoid and move with swallowing or tongue protrusion, mimicking thyroglossal duct cysts. Dermoid cysts gradually increase in size over time as sebum accumulates. Infection is uncommon, but if present can cause the cyst to rupture and lead to granulomatous inflammation.

Once a careful history and physical examination has been completed, an ultrasonogram of the lesion may aid in the delineation of the depth and approximation to the hyoid bone to plan for resection. If inflamed, dermoid lesions may require an FNA to distinguish a ruptured dermoid cyst from a thyroglossal duct cyst. If the dermoid lesion is symptomatic, enlarging, or has ruptured, a complete excision if recommended. Simple excision is adequate to remove the entire lesion; however, if the lesion is attached to the hyoid, a Sistrunk procedure should be performed to prevent inadequate excision of an atypical thyroglossal duct cyst.[25] As with prior lesions discussed, the rate of recurrence increases with incomplete resection or intraoperative rupture.[3]

Teratomas differ from dermoid cysts in that they contain all 3 germ layers and very rarely occur as neck masses. Head and neck lesions comprise fewer than 2% of all teratomas, and the most common sites are the nasopharynx and neck. Teratomas develop during the

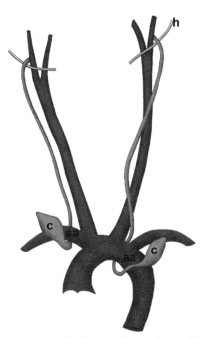

**Fig. 10.** Fourth branchial cleft anomaly. The cysts (c) are located anterior to the aortic arch (aa) on either side. The tract hooks either the subclavian artery (sa) or the aortic arch, depending on the side, and ascends to loop over the hypoglossal nerve (h). (*From* Mukherji SK, Fatterpekar G, Castillo M, et al. Imaging of congenital anomalies of the branchial apparatus. Neuroimaging Clin N Am 2000;10:75–93; with permission.)

second trimester and present as rapidly enlarging lateral or midline neck masses. Teratomas are often detected on prenatal ultrasonography, with 30% accompanied by polyhydramnios caused by esophageal obstruction.[1] If the diagnosis is made in utero a cesarean section is recommended, and an ex utero intrapartum treatment (EXIT) procedure may be required to achieve a secure airway before division of the maternal-fetal circulation.[1,2] The size of the teratoma may also lead to dysphagia and respiratory distress in the neonate. Mortality may be in excess of 80% for neonates with untreated cervical teratomas.[1] Imaging modalities such as ultrasonography, CT, or MRI may be helpful in evaluating teratomas. Neonates may require intubation, and even extracorporeal membrane oxygenation if the lesion had caused pulmonary hypoplasia. Complete surgical excision is necessary once the patient's airway has been stabilized. Malignancy has been reported in a few pediatric cases; however, all critical structures in the neck should be spared if possible.[1,26,27] Although malignant cervical teratomas in adults carry a poor prognosis despite aggressive treatment regimens, there are too few reported pediatric cases in the literature for conclusions to be drawn concerning the prognosis in infants.

## MIDLINE CERVICAL CLEFTS

Midline cervical clefts are rare congenital cervical anomalies, which are present at birth as a cutaneous ulceration with overhanging skin or cartilaginous tag in the anterior lower midline of the neck (**Fig. 11**). A sinus tract, or band, may extend downward from the skin and can connect to the sternum or mandible, or may end in a blind pouch. The

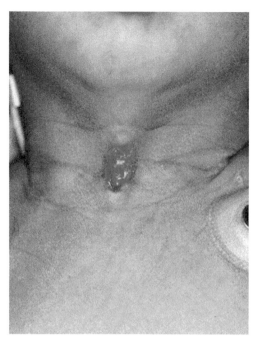

**Fig. 11.** Congenital midline cervical cleft. (*From* Foley DS, Fallat ME. Thyroglossal duct and other congenital midline cervical anomalies. Semin Pediatr Surg 2006;15(2):70–5; with permission.)

embryologic origin is unknown but is thought to be a "mesodermal fusion abnormality involving the paired branchial arches during gestational weeks 3 and 4."[3] Fibrous tissue with interwoven skeletal muscle is present. Most cases are sporadic, but can be associated with other cleft abnormalities of the tongue, lower lip, or mandible. Most are asymptomatic, but if untreated can result in neck contractures or growth deformities of the mandible or sternum.[2] Therefore, early surgical excision at the time of diagnosis is recommended, with complete excision of both the skin lesion and the subcutaneous sinus to reduce the rate of recurrence. This excision can usually be accomplished via stair-step incisions, but may require a series of Z-plasty incisions to improve the cosmetic and functional result.[3]

## REFERENCES

1. Enepekides DJ. Management of congenital anomalies of the neck. Facial Plast Surg Clin North Am 2001;9(1):131–45.
2. Flint PW, Cummings CW. Cummings otolaryngology head & neck surgery. 5th edition. Philadelphia: Mosby/Elsevier; 2010. Available at: http://www.mdconsult.com/public/book/view?title=Flint:+Cummings+Otolaryngology. Accessed March 3, 2012.
3. Foley DS, Fallat ME. Thyroglossal duct and other congenital midline cervical anomalies. Semin Pediatr Surg 2006;15(2):70–5.
4. Langman J, Sadler TW. Langman's medical embryology. 7th edition. Baltimore (MD): Williams & Wilkins; 1995.
5. Mohan PS, Chokshi RA, Moser RL, et al. Thyroglossal duct cysts: a consideration in adults. Am Surg 2005;71(6):508–11.

6. Acierno SP, Waldhausen JH. Congenital cervical cysts, sinuses and fistulae. Otolaryngol Clin North Am 2007;40(1):161–76, vii–viii.

7. Pinczower E, Crockett DM, Atkinson JB, et al. Preoperative thyroid scanning in presumed thyroglossal duct cysts. Arch Otolaryngol Head Neck Surg 1992; 118(9):985–8.

8. Pérez-Martínez A, Bento-Bravo L, Martínez-Bermejo MA, et al. An intra-thyroid thyroglossal duct cyst. Eur J Pediatr Surg 2005;15(6):428–30.

9. El Bakkouri W, Racy E, Vereecke A, et al. Squamous cell carcinoma in a thyroglossal duct cyst. Ann Otolaryngol Chir Cervicofac 2004;121(5):303–5 [in French].

10. Peretz A, Leiberman E, Kapelushnik J, et al. Thyroglossal duct carcinoma in children: case presentation and review of the literature. Thyroid 2004;14(9):777–85.

11. Ostlie DJ, Burjonrappa SC, Snyder CL, et al. Thyroglossal duct infections and surgical outcomes. J Pediatr Surg 2004;39(3):396–9 [discussion: 396–9].

12. Waldhausen JH. Branchial cleft and arch anomalies in children. Semin Pediatr Surg 2006;15(2):64–9.

13. Thomaidis V, Seretis K, Tamiolakis D, et al. Branchial cysts. A report of 4 cases. Acta Dermatovenerol Alp Panonica Adriat 2006;15(2):85–9.

14. Cochard LR, Netter FH. Netter's atlas of human embryology. 1st edition. Teterboro (NJ): Icon Learning Systems; 2002.

15. Roback SA, Telander RL. Thyroglossal duct cysts and branchial cleft anomalies. Semin Pediatr Surg 1994;3(3):142–6.

16. Arnot RS. Defects of the first branchial cleft. S Afr J Surg 1971;9(2):93–8.

17. D'Souza AR, Uppal HS, De R, et al. Updating concepts of first branchial cleft defects: a literature review. Int J Pediatr Otorhinolaryngol 2002;62(2):103–9.

18. Shrime M, Kacker A, Bent J, et al. Fourth branchial complex anomalies: a case series. Int J Pediatr Otorhinolaryngol 2003;67(11):1227–33.

19. Thomas B, Shroff M, Forte V, et al. Revisiting imaging features and the embryologic basis of third and fourth branchial anomalies. AJNR Am J Neuroradiol 2010;31(4):755–60.

20. O'Mara W, Amedee RG. Anomalies of the branchial apparatus. J La State Med Soc 1998;150(12):570–3.

21. Triglia JM, Nicollas R, Ducroz V, et al. First branchial cleft anomalies: a study of 39 cases and a review of the literature. Arch Otolaryngol Head Neck Surg 1998; 124(3):291–5.

22. Ford GR, Balakrishnan A, Evans JN, et al. Branchial cleft and pouch anomalies. J Laryngol Otol 1992;106(2):137–43.

23. Park SW, Han MH, Sung MH, et al. Neck infection associated with pyriform sinus fistula: imaging findings. AJNR Am J Neuroradiol 2000;21(5):817–22.

24. Nicollas R, Ducroz V, Garabédian EN, et al. Fourth branchial pouch anomalies: a study of six cases and review of the literature. Int J Pediatr Otorhinolaryngol 1998;44(1):5–10.

25. Türkyilmaz Z, Sönmez K, Karabulut R, et al. Management of thyroglossal duct cysts in children. Pediatr Int 2004;46(1):77–80.

26. Fichera S, Hackett H, Secola R. Perinatal germ cell tumors: a case report of a cervical teratoma. Adv Neonatal Care 2010;10(3):133–9.

27. Muscatello L, Giudice M, Feltri M. Malignant cervical teratoma: report of a case in a newborn. Eur Arch Otorhinolaryngol 2005;262(11):899–904.

# Teratomas and Ovarian Lesions in Children

Anne-Marie E. Amies Oelschlager, MD[a], Robert Sawin, MD[b],*

## KEYWORDS

- Teratoma • Ovarian lesions • Sacrococcygeal tumors • Germ cell tumors
- Ovarian cysts and tumors

## KEY POINTS

- The most common germ cell tumors are classified as teratomas and contain elements of at least 2 of the germ layers: endoderm, mesoderm, or ectoderm.
- The most common locations for teratomas vary by age; in most children's hospitals teratomas in the sacrococcygeal region are most common, followed by ovarian.
- Many of these sacrococcygeal tumors are detected by prenatal ultrasound,[1] and these fetuses should be evaluated at a high-risk perinatal center because some of these children will develop fetal hydrops, thought to be related to the large volume of excess blood flow to the tumor.
- Retroperitoneal teratomas are typically large and therefore often present as palpable masses in infancy or early childhood.
- Mediastinal teratomas may present at much later stages with chest pain or respiratory symptoms that prompt a chest x-ray.
- Cervical teratomas are uncommon neonatal lesions but are often very morbid.
- Small ovarian physiologic cysts are very common in neonatal, prepubertal, and adolescent girls and may be clinically challenging to distinguish from ovarian tumors.
- Surgical management of germ cell tumors of the ovary includes complete excision of the tumor, utmost care to preserve fertility, and appropriate staging if malignant.

Ovarian pathology in children is common and the pathology can be quite diverse. The most common benign ovarian tumor in childhood is a teratoma. In this article, we discuss the origin of these germ cell tumors followed by a complete discussion of ovarian pathology.

[a] Department of Obstetrics and Gynecology, University of Washington School of Medicine, Seattle Children's Hospital, W-7831-Adolescent Medicine, 4800 Sand Point Way Northeast, Seattle, WA 98105, USA; [b] University of Washington School of Medicine, Seattle Children's Hospital, 4800 Sand Point Way Northeast, PO Box 5371/W-7729, Seattle, WA 98145-5005, USA
* Corresponding author.
*E-mail address:* robert.sawin@seattlechildrens.org

Surg Clin N Am 92 (2012) 599–613
doi:10.1016/j.suc.2012.03.005
0039-6109/12/$ – see front matter © 2012 Elsevier Inc. All rights reserved.

## TUMORS AND MASSES OF GERM CELL ORIGIN

The term "germ cell tumor" is fairly broad and includes several different histologic types (**Fig. 1**). The origin of the term refers to the shared embryologic origin of the tumor cells from germ cells. The primordial germ cells in the developing embryo migrate from the yolk sac along the midline and paraxial regions of the embryo to the genital ridge. The development of the male or female genitals from the genital ridge depends on the presence of the SRY gene, located on the Y chromosome. In the absence of the SRY gene, an ovary will usually develop. This migration pattern along the midline explains why germ cell tumors in children occur most commonly in midline locations, or in the gonads. The totipotential cells can give rise to malignant tumors, such as embryonal carcinoma, choriocarcinoma, and endodermal sinus tumors (also known as yolk sac tumors). In children, the most common germ cell tumors are classified as teratomas and contain elements of at least 2 of the germ layers: endoderm, mesoderm, or ectoderm.

## TERATOMAS

Although most teratomas are benign (>80%), some teratomas contain immature or malignant elements, with the incidence of malignancy varying by location and age. Mature teratomas, also termed dermoid cysts, frequently contain hair, teeth, and sebum, especially in the ovaries. The most common locations for teratomas vary by age; in most children's hospitals, teratomas in the sacrococcygeal region are most common, followed by ovarian.[2] In large general hospital practice, ovarian teratomas are typically more common. The ovarian teratomas can have monodermal cell lines that result in a functional tumor, such as struma ovarii (dermoids containing thyroid tissue) and carcinoid, which resemble gastrointestinal carcinoid tumors histologically. Other common teratoma positions are midline, such as mediastinum, cervical, retroperitoneal, central nervous system (especially the pineal gland). Presenting symptoms depend on the age and location of the tumors. Regardless of location or age of the patient, a basic premise is that teratomas must be completely surgically resected if at all possible, regardless of the histology.

## SACROCOCCYGEAL TERATOMAS

Sacrococcygeal teratomas (SCTs) are typically large tumors (**Fig. 2**) and are most often obvious at birth, as more than 90% are external to the sacrum. Fewer than

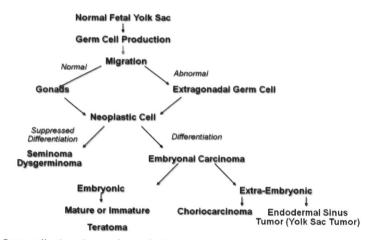

Fig. 1. Germ cell migration and neoplasia.

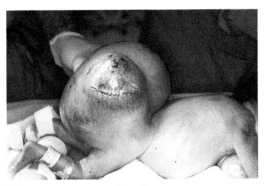

**Fig. 2.** Newborn with large sacrococcygeal teratoma.

10% of affected children have SCTs that are entirely presacral.[3] Many of these SCT tumors are detected by prenatal ultrasound,[1] and these fetuses should be evaluated at a high-risk perinatal center because some of these children will develop fetal hydrops, thought to be related to the large volume of excess blood flow to the tumor. Fetal intervention has been described for unusual cases of severe hydrops early in pregnancy. Delivery of infants with large SCTs must also be done with care, as life-threatening hemorrhage can occur if the tumor is traumatized. Complete resection of the tumor and the coccyx, most often via a posterior sacral incision, is essential to prevent recurrence. For those children who have both presacral and external tumors, a combined abdominal and posterior sacral resection is sometimes necessary. Approximately 5% of resected specimens from neonates will contain malignant elements. If complete resection has been accomplished, no adjuvant chemotherapy is necessary. Regular follow-up with physical examinations, including digital rectal examination and the serum markers alpha fetoprotein (AFP) and beta human chorionic gonadotropin (β-hCG), is necessary to monitor for recurrence. Fortunately, excellent disease-free salvage can be obtained with chemotherapy, even if the malignant tumor recurs. SCTs are also discussed under pediatric malignancies.

## OTHER NONGONADAL TERATOMA LOCATIONS

Other midline locations present at varying ages, depending on the size and the impact on surrounding organs. Retroperitoneal teratomas are typically large and therefore often present as palpable masses in infancy or early childhood. Mediastinal teratomas may present at much later stages with chest pain or respiratory symptoms that prompt a chest x-ray. Cervical teratomas are uncommon neonatal lesions but are often very morbid.[4] The larger cervical lesions can obstruct the oropharynx and result in polyhydramnios, pulmonary hypoplasia, and complete upper airway obstruction (**Fig. 3**). Thus, referral to a high-risk perinatal center is imperative so that control of the airway at the time of delivery can be optimized. Just as with SCT tumors, complete resection is the goal for all of these lesions because of the usual benign histology that makes chemotherapy ineffective.

## OVARIAN MASSES

Although teratomas are a common tumor involving the ovaries of children and young women, many other tumor types can be found in the ovaries. An understanding of the

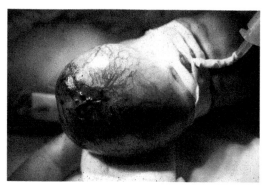

**Fig. 3.** Large cervical teratoma. Note endotracheal tube securing the airway.

ovarian development and function helps explain the differential diagnosis of these ovarian masses and their management.

## FETAL OVARIAN DEVELOPMENT

The ovary is composed of the central medulla, which contains connective tissue, blood, lymph vessels, nerves, and interstitial tissue. The cortex, or covering, contains ova, follicles, corpora lutea, corpora albicantia, and stromal cells. The cortex is covered by the tunica albuginea, which is a connective tissue layer overlaid with germinal epithelium. The fallopian tubes have fimbriae, which lie on top of the ovaries, and guide ova into the oviducts and propel them toward the uterus.

## OVARIAN PHYSIOLOGY

Because of maternal hormonal production of estradiol, placental production of chorionic gonadotropin, and fetal gonadotropins, physiologic ovarian cysts are extremely common in utero, occurring in up to 36% of fetuses at 34 to 37 weeks and 71% at 38 weeks by autopsy study of female stillborns.[5] Shortly after birth, following the withdrawal of maternal estrogen and decline of chorionic gonadotropin, gonadotropin-releasing hormone (GnRH) is secreted and there is a "mini-puberty," which occurs where the pituitary and ovary are stimulated. This GnRH activity decreases around 8 months of age and pubertal hormone production becomes quiescent until the onset of puberty. Although the ovary will decrease in size as it enters quiescence, small ovarian cysts, smaller than 9 mm, are still very common, and are seen in up to 80% of females.[6] As GnRH suppression wanes and puberty progresses, the ovaries will enlarge.[7,8] Although half of all cycles are anovulatory during the first 2 years after menarche, the hypothalamic-pituitary-ovarian axis begins to mature, resulting in 2 distinct phases: the follicular phase and the luteal phase.

### Follicular Phase

During folliculogenesis, granulosa cells begin to make estrogen and progesterone and theca cells begin to produce androgens, such as androsteinedione and testosterone. The rise in estrogen induces the pituitary to release luteinizing hormone (LH). The follicular cells produce inhibin. Most follicles that start to develop fail to ovulate and become spontaneously atretic; however, for the oocyte that does mature, the LH surge will thin the wall of the ovary resulting in rupture of the follicular cyst and ovulation with release of the oocyte, usually within 34 to 38 hours after the LH surge.

Typically, rupture of the ovarian cyst or ovulation occurs when the cyst is 2 to 3 cm in diameter; however, these cysts may be as large as 10 cm. Most will begin to spontaneously regress within 2 weeks.

### Luteal Phase

After ovulation, the granulosa cells of the follicle reorganize and produce progesterone from the stimulation by LH. The luteal phase typically lasts 13 days. Theca lutein cysts can persist in the presence of hCG, typically in response to pregnancy, but also in response to molar pregnancies or with choriocarcinoma. In the absence of pregnancy, the corpus luteum degenerates and resorbs. Corpus luteum cysts may become enlarged if internal hemorrhage into the cyst occurs, aptly named a hemorrhagic cyst. As this process repeats itself each cycle, it is not surprising that functional ovarian cysts are very common. Differentiating between functional ovarian cysts and tumors in the fetal, neonatal, prepubertal, and postpubertal child and adolescent can be clinically challenging.

## DIFFERENTIAL DIAGNOSIS OF OVARIAN CYSTS IN CHILDREN AND ADOLESCENTS

Although germ cell tumors are much more common causes of cystic and solid ovarian masses in children and adolescents, epithelial ovarian tumors, which are more common in older women, remain on the differential for younger patients. Epithelial tumors are categorized into benign, borderline, and malignant and derive of 5 different cell types: serous, mucinous, endometrioid, clear cell, and Brenner. Papillary excrescences are the hallmark of a borderline or malignant serous or mucinous cyst adenocarcinoma. Careful inspection of the peritoneal cavity is critical if there is suspicion for borderline or frank carcinoma.

Sex cord cell tumors are derived from granulosa, thecal, and Sertoli-Leydig cells. Gonadoblastoma is more commonly expected in the presence of Y chromatin. This can be identified in an evaluation for disorders of sex development, typically in girls with ambiguous genitalia, overvirilization, or with primary amenorrhea. Granulosa cell tumors produce estradiol, and therefore are associated with precocious puberty.[9]

Endometriosis, which is common in adolescents with dysmenorrhea and pelvic pain, rarely presents before puberty and infrequently results in endometriomas, also known as chocolate cysts, because of the fluid resembling chocolate syrup, in adolescence. Pedunculated myomas may present as an adnexal mass, but these are uncommon in adolescents compared with older women. Paraovarian and paratubal cysts are considered Wolffian duct remnants, and are located adjacent to the ovary in the fallopian tube or broad ligament. Finally, obstructed uterine horns found with Müllerian anomalies, may also be seen as an adnexal mass. Frequently obstructed Mullerian anomalies typically present at the time of menarche. Ectopic pregnancy, which can be fatal if not diagnosed and treated appropriately, can also cause adnexal mass and pain. Tubo-ovarian abscess, pyosalpinx, or hydrosalpinx, complications of pelvic inflammatory disease, may result in an adnexal mass, especially in the sexually active patient.

## APPROACH TO THE PATIENT
### History

#### Questions about the pregnancy
In newborn infants, the mother should be asked about a history of hypothyroidism or gestational diabetes, as these maternal conditions have been associated with fetal ovarian cysts.

### Questions about ovarian hormone production

In prepubertal children, the parent should be asked about evidence of breast development, menstrual bleeding, or recent increase in height, which can indicate estrogen excess and precocious puberty. Conversely, there should be questions about pubertal delay or amenorrhea, which can indicate gonadal dysgenesis or androgen insensitivity. In the postmenarchal patient, a careful menstrual history should be elicited to determine the age of menarche, last menstrual cycle, and if there has been a change in the menstrual pattern.

### Questions about pain

There should be careful questioning about the quality and duration of pain. Symptoms of acute onset of pain or intermittent severe pain, especially associated with vomiting, raises concern for adnexal torsion. Studies assessing symptomatology with torsion demonstrate that two-thirds of patients will have nausea and vomiting, and 75% will have right-sided pain.[10]

### Questions about sexual activity

Privately, the patient should be asked about sexual activity, contraception, and whether she has had ever been diagnosed with a sexually transmitted infection or if she has been using condoms. Often adolescents will not discuss this in the presence of a family member and therefore every effort should be made to ensure patient confidentiality and privacy with this discussion.

### Physical Examination

In the absence of pain, larger ovarian cysts may be detected by physical examination. Physical examination is useful for determining the likelihood of malignancy. Malignant tumors are more likely to be bilateral, solid, fixed, irregular, and associated with ascites than benign tumors. In prepubertal patients, vaginal examination may be limited because of the small hymenal ring. Digital and speculum vaginal examination without anesthesia should be avoided. These patients, including young adolescent patients, tolerate rectal examination much more easily. Rectal examination can assess the tumor, which often lies behind the uterus, and cul de sac nodularity, which raises the suspicion for malignancy. In sexually active and older adolescents, speculum examination can be performed to assess for signs of infection, including cervical mucopus. Bimanual examination can reveal cervical motion tenderness in the presence of peritoneal inflammation, as well as permit adnexal evaluation. Signs of an acute abdomen, including guarding, rigidity, and extreme tenderness may indicate ovarian torsion, rupture of a hemorrhagic cyst, ruptured teratoma, tubo-ovarian abscess, or ectopic pregnancy.

Assessment of systemic estrogen is performed by clinical examination of the developing breast tissue and color of the vulvar skin and vaginal mucosa, which correlates with estrogen production by the ovaries. Presence of thelarche occurring precociously, before the age of 8 in girls, can be a sign of ovarian estrogen production, either from central stimulation from gonadotropins, or from an ovarian cyst or tumor independently producing estrogen. Clitoromegaly can indicate excess testosterone production. Growth charts can be used to indicate whether there has been a recent growth spurt indicating puberty.

### Imaging

Ultrasound is the imaging modality of choice to assess the ovarian volume and presence of an ovarian cyst. Ultrasound can assess if the mass is smooth walled, unilocular or multilocular, unilateral or bilateral, and assess whether it contains solid components. Indicators of malignancy include solid components larger than 2 cm, thick septations, and papillary projections. Typically in prepubertal and adolescent patients, transabdominal ultrasound is recommended over transvaginal ultrasound, owing to patient discomfort with the vaginal ultrasound probe.

When there is suspicion for torsion, Doppler assessment of the vessels may be additive to determining the presence or absence of flow.[11] The positive predictive factor for absent venous flow for ovarian torsion is 94%. The presence of venous and arterial flow does not rule out torsion, however, and up to 60% of patients with ovarian torsion will have normal flow by Doppler evaluation.[12,13] Torsion with normal flow may occur because the torsion is intermittent, the utero-ovarian or infindibulopelvic ligament is providing collateral flow, or if the torsion only involves the paratubal cyst or the isolated fallopian tube. The absence of flow may reflect an ovary that has already undergone necrosis and cannot be salvaged but may also be found with a normal, healthy ovary. Although ultrasound and Doppler are useful for evaluation of torsion, torsion is a clinical diagnosis and the only way to definitively diagnose torsion is in the the operating room.[14]

Almost all ovaries are enlarged with torsion. Servaes and colleagues[14] described the utility of ovarian volumes for prediction of torsion and whether there is an associated tumor. In their study, the median volume of the torsed ovary was 12 times that of the normal contralateral side. Using volume ratio, in which the larger ovarian volume is divided by the contralateral ovarian volume, they found that in 70% of torsed ovaries with a volume ratio greater than 20, an ovarian mass was present. In 90% of those ovaries with a volume ratio less than 20, an internal mass was absent. Other ultrasound findings that are consistent with torsion include fluid debris in follicular cyst, which has a sensitivity of 85%, a complex mass with septations and debris, or a solid mass with peripheral cysts 8 to 15 mm in size.[15] Children and adolescents who present with lower quadrant pain or back pain may undergo alternate imaging modalities, such as magnetic resonance imaging (MRI), x-ray, or abdominal or pelvic computed tomography (CT), which may identify an ovarian mass. CT and MRI findings can be useful for evaluation of adnexal masses and torsion. CT findings in patients who were subsequently diagnosed operatively as having torsion, include abnormal fallopian tube thickening (74%), ovarian wall thickening (54%), decreased contrast enhancement of the internal solid component (50%), uterine deviation to the twisted side (61%), nonvisualized continuity of the ipsilateral gonadal vein (71%), and ascites (13%).[16,17] Ovarian teratomas may be suspected when a roentengenologic examination demonstrates a calcification. MRI has been explored as a diagnostic option for unusual or rare situations where ultrasound diagnosis is unclear, including in utero.[18] Because of concern about cost and radiation, typically ultrasound remains the first radiologic test to assess for adnexal mass.

### Laboratory Testing

The most important laboratory test that should be performed in any patient with acute pelvic pain is a urine hCG to rule out pregnancy. In addition, testing for sexually transmitted infection is especially important in a sexually active adolescent who may have pelvic inflammatory disease, hydrosalpinx, or a tubo-ovarian abscess.

Tumor markers may not be elevated with early-staged ovarian neoplasms. Tumor markers can be helpful in ovarian tumors where suspicion for malignancy is elevated, to facilitate preoperative planning for a staging procedure, and to follow for evidence of recurrence postoperatively. Germ cell tumors, such as dysgerminoma, choriocarcinoma, embryonal, immature teratoma, and mixed germ cell tumors, may have elevated levels of β-hCG, AFP, and lactase dehydrogenase (LDH). Granulosa cell tumors are associated with elevated estradiol and inhibin levels. Thecomas are associated with elevated estradiol and testosterone levels. Sertoli-Leydig cell tumors are associated with elevated testosterone and inhibin levels. CA 125 levels can be elevated with epithelial carcinoma and immature teratomas; however, caution should be used with this tumor marker, as it can be elevated with a variety of benign reasons in postpubertal patients, including endometriosis, torsion, and menses.[19,20]

## MANAGEMENT STRATEGIES

For all ages, there are several criteria that can be used as to whether a patient can qualify for observation. Given that many ovarian cysts are physiologic in nature and will spontaneously resolve, initial surgery should be reserved for patients with signs and symptoms concerning for torsion or tumor. For other patients, close observation is reasonable.

### Newborn

Even with complex masses, asymptomatic neonatal cysts can be observed and followed with serial ultrasounds. Luzzatto and colleagues,[21] in a study of 19 patients with neonatal ovarian cysts who were observed with serial ultrasounds, reported that all simple ovarian cysts resolved without intervention, on average by 3.5 months postnatal, and that 10 of 13 complex masses also spontaneously resolved, although resolution required longer, on average 8 months. Up to 16 months has been reported for complete resolution of a complex neonatal cyst.[22] Although most simple cysts are physiologic in nature in the neonatal period owing to the maternal hormones of hCG and estradiol, benign ovarian tumors, such as serous cystadenoma and ovarian lymphangiomas, have been reported in the newborn.[23] There have been no reported malignancies in newborns in multiple case series. Although most term fetuses will have ovarian cysts, and although in utero torsion is rare, it has been associated with autoamputation of the ovary, colonic stricture, and even sudden death.[24,25] Therefore, careful review of the symptoms of ovarian torsion should be reviewed with the family so that if the symptoms occur, prompt recognition and intervention can occur. If the newborn is asymptomatic; there is no solid component; there is a normal AFP, LDH, and β-hCG; and the cyst is clearly from the ovary and shrinking, then observation is appropriate with serial ultrasounds every 1 to 3 months. Another option is percutaneous drainage of the cyst. If signs or symptoms of torsion occur, if the cyst recurs or is not resolving, or if there is a diagnostic dilemma, surgical treatment may be appropriate.[26,27]

### Prepubertal

Ovarian volume will increase slowly as GnRH suppression wanes; 2-mm-diameter to 15-mm-diameter cysts are common.[8] If they are simple, reassurance is appropriate and no further ultrasound evaluation is warranted. If the cyst is larger than 2 cm, then an examination to evaluate for precocious puberty is warranted and typically a follow-up ultrasound in 4 to 6 weeks will show resolution. If there are concerning signs for a hormonally active tumor and McCune Albright is not suspected as an etiology for precious puberty, then surgical evaluation for excision of the cyst is warranted.[26]

### Adolescent

Most adolescents who present without concerning signs for torsion or malignancy will have physiologic cysts, either follicular or hemorrhagic, which will regress spontaneously without intervention. If the patient has signs or symptoms of torsion or hemodynamic compromise from rupture of a hemorrhagic cyst, then laparoscopy may be indicated. However, the vast majority of patients with follicular or hemorrhagic cysts will have mild pain and can be observed with ultrasound. Follow-up ultrasound in 6 to 12 weeks will demonstrate that the mass is decreasing in size. If the mass is persisting or if signs of worsening pain or concern for torsion arise, then surgical intervention is recommended. If the mass contains solid elements larger than 2 cm, thick septations, or papillary projections, or if there is significant associated ascites, which raises suspicion for malignancy, then surgical excision of the cyst is recommended.

## OPERATIVE INTERVENTION

In children and adolescents, there are 4 major goals to any surgical treatment of the ovaries and adnexa: (1) remove neoplastic tissue, (2) alleviate pain, (3) appropriately stage in the presence of malignancy, and (4) preserve fertility. As these patients have not completed childbearing and for many patients, most of the pathology will be benign in nature, the utmost care and caution should be used to minimize the impact on ovarian hormonal production and future fertility.

### Laparoscopy Versus Laparotomy

The most important surgical consideration is finding the appropriate plane between the cyst and the ovarian cortex to ensure complete excision (**Fig. 4**A). Laparotomy, even through a Pfannensteil incision, is associated with increased pain, longer recovery, higher incidence of infection and bleeding, and a higher rate of adhesive disease, which may affect fertility. Laparoscopy is associated with shorter hospitalization, reduced recovery time, and is more cost-effective despite increased equipment cost and increased operating time.[28–30] The benefit of laparotomy for management of an ovarian cyst is that there is a lower likelihood of rupture of the ovarian cyst during the operation. Although rupture of a benign neoplasm laparoscopically is associated with few complications, the rupture of a malignant ovarian tumor may result in upstaging the tumor; however, cyst rupture has not been associated with increased mortality with early-stage ovarian cancer.[31] There have been concerns raised about spillage of ovarian cyst contents with laparoscopy with teratomas; however, copious irrigation after spillage of the peritoneal cavity has not resulted in peritonitis.[32,33] There is a greater likelihood that with open ovarian cystectomy that an ovarian neoplasm will be more likely to be completely resected. Laberge and Levesque[34] reported an estimated recurrence rate of ovarian teratoma up to 7.6% at 2 years for laparoscopic ovarian cystectomy versus 0% estimated recurrence for laparotomy; however, a Cochrane review of

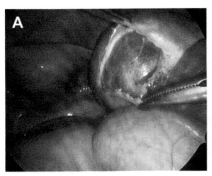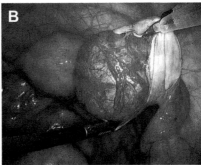

**Fig. 4.** (*A*) Laparoscopically opening the ovarian cortex and finding the plane between the ovary and the germ cell tumor. (*B*) Avoiding the fallopian tube and ovarian vessels whilst removing the teratoma intact.

randomized trials comparing laparoscopic to open ovarian cystectomy did not demonstrate any increase in recurrence of any type of benign ovarian cysts, including teratomas.[35] Although the pelvic and para-aortic lymph nodes may be palpated through a laparotomy for staging purposes, laparoscopy confers a benefit in that it allows excellent visualization of the hemidiaphragms, contralateral ovary, omentum, and liver edge. Most patients will be able to be discharged the day of surgery or postoperative day 1 after laparoscopic cystectomy or oophorectomy. Cosmesis may be especially important to adolescents and laparoscopic cystectomy is associated with significantly more satisfaction with the appearance of scars than laparotomy.

### Oophorectomy Versus Ovarian Cystectomy

Although the risk of benign neoplasm recurrence is smaller with oophorectomy versus ovarian cystectomy, removing an ovary for benign indications does potentially increase the risk of early decline in ovarian function and premature menopause. Although the contralateral ovary will compensate and provide ovarian production to promote normal puberty and menstrual cycles in adolescence, small studies indicate that after unilateral oophorectomy that women between ages 35 and 39 have a significantly increased follicle-stimulating hormone level and risk for early menopause.[36,37] Even preserving a seemingly small portion of the ovary and tube may potentially increase hormonal function for the patient, as histologic examination of the ovarian cortex maximally stretched by the tumor has demonstrated normal ovarian tissue.[38] Although oophorectomy is associated with a significant decrease in anti-Müllerian hormone levels, a measure of ovarian reserve, ovarian cystectomy, albeit less significantly, is also associated with a decrease in serum anti-Müllerian hormone levels.[39] Utmost care should be taken, especially when performing ovarian cystectomy, to preserve the ovarian vasculature and to avoid inadvertently damaging the fimbriae of the fallopian tube (**Fig. 4**B).

Intraoperatively, if torsion is encountered, then detorsion is warranted to resume blood flow to the ovary. Although spontaneous torsion of normal ovaries can occur, most often there is a cyst or tumor that has caused the torsion. Typically, time to diagnosis is the most critical factor in whether an ovary that has undergone torsion can be salvaged. Most patients presenting within 24 hours of onset of pain successfully retain their ovaries.[10] In response to the finding of multiple oophorectomy specimens with viable oocytes histologically where intraoperatively the ovaries appeared black blue in color, however, Galinier and colleagues followed 9 patients with ovarian torsion where the ovaries appeared nonviable intraoperatively and underwent simple detorsion. Of the 9, 1 patient was lost to follow-up, 2 ovaries were viable at a second look but oophorectomy was performed for neoplasm, and 5 ovaries were demonstrated to be follicular by follow-up ultrasound.[40] Oelsner and colleagues reported that of 92 patients with ovarian torsion and ischemic or necrotic adnexa, that sonographic function was demonstrated in 85 of the 92 by 3 months. Five (71%) of the 7 without demonstrated sonographic ovarian function had cystectomy at the time of detorsion. Of the 31 who had detorsion and immediate cystectomy, 16% of patients had ovarian dysfunction versus 7% of the overall cohort.[29,41] Therefore, performing an immediate ovarian cystectomy at the time of torsion may compromise ovarian function more than observation with interval cystectomy for persistent ovarian cysts. Current research supports considering immediate laparoscopic detorsion and cyst aspiration or fenestration in the situation of acute torsion with a physiologic cyst, with follow-up ultrasound to evaluate for persistence of a cyst, even if the ovary appears black blue. If the cyst persists despite observation, then a cystectomy can be performed later when the ovarian tissue is less ischemic and where clearer planes between the cyst and the ovarian cortex can be identified. Although there has been concern about this algorithm in the possible delay in diagnosis and management of an ovarian malignancy, malignant tumors are less likely to undergo torsion than benign tumors.[42,43] In a meta-analysis of ovarian torsion, only 9 (1.5%) of 593 patients who underwent surgery for ovarian torsion were found to have a malignancy. The most common neoplasms with torsion are mature teratoma (24%), serous cystadenoma (8%), and fibroma (0.3%).[36,37] Concern about embolic phenomena occurring with unwinding has been unfounded and indeed no cases have been noted for pediatric and adolescent patients.[42]

### Recurrent Torsion and Oophoropexy

Although the exact risk of recurrent ipsilateral torsion is unknown, there is an estimated 5% risk of recurrent torsion if cystectomy is not performed at initial unwinding. If there is no underlying pathology, approximately 11% of patients may have spontaneous recurrence of torsion, potentially on the contralateral side. If an oophorectomy is performed for the first episode of torsion, there is a risk of castration after second torsion on the contralateral side.[41,44–46] This has led several surgeons to advocate for oophoropexy to prevent recurrent torsion. Although oophoropexy does prevent recurrence of torsion and decreases the risk of castration with subsequent torsion, it can alter the adnexal blood supply and distort tubal anatomy, which may decrease ovarian function and fertility.[44,47–49] Oophoropexy techniques include shortening of the utero-ovarian ligament; fixation of the ovary to the pelvic sidewall, uterus, or uterosacral ligaments; or utero-ovarian ligament plication to the round ligament. Typically, permanent suture, such as prolene, is used for this procedure. Currently oophoropexy is recommended in patients with recurrent torsion of a normal ovary, previous oophorectomy for torsion without mass, or a grossly abnormal attachment.

### Staging of Malignancy

Operative staging of ovarian malignancies in children and adolescents differs from ovarian carcinoma staging in adults because preservation of fertility is critical and because often germ cell malignancies, which predominate in this age, are more chemosensitive than epithelial ovarian adenocarcinomas. The staging of pediatric ovarian germ cell and sex cord tumors follows the recommendations from Billmire (**Table 1**).[50] The Children's Oncology Group has recommended the following for complete surgical

**Table 1**
**Children's Oncology Group staging of ovarian germ cell tumors in children and adolescents**

| Stage | Extent of Disease | Peritoneal Washings | Lymph Node Involvement | Tumor Markers |
|-------|-------------------|---------------------|------------------------|---------------|
| I | Limited to ovaries | Negative | Negative | Normal after appropriate half-life |
| II | | Negative | Microscopic positive | Positive or negative |
| III | Contiguous viscera involved (omentum, intestine, bladder) | Positive | Greater than 2 cm, gross residual or biopsy only | Positive or negative |
| IV | Distant metastases, including liver | | | |

**Table 2**
**International Federation of Gynecology and Obstetrics (FIGO) staging of ovarian cancer**

| Stage | Extent of Disease | Lymph Node Involvement | Peritoneal Washings |
|-------|-------------------|------------------------|---------------------|
| I | Growth limited to the ovaries | | Positive or negative |
| II | Pelvic extension of disease | | Positive or negative |
| III | Disease limited to pelvis | Inguinal or retroperitoneal | Positive or negative |
| IV | Distant metastases | | |

staging of germ cell and sex cord tumors in those younger than age 21: (1) collecting cytology from pelvic washings or ascites on entry into the peritoneal cavity; (2) close inspection of the peritoneal cavity for evidence of peritoneal implants, and if present, biopsy or excision of lesions; (3) palpation or examination of pelvic lymph nodes with sampling of enlarged or firm nodes; (4) inspection of the omentum with removal of adherent or abnormal areas; (5) inspection of the opposite ovary with biopsy of abnormal areas; and (6) complete resection of the involved ovary, including the fallopian tube if involved. Staging for epithelial ovarian adenocarcinomas follow the International Federation of Gynecology and Obstetrics staging (**Table 2**).[51] Although routine lymphadenectomy has been recommended for staging of epithelial ovarian carcinomas, it has not demonstrated a survival benefit for those with germ cell malignancies.[52]

### Outcomes for Malignancy

With the advent of cisplatin, vinblastine, and bleomycin chemotherapy for germ cell malignancies, survival for children and adolescents is 97%.[53] With immature teratomas, complete surgical excision by unilateral salpingo-oophorectomy has a 97.8% event-free survival at 3 years.[54] For most patients with stage I immature teratoma, close observation is reasonable given that survival rates are very high and risk of chemotherapy to gonadal function may be significant. Unfortunately, intraoperative frozen section may not be as accurate for germ cell tumors as for other epithelial ovarian cancers. Although there have been small case series of patients diagnosed with immature teratomas who underwent ovarian cystectomy without removal of the ovary, there are insufficient data to suggest that cystectomy alone is adequate treatment for immature ovarian germ cell tumors.[55]

### SUMMARY

In summary, germ cell tumors occur most frequently in children and adolescents, and surgeons who care for younger patients should be prepared to manage these interesting tumors. In the case of antenatally diagnosed tumors or those at high risk for malignancy, consideration should be given to refer to a tertiary care center if the surgeon is not experienced at resection and staging recommendations. Regardless of location or age of the patient, teratomas should be completely resected, including in the ovary, using minimally invasive and fertility-preserving techniques whenever possible.

### REFERENCES

1. Gucciardo L, Uyttebroek A, De Wever I, et al. Prenatal assessment and management of sacrococcygeal teratoma. Prenat Diagn 2011;31(7):678–88.

2. DeBacker A, Madern GC, Pieters R, et al. Influence of tumor site and histology on long term survival in 193 children with extracranial germ cell tumors. Eur J Pediatr Surg 2008;18(1):1–6.
3. Altman RP, Randolph JG, Lilly JR. Sacrococcygeal teratoma: American Academy of Pediatrics Surgical Section Survey-1973. J Pediatr Surg 1974;9(3):389–98.
4. Tonni G, De Felice C, Centini G, et al. Cervical and oral teratoma in the fetus: a systematic review of etiology, pathology, diagnosis, treatment and prognosis. Arch Gynecol Obstet 2010;282(4):355–61.
5. deSa DJ. Follicular ovarian cysts in stillbirths and neonates. Arch Dis Child 1975; 50(1):45–50.
6. Cohen HL, Shapiro MA, Mandel FS, et al. Normal ovaries in neonates and infants: a sonographic study of 77 patients 1 day to 24 months old. AJR Am J Roentgenol 1993;160(3):583–6.
7. Razzaghy-Azar M, Ghasemi F, Hallaji F, et al. Sonographic measurement of uterus and ovaries in premenarcheal healthy girls between 6 and 13 years old: correlation with age and pubertal status. J Clin Ultrasound 2011;39(2):64–73.
8. Herter LD, Golendziner E, Flores JA, et al. Ovarian and uterine sonography in healthy girls between 1 and 13 years old: correlation of findings with age and pubertal status. Am J Roentgenol 2002;178(6):1531–6.
9. Fleming NA, de Nanassy J, Lawrence S, et al. Juvenile granulosa and theca cell tumor of the ovary as a rare cause of precocious puberty: case report and review of literature. J Pediatr Adolesc Gynecol 2010;23(4):e127–31.
10. Rousseau V, Massicot R, Darwish AA, et al. Emergency management and conservative surgery of ovarian torsion in children: a report of 40 cases. J Pediatr Adolesc Gynecol 2008;21(4):201–6.
11. Albayram F, Hamper UM. Ovarian and adnexal torsion: spectrum of sonographic findings with pathologic correlation. J Ultrasound Med 2001;20(10):1083–9.
12. Ben-Ami M, Perlitz Y, Haddad S. The effectiveness of spectral and color Doppler in predicting ovarian torsion: a prospective study. Eur J Obstet Gynecol Reprod Biol 2002;104(1):64–6.
13. Pena JE, Ufberg D, Cooney N, et al. Usefulness of Doppler sonography in the diagnosis of ovarian torsion. Fertil Steril 2000;73(5):1047–50.
14. Servaes S, Zurakowski D, Laufer MR, et al. Sonographic findings of ovarian torsion in children. Pediatr Radiol 2007;37(5):446–51.
15. Kiechl-Kohlendorfer U, Maurer K, Unsinn K, et al. Fluid-debris level in follicular cysts: a pathognomonic sign of ovarian torsion. Pediatr Radiol 2006;36:421–5.
16. Lee JH, Park SB, Shin SH, et al. Value of intra-adnexal and extra-adnexal computed tomographic imaging features diagnosing torsion of adnexal tumor. J Comput Assist Tomogr 2009;33(6):872–6.
17. Hiller N, Appelbaum L, Simanovsky N, et al. CT features of adnexal torsion. AJR Am J Roentgenol 2007;189(1):124–9.
18. Nemec U, Nemec SF, Bettelheim D, et al. Ovarian cysts on prenatal MRI. Eur J Radiol 2011. [Epub ahead of print].
19. McDonald JM, Doran S, DeSimone CP, et al. Predicting risk of malignancy in adnexal masses. Obstet Gynecol 2010;115(4):687–94.
20. McCarthy JD, Erickson KM, Smith YR, et al. Premenarchal ovarian torsion and elevated CA-125. J Pediatr Adolesc Gynecol 2010;23(1):e47–50.
21. Luzzatto C, Midrio P, Toffolutti T, et al. Neonatal ovarian cysts: management and follow-up. Pediatr Surg Int 2000;16(1–2):56–9.
22. Kwak DW, Sohn YS, Kim SK, et al. Clinical experiences of fetal ovarian cyst: diagnosis and consequence. J Korean Med Sci 2006;21(4):690–4.

23. Jallouli M, Trigui L, Gouiaa N, et al. Neonatal ovarian lymphangioma. J Pediatr Adolesc Gynecol 2011;24(1):e9–10.

24. Karmazyn B, Steinberg R, Ziv N, et al. Colonic stricture secondary to torsion of an ovarian cyst. Pediatr Radiol 2002;32(1):25–7.

25. Fitzhugh VA, Shaikh JR, Heller DS. Adnexal torsion leading to death of an infant. J Pediatr Adolesc Gynecol 2008;21(5):295–7.

26. Brandt ML, Helmrath MA. Ovarian cysts in infants and children. Semin Pediatr Surg 2005;14(2):78–85.

27. Strickland JL. Ovarian cysts in neonates, children and adolescents. Curr Opin Obstet Gynecol 2002;14(5):459–65.

28. Vilos GA, Alshimmiri M. Cost-benefit analysis of laparoscopic versus laparotomy for benign tuboovarian disease. J Am Assoc Gynecol Laparosc 1995;2(3): 299–303.

29. Cohen SB, Wattiez A, Seidman DS, et al. Laparoscopy versus laparotomy for detorsion and sparing of twisted ischemic adnexa. JSLS 2003;7(4):295–9.

30. Yuen PM, Yu KM, Yip SK, et al. A randomized prospective study of laparoscopy and laparotomy in the management of benign ovarian masses. Am J Obstet Gynecol 1997;177(1):109–14.

31. Lécuru F, Desfeux P, Camatte S, et al. Stage I ovarian cancer: comparison of laparoscopy and laparotomy on staging and survival. Eur J Gynaecol Oncol 2004;25(5):571–6.

32. Lin P, Falcone T, Tulandi T. Excision of ovarian dermoid cyst by laparoscopy and by laparotomy. Am J Obstet Gynecol 1995;173(3 Pt 1):769–71.

33. Zanetta G, Ferrari L, Mignini-Renzini M, et al. Laparoscopic excision of ovarian dermoid cysts with controlled intraoperative spillage. Safety and effectiveness. J Reprod Med 1999;44(9):815–20.

34. Laberge PY, Levesque S. Short-term morbidity and long-term recurrence rate of ovarian dermoid cysts treated by laparoscopy versus laparotomy. J Obstet Gynaecol Can 2006;28(9):789–93.

35. Medeiros LR, Fachel JM, Garry R, et al. Laparoscopy versus laparotomy for benign ovarian tumours. Cochrane Database Syst Rev 2005;3:CD004751.

36. Cooper GS, Thorp JM. FSH levels in relation to hysterectomy and to unilateral oophorectomy. Obstet Gynecol 1999;94(6):969–72.

37. Cramer DW, Xu H, Harlow BL. Does "incessant" ovulation increase risk for early menopause? Am J Obstet Gynecol 1995;172(2 Pt 1):568–73.

38. Maneschi F, Marasá L, Incandela S, et al. Ovarian cortex surrounding benign neoplasms: a histologic study. Am J Obstet Gynecol 1993;169:388–93.

39. Chang HJ, Han SH, Lee JR, et al. Impact of laparoscopic cystectomy on ovarian reserve: serial changes of serum anti-Müllerian hormone levels. Fertil Steril 2010; 94(1):343–9.

40. Galinier P, Carfagna L, Delsol M, et al. Ovarian torsion. Management and ovarian prognosis: a report of 45 cases. J Pediatr Surg 2009;44(9):1759–65.

41. Oelsner G, Cohen SB, Soriano D, et al. Minimal surgery for the twisted ischaemic adnexa can preserve ovarian function. Hum Reprod 2003;18(12):2599–602.

42. Guthrie BD, Adler MD, Powell EC. Incidence and trends of pediatric ovarian torsion hospitalizations in the United States, 2000-2006. Pediatrics 2010;125(3):532–8.

43. Oltmann S, Fischer A, Barber R, et al. Pediatric ovarian malignancy presenting as ovarian torsion: incidence and relevance. J Pediatr Surg 2010;45:135–9.

44. Ozcan C, Celik A, Ozok G, et al. Adnexal torsion in children may have a catastrophic sequel: asynchronous bilateral torsion. J Pediatr Surg 2002;37(11): 1617–20.

45. Beaunoyer M, Chapdelaine J, Bouchard S, et al. Asynchronous bilateral ovarian torsion. J Pediatr Surg 2004;39(5):746–9.
46. Dunnihoo D. Bilateral torsion of the adnexa: a case report and a review of the world literature. Obstet Gynecol 1984;64:555–95.
47. Cass DL. Ovarian torsion. Semin Pediatr Surg 2005;14(2):86–92.
48. Crouch NS, Gyampoh B, Cutner AS, et al. Ovarian torsion: to pex or not to pex? Case report and review of the literature. J Pediatr Adolesc Gynecol 2003;16(6): 381–4.
49. Abeş M, Sarihan H. Oophoropexy in children with ovarian torsion. Eur J Pediatr Surg 2004;14(3):168–71.
50. Billmire D, Vinocur F, Rescorla B, et al. Outcome and staging evaluation in malignant germ cell tumors of the ovary in children and adolescents: an intergroup study. J Pediatr Surg 2004;39(3):424–9.
51. Pecorelli S, Benedet JL, Creasman WT, et al. FIGO staging of gynecologic cancer. 1994-1997 FIGO Committee on Gynecologic Oncology. International Federation of Gynecology and Obstetrics. Int J Gynaecol Obstet 1999;65(3): 243–9.
52. Mahdi H, Swensen RE, Hanna R, et al. Prognostic impact of lymphadenectomy in clinically early stage malignant germ cell tumour of the ovary. Br J Cancer 2011; 105(4):493–7.
53. Dimopoulos MA, Papadimitriou C, Hamilos G, et al. Treatment of ovarian germ cell tumors with a 3-day bleomycin, etoposide, and cisplatin regimen: a prospective multicenter study. Gynecol Oncol 2004;95(3):695–700.
54. Marina NM, Cushing B, Giller R, et al. Complete surgical excision is effective treatment for children with immature teratomas with or without malignancy elements: a Pediatric Oncology Group/Children Cancer Group intergroup study. J Clin Oncol 1999;17(7):2137–43.
55. Beiner M, Gotlieb W, Korach Y, et al. Cystectomy for immature teratoma of the ovary. Gynecol Oncol 2004;93:381–4.

# Pediatric Chest I

## Developmental and Physiologic Conditions for the Surgeon

Christopher Guidry, MD[a], Eugene D. McGahren, MD[b],*

### KEYWORDS

- Pediatric chest • Pediatric mediastinum • Pediatric thorax anatomy
- Pediatric thorax surgery

### KEY POINTS

- The mediastinum, pleura, and lungs are a collection of complex organs interacting in a constant and literally fluid manner.
- A pneumothorax results from the separation of the visceral pleura of the lung from the parietal pleura of the chest wall.
- Surgical management of congenital and acquired conditions of the pediatric thorax is predicated on the understanding of anatomical and physiologic development, appropriate anatomical relationships, and appropriate surgical principles concerning the thorax.

This article addresses basic anatomic considerations of the chest and describes common conditions of the lungs, pleura, and mediastinum that affect children. Treatment of malignant conditions and management of congenital diaphragmatic hernia and congenital chest wall deformities are addressed in other articles by Ken Azarow elsewhere in this issue.

### ANATOMY

The mediastinum, pleura, and lungs are a collection of complex organs interacting in a constant and literally fluid manner. The mediastinum comprises the central portion of the thoracic cavity. Its boundaries are the sternum anteriorly, the vertebral column posteriorly, and the medial parietal pleural surfaces of the right and left lungs laterally. The mediastinum is sometimes described as having 4 compartments: superior, anterior, middle, and posterior.[1] However, clinically, lesions are usually described as being

[a] Department of General Surgery, University of Virginia Health System, Box 800709, Charlottesville, VA 22908, USA; [b] Division of Pediatric Surgery, University of Virginia Children's Hospital, University of Virginia Health System, Box 800709, Charlottesville, VA 22908, USA
* Corresponding author.
*E-mail address:* edm6k@virginia.edu

Surg Clin N Am 92 (2012) 615–643
doi:10.1016/j.suc.2012.03.013
0039-6109/12/$ – see front matter © 2012 Elsevier Inc. All rights reserved.
surgical.theclinics.com

within 1 of 3 compartments: anterior, middle, and posterior. In this schema, the superior compartment is subsumed into the other compartments. The anterior mediastinum is bounded by the sternum anteriorly, the diaphragm inferiorly, the trachea,
great vessels, and pericardium posteriorly, and the pleurae and lungs laterally. The
anterior compartment contains the thymus, lymphoid structures, and nerves and
vessels. The middle mediastinum is bounded by the anterior and posterior limits of
the pericardium. It contains the trachea, main-stem bronchi, the heart and great
vessels, and hilar lymph nodes. The posterior mediastinum is bounded inferiorly by
the diaphragm, anteriorly by the pericardium, and posteriorly by the vertebral column.
It contains the aorta, thoracic esophagus, and the sympathetic nerve chain (**Fig. 1**).[1,2]

The right and left pleural spaces are separate entities. They envelop each lung as they
extend from the lateral aspects of the mediastinum. The parietal pleura lines the thoracic
wall and is continuous with the visceral pleura as it adheres intimately to the pulmonary
surface. A thin layer of mesothelial cells and fluid is interposed between the 2 surfaces
as they adhere to each other. In some areas, the parietal pleura may fold onto itself until
the lung intercedes during inspiration. These areas are found inferiorly along the edges
of the diaphragm, in the costodiaphragmatic sinus, and in a small cleft behind the

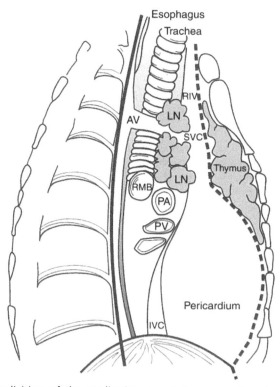

**Fig. 1.** Anatomic division of the mediastinum: anterior compartment extends from the
sternum to the *dotted line* anterior to the pericardium. Middle mediastinum extends posteriorly to the anterior border of the vertebrae (*solid line*). AV, azygous vein; IVC, inferior vena
cava; LN, lymph node; PA, pulmonary artery; PV, pulmonary vein; RIV, right internal jugular
vein; RMB, right main-stem bronchus; SVC, superior vena cava. (*From* Tovar JA. Mediastinal
tumors. In: Holcomb III GW, Murphy JP, editors. Ashcraft's pediatric surgery. 5th edition.
Philadelphia: Saunders; 2010. p. 322; with permission.)

sternum known as the costomediastinal sinus. The parietal pleura receives its blood supply from the intercostal, internal mammary, superior phrenic, and anterior mediastinal arteries. Corresponding veins drain the parietal pleura into the systemic veins. The visceral pleura receives its perfusion from bronchial and pulmonary artery radicals. Venous drainage is only to the pulmonary circulation. The parietal pleura receives sensory innervation from the intercostal and phrenic nerves, resulting in relatively precise sensory localization. The visceral pleura receives vagal and sympathetic innervation and has less precise sensory localization.[1,3]

The systemic and pulmonary vasculature and the lymphatic circulation interact to maintain a relatively constant amount of pleural fluid, which is evenly distributed within the pleural space.[1,4,5] Most pleural fluid is formed from the systemic circulation. It then travels along pressure gradients in the pleural space until it is primarily resorbed by parietal pleural lymphatics. Increase of systemic venous pressure or lymphatic pressure results in excessive accumulation of pleural fluid either by increased production (venous congestion) or decreased absorption (lymphatic congestion). Normally, there is little interchange between pleural and pulmonary fluids. However, pulmonary edema can contribute to an increase in pleural fluid by presenting a greater amount of fluid to the visceral pleura from the pulmonary parenchyma itself.[1,6]

In children, the lungs and airways are not fully developed at birth. In the postnatal period, the number of immature alveoli continues to increase. They subsequently enlarge into mature alveoli. The area of the air-blood interface continues to increase as alveoli and capillaries multiply. These changes continue until at least the eighth postnatal year. Only about 50 million alveoli (one-sixth of the adult number) are present at birth. The structural integrity of the airway improves after birth as the flexible cartilage of the infant's larynx and trachea becomes more rigid.[1,7]

## PLEURA AND LUNGS
### Pneumothorax

A pneumothorax results from the separation of the visceral pleura of the lung from the parietal pleura of the chest wall. Air accumulates in this space. If the air accumulates under pressure, a tension pneumothorax ensues. A pneumothorax may occur spontaneously or as the result of trauma, surgery, or a therapeutic intervention. Pulmonary volume, compliance, and diffusing capacity are compromised and if the pneumothorax is substantial, hypoxia may result secondary to ventilation-perfusion mismatch. A normal lung may be able to compensate for this situation. Children with underlying chronic pulmonary disease may suffer relatively smaller pneumothoraces secondary to diminished elastic recoil of their lungs, but the symptomatic consequences may be more significant because of their small margin of pulmonary reserve.[8,9]

Many pneumothoraces experienced by children are spontaneous. Most of these spontaneous pneumothoraces occur in the adolescent age group. The typically affected adolescent is 14 to 18 years old, male, tall, and thin. Few of these youngsters are smokers.[10,11] Spontaneous pneumothorax often occurs in the absence of any underlying disease. However, it may result from an underlying condition such as a congenital or acquired bleb, familial tendency, pneumonia with pneumatocele or abscess, tuberculosis, pleuropulmonary blastoma, osteochondroma, or cystic adenomatoid malformation.[8,12–17]

Pneumothorax is also common in the infant population. Symptomatic pneumothorax is estimated to occur in 0.08% of all live births, and in 5% to 7% of infants with a birth weight 1500 g or less. Typical risks include respiratory distress syndrome, meconium aspiration, pulmonary hypoplasia, continuous positive airway pressure, and mechanical ventilation. Risks may be lowered by the use of surfactant and synchronized and low-volume ventilation.[18–21]

Pneumothorax from trauma may result from a tear in the pleura, esophagus, trachea, or bronchi. Iatrogenic causes include mechanical ventilation, thoracentesis, central venous catheter insertion, bronchoscopy, or cardiopulmonary resuscitation.[8,12–14]

Spontaneous pneumothorax most commonly presents with chest pain. Accompanying symptoms may also include back or shoulder pain, dyspnea, and cough. In the trauma setting, pneumothorax is routinely screened for. But the presence of the signs and symptoms noted earlier should raise suspicion for pneumothorax. In any infant or child who is already being ventilated, any decline in respiratory status should also raise suspicion for pneumothorax.[8,10,11,13,21]

Severe dyspnea or respiratory insufficiency should alert the provider to the presence of a tension pneumothorax. Physical examination of a patient with pneumothorax reveals diminished breath sounds on the affected side of the chest. The trachea may be shifted away from the side of a tension pneumothorax. Pneumothorax should be visible on a chest radiograph and is enhanced if the radiograph is taken at end expiration. It is common practice for the size of a pneumothorax to be described as a proportion of the chest field on an upright radiograph. However, the volume loss of the lung is greater than such a description because pulmonary volume is lost in 3 dimensions.

The factors that determine the proper management of pneumothorax include the initial size, signs and symptoms, ongoing expansion, presence of tension, and any contributing underlying condition, A spontaneous unilateral pneumothorax that is asymptomatic and less than 15% to 20% of the chest volume can usually be followed by observation alone.[8,10,11,14] Pleural air reabsorbs at a rate of 1.25% per day, but this can be hastened by breathing supplemental oxygen.[8,22] Options for treatment of a small pneumothorax include thoracentesis, placement of a Heimlich valve, or placement of a pigtail catheter.[10,11,23–25] However, if air is continuously aspirated, the pneumothorax persists, symptoms are initially significant or not relieved by the initial maneuvers, or the presenting pneumothorax is large in size, a standard chest tube should be inserted.

A tension pneumothorax requires emergent placement of a chest tube. If a tube is not immediately available or if the patient's condition deteriorates during preparation for placement, a large-bore (14-gauge) needle should be placed just over the rib in the anterior second intercostal space in the midclavicular line to relieve the tension. A chest tube can then be placed.

Pneumothoraces in infants, particularly infants being ventilated, may sometimes be treated expectantly by keeping ventilator settings low, by using an oscillatory ventilator, and by keeping the affected side down. Most commonly, needle aspiration or chest tube drainage is required. Neonates are most prone to injuries from chest tubes that can result in lung tears, phrenic nerve injury, chylothorax and pericardial effusions.[21,26] Fibrin glue has been used in infants to try to seal pneumothoraces. However, this treatment carries risks of hypercalcemia, bradycardia, diaphragm paralysis, and skin necrosis.[26,27]

In a posttraumatic pneumothorax, large or persistent air leaks may indicate damage to the airway or the esophagus. Appropriate diagnostic studies using an esophagogram, bronchoscopy, esophagoscopy, thoracoscopy, or thoracotomy should be undertaken and direct repair of the injury, if present, performed. If the air leak is the result of lung parenchymal injury, chest tube drainage is usually corrective.

If a spontaneous pneumothorax occurs for the first time, initial treatment is usually limited to one of the types of chest drainage noted earlier. A recent study assessing cost and morbidities of treatment options advocates against aggressive surgical intervention as a primary treatment of spontaneous pneumothorax.[28] Pneumothorax recurs with a frequency of 50% to 60% after the first episode in children.[11,29-31] If a persistent air leak is present, or if the pneumothorax recurs after removal of the chest tube, then further surgical intervention is warranted.[10,11,28,31,32] Such intervention is now typically performed using a video-assisted thoracoscopic (VATS) technique.[27,33-37]

Once a VATS procedure is undertaken, the goal is to remove any resectable lung disease if present and perform pleurodesis. Blebs and cysts can usually be removed with a stapled or ligated wedge resection. Fibrin glue or absorbable mesh, or both, are sometimes used to reinforce the resected area.[37,38] Pleurodesis can be undertaken using an instilled agent, mechanical abrasion with a bovie pad or sponge, or both. The most commonly used pleurodesis agent is USP purified talc. A recent study in adults suggested that talc may have systemic distribution and may rarely produce acute respiratory distress syndrome (ARDS).[39] However, multiple other reports have advocated the safety of talc.[40-43] Treatment with talc has been shown to be particularly effective in treating pneumothoraces in children with cystic fibrosis.[44] Other agents such as silver nitrate, quinacrine, iodized oil, minocycline, doxycycline, and hypertonic glucose have also been reported as potential agents, but are not commonly used.[31,44-49] The results of VATS pleurodesis for pneumothorax have been excellent, and complications of the technique are uncommon.[10,11,32,50,51]

### Empyema

Empyema refers to the accumulation of infected fluid in the pleural space. In children, empyema is most commonly secondary to an underlying pneumonia. Other causes may include perforation of the esophagus or tracheobronchial tree, spontaneously or from trauma, and spread of infection from retropharyngeal, mediastinal, or paravertebral spaces. These latter causes are less common in children than in adults.[52-54] In 1962, the American Thoracic Society described what are still considered the 3 classic stages of empyema.[55] The first stage, or the exudative stage, lasts for about 24 to 72 hours. It is characterized by an accumulation of thin pleural fluid and is amenable to drainage by thoracentesis. The second stage is the fibrinopurulent stage. This stage lasts 7 to 10 days and is characterized by the formation of a thicker, more fibrinous fluid with loculations. The lung loses its mobility in this stage. The third stage is the organizing stage. This stage usually occurs about 2 to 4 weeks after the onset of the empyema. A pleural peel forms and the lung becomes entrapped.

Historically, the most common organisms causing empyema have varied. *Streptococcus pyogenes*, *Staphylococcus aureus*, and *Haemophilus influenzae* were most common before the advent of antibiotics. Subsequent offending organisms then emerged depending on the nature of antibiotics developed.[56] Currently, *Streptococcus pneumoniae* along with other streptococcal species, and *Staphylococcus aureus*, including methicillin-resistant *Staphylococcus aureus*, are the leading causative organisms of empyema.[52,57-61] The incidence of *Streptococcus pneumoniae* is increasing despite the use of pneumococcal vaccine.[62]

Children with empyema most commonly present with fever. Other symptoms include cough, respiratory insufficiency, chest pain, and sometimes abdominal pain.[59] Physical signs may include dullness on chest percussion, tactile and vocal fremitus, decreased breath sounds, rales, and a pleural friction rub.[56,63] A chest radiograph reveals a density on the affected side of the chest that reflects pleural fluid accumulation and thickening as well as parenchymal compression. In advanced empyema, there may be shifting of the mediastinum to the contralateral side, and there may be air-fluid levels in a loculated area, or in a lung abscess. Transthoracic ultrasonography or a chest computed tomography (CT) scan can better determine the degree of pleural thickening, fluid loculation, and lung consolidation (**Fig. 2**).[64–66] The diagnosis of empyema is confirmed by thoracentesis. The fluid is characteristically turbid and may be thick during the later stages of the infection. Laboratory analysis reveals a specific gravity greater than 1.016, protein greater than 3 g/dL, lactate dehydrogenase (LDH) level greater than 200 U/L, pleural fluid protein/serum protein ratio greater than 0.5, pleural fluid LDH/serum LDH ratio greater than 0.6, and white blood cell count higher than 15,000/mm³. Fibrin clots may also be present.[63]

Once the diagnosis of empyema is made, and if fluid is obtained before the initiation of treatment, antibiotic therapy can be targeted toward the offending organism. However, it is common in children for antibiotics to be started without a fluid sample. If fluid is obtained after this point, it is often unrevealing. It is possible to treat pneumonia with a small to moderate empyema with antibiotics alone.[67] However, if a child is showing respiratory insufficiency, or if antibiotic treatment is not showing progress in resolving fever or symptoms such as pain within the first few days, then the empyema should be drained. As complete a drainage of the empyema as possible should be accomplished either by thoracentesis, tube thoracostomy with or without fibrinolytic agents, or thoracoscopic drainage. Thoracotomy is rarely needed for the treatment of empyema. In general, the longer the prehospital or pretreatment illness has persisted, the more involved the interventions that are needed may be.[52,57,68–70]

There is debate within the literature about the optimal drainage procedure for empyema. The surgical objective is to remove as much of the infected pleural fluid and debris as possible, to break up any loculations, and to free the lung to expand and to fill the pleural space. The lung expansion allows better clearance of infection from the lung parenchyma itself. Unlike adults, children rarely develop any chronic constricting pleural rinds with appropriate therapy. Children usually need sedation or anesthesia for any type of invasive procedure such as thoracentesis or chest tube placement. This situation has led some investigators to advocate VATS-assisted drainage early in the patient's course (**Fig. 3**). It is believed that this strategy leads to a faster, more complete evacuation of the chest, a faster resolution of symptoms, and a decreased length of stay compared with other interventions. In addition, it may prevent multiple procedures in the case of failed initial therapy with thoracentesis or thoracostomy with or without fibrinolysis.[57,71–79] Others believe that thoracostomy

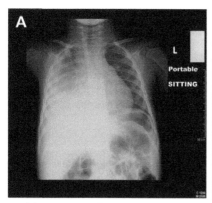 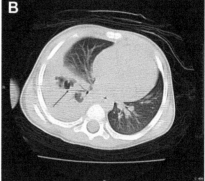

**Fig. 2.** (*A*) Empyema of right chest; density reflects pleural fluid accumulation, pleural thickening, and parenchymal compression. (*B*) CT image of right chest empyema; arrow denotes compressed lung parenchyma and pneumatoceles within lower lobe.

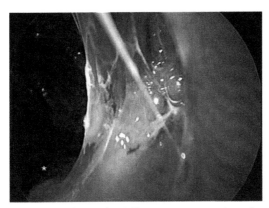

**Fig. 3.** This thoracoscopic view shows the inflammatory septations that can develop after the development of an empyema. These septations often result in loculations of the fluid, which makes chest tube drainage alone ineffective. Note the collapsed lung (*asterisk*) as a result of this inflammatory material. (*From* Rodgers BM, Michalsky MP. Acquired lesions of the lung and pleura. In: Holcomb III GW, Murphy JP, editors. Ashcraft's pediatric surgery. 5th edition. Philadelphia: Saunders; 2010. p. 291; with permission.)

with fibrinolysis, using agents such as streptokinase, urokinase, or tissue plasminogen activator, is as effective as VATS drainage in most cases, and that it may be more cost-effective with less morbidity than VATS.[52,57,79–81] However, only 1 prospective study of these 2 modes of therapy has been performed.[57] A position paper by the American Pediatric Surgical Association in 2009 suggests an algorithm for treatment of empyema (**Fig. 4**). The algorithm indicates that simple empyemas present for 5 days or less may be treated with catheter drainage alone. Empyemas that are loculated or present for greater than 5 days may be initially addressed with VATS or with chest tube placement with fibrinolytic therapy. The need for a prospective study in this regard is acknowledged in this article.[52]

Radiographic resolution of empyema typically lags behind clinical response. Therefore, persistent findings of radiographic abnormalities should not be an indication for repeat or further intervention if the child is clinically recovering. If a lung abscess develops, treatment may require pneumonostomy, wedge resection, or lobar resection.[82–84] After a child has clinically recovered from an empyema, it is advisable to follow serial chest radiographs over time until the lung fields return to normal to be sure there were no previously unknown inciting causes of the infection such as congenital cystic adenomatoid malformation (CCAM) or sequestration. With prompt and appropriate therapy, the overall outcome for children with empyema is excellent. Pulmonary function after recovery is usually clinically normal. However, some investigators have found mild restrictive or obstructive disease on follow-up spirometry.[85,86]

### Chylothorax

Chylothorax is the accumulation of lymphatic fluid within the pleural space. Congenital chylothorax is reported to be the most common cause of pleural effusion in neonates. In this age group, it is believed to be caused by abnormalities in the development of the lymphatic system such as lymphangiomatosis or lymphangiectasia. It may be present prenatally on ultrasonography and is sometimes associated with fetal hydrops. Prenatal chylothorax is a lethal condition and may require prenatal intervention such as thoracoamniotic shunting.[87–90] Another major cause of chylothorax in

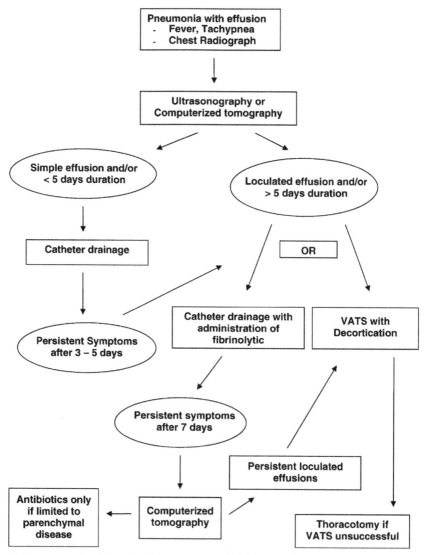

**Fig. 4.** Proposed algorithm for the treatment of children with pneumonia and parapneumonic effusions or empyema. (*From* Kokoska ER, Chen MK, The New Technology Committee. Position paper on video-assisted thoracoscopic surgery as treatment of pediatric empyema. J Pediatr Surg 2009;44:292; with permission.)

infants and children is injury to lymphatic channels as a result of an operative procedure, most typically for cardiac anomalies but also after repair of congenital diaphragmatic hernia, amongst other conditions. The incidence of chylothorax after thoracic surgery in children reportedly ranges from 0.25% to 0.9%.[91–93] The incidence after repair of congenital diaphragmatic hernia is 5% to 10%.[94–96] Other causes of chylothorax in children are malignancy, particularly neuroblastoma and lymphoma, occlusion or thrombosis of the upper central venous system, hypothyroidism, a variety of syndromes, and traumatic injury caused by either blunt or penetrating thoracic trauma or child abuse.[87,97–100] If an older child presents with chylothorax but has no history of trauma or operation, an intrathoracic tumor should be suspected and investigated with chest CT or magnetic resonance imaging (MRI).

Chylothorax typically presents with respiratory insufficiency, although it may also be first recognized as the incidental finding of a pleural effusion on an imaging study of the chest. As noted earlier, it may also be found on prenatal ultrasonography. The diagnosis of chylothorax is confirmed by evaluating the pleural fluid. Chyle is usually milky, but may be serosanguinous or straw-colored in children who are receiving no enteral fats, such as those who have just undergone surgery. One recent report defines chylothorax as having the following characteristics: more than 1000 leukocytes/mL (>70% lymphocytes), triglycerides greater than 100 mg/dL; protein greater than 20 g/L; sterile culture, positive Sudan III (a fat-soluble dye) staining of the fluid from enterally fed patients.[101] Loss of significant volumes of chyle from the pleural space results in a substantial loss of protein and lymphocytes. These losses must be monitored closely and replaced to avoid severe nutritional deficits in affected children.

Initial treatment of chylothorax is nonoperative, with about 70% to 80% of patients responding appropriately.[101–104] The pleural space is drained by thoracentesis or placement of a chest tube to relieve symptoms and facilitate closure of the lymphatic leak. Administering a diet that principally contains medium-chain triglycerides can diminish lymphatic flow through the thoracic duct. These fats are absorbed directly into the portal venous system, unlike long chain fatty acids, which are absorbed through the intestinal lymphatics. If chyle drainage persists, the patient can be placed on total parental nutrition, with cessation of enteral intake. If these measures fail to significantly reduce or eliminate lymphatic drainage within a few days, administration of octreotide, an analogue of somatostatin, may be helpful. This procedure can also be used in conjunction with the interventions noted earlier. It is uncertain how octreotide inhibits lymphatic flow, but it may act directly on somatostatin receptors in the splanchnic circulation to reduce lymph fluid production and thereby reduce its passage through the thoracic duct. It may also reduce the volume and protein content of lymph fluid within the thoracic duct by reducing gastric, pancreatic, and bile secretions.[87] No prospective study has been performed to evaluate the efficacy of somatostatin or octreotide in treating chylothorax.[105] However, there are multiple reports of the efficacy of somatostatin and octreotide in this regard.[87,102,104,106–110] Other reports indicate no particular success with these agents.[92,111]

If nonoperative treatment fails to resolve a chylothorax, surgical intervention is indicated. Options include ligation of the thoracic duct, embolization of the thoracic duct, pleurodesis or pleurectomy, sealing the area of leakage with fibrin glue, or the use of a pleural-peritoneal shunt. Thoracotomy or thoracoscopic technique may be used when appropriate.[112–119]

The timing of surgical intervention has been a matter of debate. Contemporary reports recommend intervention at as early as 5 to 7 days, particularly if less invasive procedures such as thoracoscopy or pleuroperitoneal shunts are to be used.[115,118,120] This situation is especially true if the child has increased right-heart pressures or central venous thrombosis. Such children are unlikely to respond to nonoperative treatment.[115]

## CCAM

CCAM is a rare anomaly with potentially serious clinical implications. These lesions are also referred to as congenital pulmonary airway malformations. The terminology still seems unsettled in the literature and therefore the more traditional CCAM terminology is used in this section. The reported incidence of CCAM is between 1:25,000 and

1:35,000 live births and it is the most common congenital cystic lung lesion. These lesions are usually confined to a single lobe and are more commonly left sided (**Fig. 5**).[121,122] Bilateral lesions are rare.[123] There is an 18% rate of associated abnormalities, which include renal agenesis and cardiac anomalies.[121] The differential diagnosis includes pulmonary sequestration, bronchogenic cyst, congenital lobar emphysema (CLE), enteric duplication, and congenital diaphragmatic hernia.[124]

Embryologically, CCAMs are believed to arise from a derangement of lung maturation at the level of the terminal bronchioles, leading to suppression of alveolar development and disorganized proliferation, resulting in cyst formation.[121–123] Although clinically distinct from pulmonary sequestrations, hybrid lesions do exist that contain features of both CCAM and sequestrations. These lesions usually meet criteria for CCAM but also have a supplemental systemic arterial supply. This discovery has led many investigators to suggest that CCAM and sequestrations may represent a spectrum of the same embryologic process.[125]

CCAMs are generally classified by cyst size and histology. The Stocker classification system is the most commonly used means of description. Type 0 consists of small solid lungs and is incompatible with life. Type I (most common) consists of single or multiple cysts of greater than 1 cm in diameter lined with pseudostratified epithelium, mucus-secreting cells, and prominent cartilage.[126] Type II is defined as having multiple cysts, all less than 1 cm in diameter, composed of cylindrical or cuboidal epithelium with prominent smooth or striated muscle. Type III is grossly solid but microcystic, lined by cuboidal epithelium and often intricately folded.[125] Type IV consists of large cysts lined with flattened epithelium surrounded by loose mesenchymal tissue. Types I and IV are considered to have a favorable prognosis. The remaining types have a poorer prognosis because of increased rates of other associated anomalies.[126]

The increasing use and sophistication of prenatal Doppler ultrasonography (DUS) has led to an increase in the reported diagnosis of CCAM. Lung malformations may be detected by DUS as early as 18 to 20 weeks' gestational age with a sensitivity of 76% to 81%.[122,125,127] Although definitive diagnosis of a specific lung lesion is uncertain on DUS, a CCAM typically appears as large macrocystic lesions or as a solid, echogenic-appearing mass. If a systemic feeding vessel is identified, then the mass is more likely a pulmonary sequestration or hybrid lesion.[123] Some CCAMs may appear to regress or involute on serial DUS. Postnatal chest radiography may show a mass,

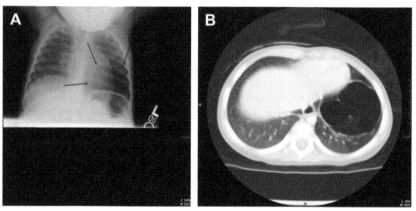

**Fig. 5.** (A) Chest radiograph depicts CCAM (*arrows*) in left lower lung field. (B) CT image shows the CCAM in (A) to involve the left lower lobe.

a cystic lesion, or hyperinflation, or may be normal.[125,128] Even if a lesion appears to resolve on DUS, or is not seen on postnatal chest radiography, these lesions are usually identified with postnatal CT or MRI, which have been reported to have a 100% specificity in these cases.[122,123,125,129] Such imaging should be performed in all asymptomatic infants within the first 6 to 12 months of life, or sooner in symptomatic infants. This imaging is helpful in identifying the extent of the lesion for operative planning. There is little evidence to suggest that lesions present postnatally involute further.[123,124]

Although most patients are born with few or no symptoms from their lesion, CCAMs may grow large enough to cause significant impairment both prenatally and postnatally.[122,128,129] Prenatally, the lesion may present with polyhydramnios, hydrothorax, or hydrops fetalis.[123,129,130] Compression of the fetal esophagus by a large intrathoracic mass interferes with fetal swallowing and produces polyhydramnios. Cardiac and vena cava compression caused by significant mediastinal shift by a large CCAM may lead to hydrops fetalis. Adzick and colleagues[123] have reported that a cystic adenomatoid volume ratio (CVR) greater than 1.6 is predictive of an increased risk of hydrops. The CVR is calculated by dividing CCAM volume by head circumference. Patients presenting with, or at risk for, development of hydrops may be considered for fetal intervention consisting of fetal pulmonary lobectomy or ex utero intrapartum therapy. Fetal hydrothorax may be amenable to thoracoamniotic shunting.[123,124,130] Postnatally, patients may be asymptomatic or present with cough, respiratory distress, recurrent infection, pneumothorax, or malignant degeneration.[122,125,127,128] Although rare, CCAMs have been associated with pulmonary malignancy.[128] Pleuropulmonary blastoma, bronchioloalveolar carcinoma, pulmonary rhabdomyosarcoma, and mesenchymoma have all been described as arising within CCAMs.[122,125,127,128,131–133] Pleuropulmonary blastoma has been shown to present more commonly in infants and young children, whereas older children and adults are more often diagnosed with bronchioloalveolar carcinoma.[125,127,133] Type I CCAM is associated with bronchioloalveolar carcinoma, whereas type IV shows histologic overlap with pleuropulmonary blastoma.[126,134] The overall risk of malignant transformation seems to be 2% to 4%.[132]

Patients presenting with acute respiratory distress shortly after birth should undergo urgent resection of the CCAM once stable. Acute treatment of severely symptomatic neonates may include emergent chest decompression with tube thoracostomy.[124] Most investigators agree that asymptomatic patients should undergo surgical resection on an elective basis at around 3 to 12 months of age, although the rate of infection begins to increase after 7 months of age.[121,127,129] Anatomic lobectomy via standard thoracotomy or with a thoracoscopic approach is the standard of care.[122,124,133,135] Thoracoscopy may generally be better tolerated and may result in better postoperative pain control, shorter hospital stay, a lower respiratory complication rate, and a lower risk of later chest wall deformity than thoracotomy.[124,135] Conversion from thoracoscopic to open resection is directly correlated with previous episodes of pneumonia as a result of the development of adhesions within the pleural space.[135] Pulmonary segmentectomy may be performed but carries a risk of failing to remove all of the abnormal tissue, thereby leaving a residual risk of infection and malignancy.[122,125,133] Early resection has the added benefit of allowing for compensatory lung growth and development.[122,125,129] Resection is indicated both to prevent symptoms but also to avoid malignant degeneration.[124,132,133] The long-term outcome for patients with completely resected CCAM is excellent.[128,129]

### Pulmonary Sequestration

Pulmonary sequestration is a rare congenital malformation of the respiratory tract. It is defined as a mass of nonfunctioning pulmonary tissue that lacks a definitive connection to the tracheobronchial tree and has a systemic arterial supply of variable origin.[136,137] Classically, these lesions are subdivided into 2 types: intralobar and extralobar pulmonary sequestrations. Intralobar sequestrations are located within the same investing visceral pleura as the adjacent normal lung tissue (**Fig. 6**). Extralobar sequestrations have their own visceral pleura, which physically separate them from the nearby normal tissue. Incidence is 0.15% to 6.4%.[138] The differential diagnosis for this pulmonary malformation includes CCAM, bronchogenic cyst, CLE, teratoma, enteric duplication, and neural crest tumors.[136,139,140]

Embryologically, normal lung development begins at about 4 weeks' gestation with the emergence of the tracheal bud from the ventral aspect of the primitive foregut. The tracheal bud progresses in a caudad direction and eventually bifurcates to form the primary bronchial buds. The tracheoesophageal septum forms to separate developing lung from the foregut and thus defines the trachea and esophagus as separate structures.[141] Multiple generations of bifurcation lead to the development of the normal tracheobronchial tree and are intimately associated with similar branching of the developing pulmonary arteries. Pulmonary sequestrations are believed to arise as supernumerary lung buds that develop caudally to the main lungs. Because these extra lung buds are typically not associated with normal pulmonary artery development, they develop a separate systemic blood supply.[139] If this process occurs before the development of the visceral pleura, then the aberrant pulmonary tissue becomes invested in the same visceral pleura as the normal lung tissue and is termed intralobar. If the process occurs after the development of the pleura, the sequestration develops its own visceral pleura and is termed extralobar. The arterial supply usually arises directly off the aorta and may arise from below the diaphragm in 20% of cases. The venous drainage displays more variation. Venous drainage may be via the pulmonary veins, vena cava, azygous or hemiazygous veins, or a combination of some or all of these.[136,139]

Intralobar sequestrations are the most common type (75%) and are typically located in the medial and posterior left lower lobe.[138] Intralobar sequestrations have a low rate of associated anomalies. During childhood, these lesions may present with recurrent

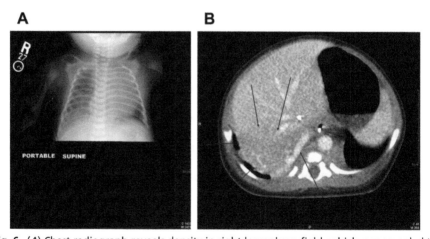

**Fig. 6.** (A) Chest radiograph reveals density in right lower lung field, which was revealed to be an intralobar pulmonary sequestration. (B) CT image shows the intralobar sequestration shown in (A) within the arrows on the patient's right outlining the lesion. The most medial arrow indicates a systemic artery to the sequestration that arises from the aorta.

respiratory infections as a result of both compression of the adjacent lung tissue as well as inadequate pulmonary toilet through the pores of Kohn. Intralobar lesions have an infection rate reported as high as 91%.[137] Symptoms may progress to lung abscess and hemoptysis if unrecognized. In 10% of intralobar sequestrations, there is a connection to the esophagus, which also predisposes to recurrent infection.[136]

Extralobar sequestrations make up about 25% of all sequestrations.[140] Patients with extralobar sequestrations have a high rate of associated anomalies and therefore are generally diagnosed at an earlier age than patients with intralobar lesions. Up to 40% of patients have some other associated anomaly, including vertebral and chest wall deformities, hindgut duplications, bronchogenic cysts, CCAM, and congenital cardiac malformations.[136,138] A total of 5% to 15% of patients with congenital diaphragmatic hernia have an associated extralobar sequestration. As indicated by their embryologic origin, up to 15% of these lesions are located within or below the diaphragm, with up to 10% being located within the abdominal cavity.[139] The most common location for an intra-abdominal extralobar sequestration is the left suprarenal area.[136] Air within an extralobar sequestration or a history of feeding intolerance should prompt a search for a connection to the gastrointestinal tract (including the stomach), which may, although it is uncommon, serve as a source of infection.[137,138] The overall infection rate for extralobar lesions is reported as low as 14%.[137] Patients may also present with swallowing difficulties, respiratory distress, high-output congestive heart failure, or back pain from torsion.[136,138]

Prenatal DUS is identifying pulmonary sequestrations with increasing frequency. These lesions typically appear well defined, echogenic, homogeneous, and often with a definable systemic arterial supply.[136,137] Postnatally, chest radiograph may be normal or show a mass. Sequestrations with cystic components should raise the suspicion of an associated CCAM within the lesion.[137,142] Air within the lesion may arise from an anomalous connection with foregut structures or from the pores of Kohn, if the lesion is intralobar. MRI and CT are also helpful for establishing the diagnosis and may show a systemic artery not seen on DUS. These imaging modalities are most beneficial for defining anatomy before surgical intervention. Of paramount importance is identifying both arterial and venous drainage from the sequestration before resection. MRI or CT should also be performed in the case of a disappearing lung lesion on DUS. Several reports have indicated that some lesions seen on DUS may seem to regress spontaneously. This situation is believed to be a result of vascular compromise or spontaneous decompression into the adjacent tracheobronchial tree.[137,141,142] However, many of these lesions may still be identified postnatally with MRI or CT. A Gastrografin swallow study or esophagogastroduodenoscopy may be helpful in identifying a connection to the esophagus or stomach. Because of significant overlap between sequestrations and other congenital pulmonary lesions on imaging, a definitive diagnosis may not be possible based purely on imaging data. If a suspected sequestration is in the left suprarenal area, it is important to rule out a neural tumor by obtaining urinary catecholamines.[139]

Sequestrations may present in the fetal period with polyhydramnios, hydrops fetalis, mediastinal shift, or hydrothorax.[137] Compression of the esophagus or fetal stomach, the vena cava, or mediastinal shift may lead to polyhydramnios and potential preterm labor. Pulmonary sequestration associated with hydrops is considered potentially lethal. The role for amniocentesis in this setting is unclear. Patients may be considered for fetal intervention if they are between 24 and 30 weeks' gestation and there is the presence of hydrops. Pulmonary sequestration with associated hydrothorax has a 22% reported survival rate and fetuses showing this should be considered for thoracoamniotic shunting.[136] Postnatally, the degree of associated pulmonary hypoplasia in the remaining lung tissue and the nature of other congenital anomalies, if present, are the main determinates of outcome.

All symptomatic lesions require surgical excision.[142] Generally, all intralobar lesions and lesions with a cystic component must also be excised.[137] Most investigators suggest that all lesions should be excised by 6 months to 1 year of age both for diagnostic purposes as well as to avoid the risk of infection and malignant degeneration. The latter is a low risk, and is likely a result of the presence of other pathologic tissue in the presence of an intralobar sequestration.[137,140,142] Any infection should be adequately treated before excision.[137] Surgical excision requires careful dissection of the vascular stalk, with ligation of the feeding vessels. The aberrant arteries tend to be large, elastic, and thin walled. Exsanguination may occur if a large feeding vessel of infradiaphragmatic origin retracts below the diaphragm before achieving adequate vascular control.[138] Classically, intralobar lesions are removed via thoracotomy and require a segmental lung resection at minimum. Large intralobar lesions may be best served by lobectomy. The short-term loss of normal pulmonary tissue is offset by compensatory lung growth from the remaining lung. Thoracoscopic approaches are also safe and are associated with decreased postoperative pain, faster recovery, and a lower rate of chest wall deformity.[137,142] Extralobar sequestrations may be removed without any damage to the adjacent lung. Diaphragmatic or intra-abdominal sequestrations may require laparoscopy or laparotomy for adequate excision.[139,140] In the rare case of bilateral sequestrations, bilateral excision may be performed during the same procedure, sometimes from 1 side, or as a staged procedure.[143] Embolization procedures have also been described via both the femoral and umbilical route. This approach may be best used for patients who are not stable enough to undergo resection, such as those in high-output heart failure.[136,142]

## CLE

CLE is a condition characterized by hyperinflation of otherwise normal alveoli. Most cases are discovered either prenatally, or within the first 6 months of life. Traditionally, this condition has been most commonly recognized in White men, with a male/female ratio ranging from 2:1 to 3:2 reported.[144–146] This finding has supported a theory that there may be a genetic cause for this condition. However, a series of 21 non-White Arab children with this condition reported in 2001[147] has brought this theory into question.

The left upper lobe is the most common location of CLE. The right upper and middle lobes are the next most commonly involved. The lower lobes are not commonly affected.[144,145,148] This latter point may help in differentiating CLE from CCAM when there is an abnormal degree of lucency in a lower lung field. Causes of CLE are believed to be both intrinsic and extrinsic. Intrinsic causes include bronchial cartilage dysplasia, deficiency, or atresia, bronchial mucosal proliferation, bronchial torsion, and granulation tissue or inspissated meconium or mucus within a bronchus. External causes include compression from aberrant vascular structures, hilar lymph nodes, or mediastinal cysts. A condition known as polyalveolar lobe, in which there is a proliferation of expanded alveoli within a lung lobe, may be a cause of some cases of CLE. About 50% of children have no identifiable inciting cause.[144–146,149–152]

CLE can be suspected by the appearance of cystic changes in a fetal lung on prenatal ultrasonography. However, a diagnosis of CLE is not possible because abnormal cystic lesions seen on such studies may also represent CCAM, lung sequestration, or congenital diaphragmatic hernia. Cystic changes seen prenatally may appear to diminish in size or even disappear. However, postnatal imaging is imperative to further assess the nature of the lesions seen. It cannot be presumed that they have resolved.[137,148,153]

Presenting symptoms and signs of CLE may include dyspnea, tachypnea, wheezing, cyanosis, and tachycardia. Symptoms are not commonly present at birth, and typically progress gradually. However, they can progress rapidly in some instances, particularly in infants. Rapid progression of symptoms is not common in older children.[144]

A chest radiograph shows a hyperlucency in the area of the involved lung lobe. The presence of some lung markings helps to differentiate this finding from that of tension pneumothorax. There is often mediastinal and tracheal shift and herniation of the lung across the midline. CT or MRI can further delineate the involved anatomy and also reveal obstructing lesions of the involved bronchus such as enlarged lymph nodes, a mediastinal cyst, or an aberrant vascular structure (**Fig. 7**). Once CLE is believed to be present, bronchoscopy may also be useful in determining the cause of the CLE. Flexible bronchoscopy may be better than rigid bronchoscopy in a controlled setting so as to minimize the use of positive pressure. Identification of abnormal bronchial anatomy may reinforce the diagnosis of CLE as opposed to an intrinsic parenchymal disease. In addition, if inspissated meconium, mucus, or granulation tissue is found, the potential exists to relieve the obstruction and resolve the CLE. Evaluation of CLE should also include an investigation for any congenital heart anomalies because they present in 10% to 20% of children with CLE.[144,146]

It is important not to confuse CLE with tension pneumothorax in a symptomatic patient, because placement of a chest tube into an emphysematous lobe may exacerbate the symptoms. In addition, if intubation is required, positive pressure should be kept at a minimal level so as to minimize further expansion of the involved lobe and avoid worsening pulmonary compromise. Management of CLE has most commonly involved removal of the involved lobe. Although this goal has been accomplished successfully using thoracoscopic technique, other investigators have favored an open technique because of the overexpanded lobe and the difficulty this presents with visualization during thoracoscopic technique. Removal of a lung lobe can be accomplished safely in any age group and is tolerated well.[137,144,154,155] Some

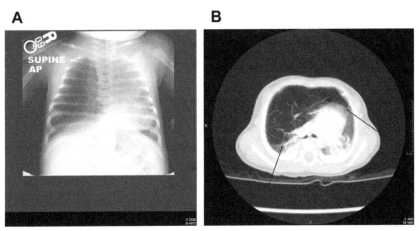

**Fig. 7.** (*A*) Hyperexpanded right lung shows lung markings throughout, indicating CLE in this infant. The mediastinum is shifted to the left. (*B*) CT image of the CLE (*arrows*) shown in the radiograph in (*A*); this lesion involved the right upper and middle lobes.

investigators have advocated observation of patients who are asymptomatic. This practice has been successful in the short-term in a few series.[137,147,148,156] However, others have suggested that lung lobes that seem to harbor CLE may contain other disease, such as CCAM, that places the patient at risk. There have been reports of patients having lobectomies for a diagnosis of symptomatic CLE only to have other pathologic tissue, such as that indicating CCAM, found within the specimen. Furthermore, if lung lobe removal is needed beyond the infant and toddler years, a window for compensatory lung growth may be lost. Long-term follow-up involves repeated radiologic studies that may present potential risk. In general, long-term results of nonoperative management beyond childhood are not known.[146,148,151,157]

### Esophageal Atresia and Tracheoesophageal Fistula

Esophageal atresia and tracheoesophageal fistula (EA-TEF) refer to a constellation of anomalies that result from improper embryogenesis of the foregut. Historically, these lesions were believed to be caused by inappropriate fusion of invaginating lateral longitudinal ridges, which created a septum dividing the foregut into the trachea and the esophagus. However, more modern evidence suggests that foregut development is more intimately involved with the respiratory tract development itself. Adriamycin-induced EA-TEF in rats suggests that the fistula and lower esophagus is of respiratory origin. Another theory holds that abnormalities in signaling of the organ differentiation-promoting glycoprotein, sonic hedgehog, play a role in these esophageal anomalies. Therefore, further understanding is needed about the origin of these anomalies.[158-161]

EA-TEFs affect males and females equally and occur in about 1 per 3000 to 5000 live births. Infants affected by EA-TEF are premature in 35% of cases. A variety of anatomic areas are known to have a high incidence of anomalies in infants born with EA-TEF. This constellation was originally given the acronym VATER association. This term was later expanded to include the recognized increased incidence of congenital cardiac anomalies and therefore was denoted VACTERL: V, vertebral; A, anorectal; C, cardiac; TE, tracheoesophageal; R, renal; L, limb; lumbar. EA-TEF may also be associated with a variety of other conditions, including Down syndrome, Di George sequence, polysplenia, Pierre-Robin sequence, Fanconi syndrome and the CHARGE association (coloboma, heart defects, atresia choanae, developmental retardation, genital hypoplasia, ear deformities).[158,162,163]

The presence of EA-TEF, when not an isolated fistula, may occasionally be detected on prenatal ultrasonography. Findings of a small stomach, polyhydramnios, or upper pouch dilation may be evident.[164] Fetal MRI may be a useful tool in showing EA-TEF prenatally when suspected.[165] Delivery method is based on the obstetric needs of the mother and baby, but delivery at a tertiary care center is typically desired.

EA-TEFs are typically classified into 5 basic types, although many variations may exist.[166] The 5 types and their relative incidences are shown in **Fig. 8**. Type C is the most common. Type D may occur more frequently than originally believed because many of what are believed to be recurrent TEFs after repair of type C EA-TEF are missed proximal fistulae of type D.[158,167]

Symptoms of EA-TEF are usually evident at birth. If esophageal atresia is present, the infant often shows excessive drooling at birth. Any attempt at feeding results in regurgitation and choking. Aspiration may result in cyanosis and respiratory distress. An attempt to pass an orogastric tube results in resistance. If a distal fistula is present, the abdomen may become distended because of inspired air filling the stomach through the fistula. This situation may be exacerbated by any positive pressure generated by hand-mask ventilation, or positive pressure ventilation through an

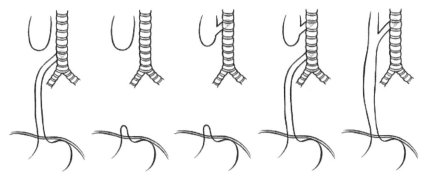

**Fig. 8.** Classification of esophageal atresia or tracheoesophageal fistula (from *left* to *right*): type C, esophageal atresia with distal tracheoesophageal fistula (85%); type A, esophageal atresia without fistula (8%); type B, esophageal atresia with proximal fistula (1%); type D, esophageal atresia with proximal and distal fistulae (2%); type E, tracheoesophageal fistula (H-type) without atresia (4%). (*Adapted from* Bax K. Esophageal atresia and tracheoesophageal malformations. In: Holcomb III GW, Murphy JP, editors. Ashcraft's pediatric surgery. 5th edition. Philadelphia: Saunders; 2010. p. 346; with permission.)

endotracheal tube. In addition, pulmonary compromise may result from reflux of gastric contents into the airway through a distal fistula, or from spill-over of saliva from the proximal atretic pouch. A chest radiograph that includes the neck shows the end of a tube placed through the mouth or nose into the esophagus to be at the level of the lower neck or proximal thorax. Instillation of a small amount of air can help outline the proximal atretic esophageal pouch. An abdominal radiograph shows the presence of air in the intestine if there is a distal TEF. However, the absence of air typically indicates the presence of isolated esophageal atresia. This finding is the same in the rare instance of esophageal atresia with only a proximal fistula. The length of the proximal pouch, and the presence or absence of a proximal fistula, can be determined by instillation of 0.5 to 1 mL of thin barium under direct fluoroscopic vision (**Fig. 9**). A proximal fistula can also be assessed for using bronchoscopy at the time of surgery if necessary.

Isolated TEF without EA is usually a delayed diagnosis because the esophagus is intact, and babies often tolerate early feeds. However, these babies tend to have frequent coughing with feeding and are prone to recurrent respiratory infections. The diagnosis can be established by a contrast esophagogram. However, it is important to specifically discuss with the radiologist that an isolated TEF is being sought because the baby must be prone, and possibly in a small amount of Trendelenburg position, to define this fistula with the contrast. This radiographic strategy is used because the fistula typically courses from the esophagus in a cephalad direction to the trachea. Bronchoscopy or esophagoscopy may be required if suspicion remains high and the contrast study is negative.

When EA or TEF is established, further workup is required to assess for any of the anomalies of the VACTERL association. Evaluation should include a thorough physical examination, looking particularly for any anorectal anomalies, a cardiac echo, a renal echo, chromosomal studies, and appropriate plain radiographs to assess the vertebral column and limbs as needed.

In the preoperative period, the infant should be positioned in a semiupright position. A suction catheter should be placed in the atretic esophageal pouch, and intravenous fluids and antibiotic coverage should be provided. It is preferable to avoid intubation if

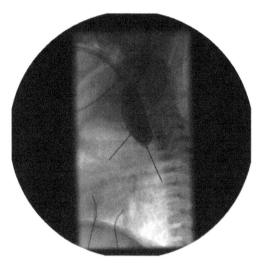

**Fig. 9.** The atretic proximal pouch of esophageal atresia is outlined by instillation of thin barium (*arrows*) under direct fluoroscopy. No proximal fistula is found.

possible, but if intubation is required for airway support, it is desirable to keep the positive pressure as low as possible, and even allow the baby to breathe on its own if possible. In the rare instance that an infant's respiratory status is unduly compromised by abdominal distention, an emergent gastrostomy tube can be placed for decompression.

Operative intervention can usually be undertaken in an elective or semielective manner. The particular operation is determined by the lesion present. Type C and type D anomalies can usually be repaired primarily. The traditional approach has been via a right-sided thoracotomy through the fourth intercostal space. A muscle-splitting incision may preserve most or all of the latissimus dorsi and serratus anterior muscles and reduce the incidence of muscle atrophy and scoliosis. A retropleural dissection facilitates exposure. The fistula (or fistulae) is divided and a primary anastomosis of the esophagus is accomplished with a single layer of suture. This repair has also been accomplished via a thoracoscopic technique.[168] The repair can be assessed at 5 to 7 days postoperatively with an esophagogram. If there is no leak, and the anastomosis is acceptably patent, feeding by mouth can begin and any chest drainage tubes can be removed.

Occasionally, a right-sided aortic arch may be discovered on preoperative cardiac echo, or at operation. Repair can be undertaken either through a right-sided or left-sided approach. However, these infants are prone to having a long-gap atresia, double aortic arch, or other arch anomalies.[169,170] If a long-gap atresia is found at operation for a type C or D lesion, it is best to divide the fistula(e), attach the lower esophagus to the prevertebral fascia, and place a gastrostomy feeding tube. The infant can then be supported with a suction catheter in the proximal pouch and gastrostomy feeds for the next 8 to 12 weeks. The 2 ends of the esophagus typically grow closer together over this time, or at least grow stronger, thereby optimizing the opportunity to use the native esophagus at final repair. Some investigators advocate techniques of bougienage of the proximal pouch and bolus feeding of the stomach to stretch the esophagus at both ends as much as possible. Techniques at operation for maximizing esophageal length include mobilizing both the proximal and distal esophageal limbs, and circular or spiral myotomy for the proximal limb. External traction on the proximal and distal limbs has also been reported. If the esophagus cannot be approximated, operative strategies can include gastric pull-up, gastric tube formation, and colon interposition.[171–178]

Operative strategy for isolated esophageal atresia, or EA with proximal TEF (types A and B), is the same as that for long-gap atresia found with type C or D, as described earlier. Types A and B commonly have a long gap between the 2 ends of the esophagus. If a proximal fistula is present, bronchoscopic and esophagoscopic evaluation can localize it, and the fistula may be divided through the neck.

Isolated TEF can usually be repaired through a neck approach. Bronchoscopy is used to place a ureteral catheter through the fistula into the esophagus. The infant is then intubated, and the catheter is retrieved via esophagoscopy. The catheter is then used to localize the fistula by both traction and fluoroscopic examination. Care must be taken to preserve the recurrent laryngeal nerves during the division of an isolated TEF and the subsequent repairs of the esophagus and trachea. Surgical division may be accomplished via a thoracoscopic technique.[179] Obliteration of an isolated TEF using a yttrium aluminum garnet laser or electrocautery has also been described.[180]

Prognosis for outcomes from EA-TEF repairs has been classified in many ways, and with modifications, over the years. The Waterston and Spitz classifications have based prognosis primarily on birth weight and the presence or absence of cardiac disease. Overall, survival has improved markedly over the years, and in general, with modern intensive care unit support and surgical technique and strategies, outcomes are favorable, rendering these classifications potentially obsolete.[158]

Complications of repair of EA or TEF include (with reported ranges) leak (5%–20%), stricture (6%–40%), dysphagia (50%–75%), reflux (30%–60%), recurrent fistula (10%), chest wall deformity (5%), and scoliosis (5%).[181,182] Esophageal motility is not normal in patients with esophageal atresia, and parents must be counseled to provide food that infants and children can chew and swallow well. Strictures can usually be balloon-dilated under fluoroscopic guidance. The advantage of this strategy over bougienage is that the dilation is performed under direct vision with controlled pressures, and any leak can be studied immediately.[183,184] Recurrent fistulae have traditionally been repaired via thoracotomy, sometimes using a pericardial, pleural, or azygous vein flap. However, recurrent fistula rates after thoracotomy for initial recurrence approach 20%.[185–187] Successful closure of a recurrent fistula using a bronchoscopic technique has been described.[188]

Increasing information is being gathered regarding the long-term outcomes of EA-TEF repairs because some of the patients repaired in the early days of these repairs are now adults. Many of these patients have symptoms of gastroesophageal reflux, dysphagia, and occasional compromised passage of food. They have learned to accommodate this in many instances. In addition, endoscopic studies have shown that some patients do have inflammatory or metaplastic changes in their esophageal mucosa. However, there are no reports linking any increase in esophageal cancer to patients having undergone EA-TEF repair.[179,189–191] In addition, when symptoms have been recognized in these patients, they seem to dissipate noticeably in many patients over the long-term.[181,182]

## REFERENCES

1. McGahren ED, Rodgers BM. Mediastinum and pleura. In: Oldham KT, Colombani PM, Foglia RP, et al, editors. Principles and practice of pediatric surgery. Philadelphia: Lippincott Williams & Wilkins; 2005. p. 929–49.

2. Tova JA. Mediastinal tumors. In: Holcomb GW III, Murphy JP, editors. Ashcraft's pediatric surgery. 5th edition. Philadelphia: Saunders; 2010. p. 345–61.

3. Davis RD, Oldham HN, Sabiston DC. The mediastinum. In: Sabiston DC, Spencer FC, editors. Surgery of the chest. 6th edition. Philadelphia: WB Saunders; 1995. p. 576–612.

4. Agostoni E, D'Angelo E. Pleural liquid pressure. J Appl Physiol 1991;71: 393–403.

5. Wang PM, Lai-Fook SJ. Upward flow of pleural liquid near lobar margins due to cardiogenic motion. J App1 Physiol 1992;73:2314–9.

6. Wiener-Kronish JP, Broaddus VC. Interrelationships of pleural and pulmonary interstitial liquid. Annu Rev Physiol 1993;55:209–26.

7. Dunnill MS. Postnatal growth of the lung. Thorax 1962;17:329–33.

8. Cohen RG, DeMeester TR, Lafontaine E. The pleura. In: Sabiston DC, Spencer FC, editors. Surgery of the chest. 6th edition. Philadelphia: WE Saunders; 1995. p. 523–75.

9. Ravitch MM. Mediastinal cysts and tumors. In: Welch KJ, Randolph JG, Ravitch MM, et al, editors. Pediatric surgery. 4th edition. Chicago: Year Book Medical Publishers; 1986. p. 602–18.

10. Shih CH, Yu HW, Tseng YC, et al. Clinical manifestations of primary spontaneous pneumothorax in pediatric patients: an analysis of 78 patients. Pediatr Neonatol 2011;52:150–4.

11. Seguier-Lipszyc E, Elizur A, Klin B, et al. Management of primary spontaneous pneumothorax in children. Clin Pediatr 2011;50(9):797–802.

12. Benteur L, Canny G, Thorner P, et al. Spontaneous pneumothorax in cystic adenomatoid malformation. Chest 1991;99:1292–3.

13. Davis AM, Wensley DF, Phelan PD. Spontaneous pneumothorax in pediatric patients. Respir Med 1993;87:531–4.

14. Kemp JS, Seilheimer DK. Diseases of the pleura. In: Oski FA, editor. Principles and practice of pediatrics. 1st edition. Philadelphia: JB Lippincott; 1990. p. 1378.

15. Teeratakulpisarn J, Wiangnon S, Srinakarin J, et al. Pleuropulmonary blastoma in a child presenting with spontaneous pneumothorax. J Med Assoc Thai 2003; 86(4):385–91.

16. Numanami H, Tanaka M, Hashizume M, et al. Pleuropulmonary blastoma in a 12-year-old boy presenting with pneumothorax. Jpn J Thorac Cardiovasc Surg 2006;54:504–6.

17. Khosia A, Parry RL. Costal osteochondroma causing pneumothorax in an adolescent: a case report and review of the literature. J Pediatr Surg 2010; 45(11):2250–3.

18. Trevisanuto D, Doglioni N, Ferrarese P, et al. Neonatal pneumothorax: comparison between neonatal transfers and inborn infants. J Perinat Med 2005;33(5): 449–54.

19. Faranoff AA, Stoll BJ, Wright LL, et al. Trends in neonatal morbidity and mortality for very low birth weight infants. Am J Obstet Gynecol 2007;196(2):e1–8.

20. Horbar JD, Carpenter JH, Buzas, et al. Collaborative quality improvement to promote evidence based surfactant for preterm infants: a cluster randomized trial. BMJ 2004;329(7473):1004–11.

21. Litmanovitz I, Carlo WA. Expectant management of pneumothorax in ventilated infants. Pediatrics 2008;122(5):e975–9.

22. Zierold D, Lee SL, Subramanian S, et al. Supplemental oxygen improves resolution of injury-induced pneumothorax. J Pediatr Surg 2000;35:998–1001.

23. Vernejoux JM, Raherison C, Combe P, et al. Spontaneous pneumothorax: pragmatic management and long-term outcome. Respir Med 2001;95:857.

24. Gammie JS, Banks MC, Fuhrman CR, et al. The pigtail catheter for pleural drainage: a less invasive alternative to tube thoracostomy. JSLS 1999;3:57.

25. Noemi T, Hannukainen J, Aarnio P. Use of the Heimlich valve for treating pneumothorax. Ann Chir Gynaecol 1999;88:36.

26. Poenaru D, Yazbeck S, Murphy S. Primary spontaneous pneumothorax in children. J Pediatr Surg 1994;29:1183–5.

27. Cook CH, Melvin WS, Groner JI, et al. A cost-effective thoracoscopic treatment strategy for pediatric spontaneous pneumothorax. Surg Endosc 1999;13:1208–10.

28. Butterworth SA, Blair GK, LeBlanc JG, et al. An open and shut case for early VATS treatment of primary spontaneous pneumothorax in children. Can J Surg 2007;50:171–4.

29. Qureshi FG, Sandulache VC, Richardson W, et al. Primary vs delayed surgery for spontaneous pneumothorax in children: which is better? J Pediatr Surg 2005;40:166–9.

30. Bialas RC, Weiner TM, Phillips JD. Video-assisted thoracic surgery for primary spontaneous pneumothorax in children: is there an optimal technique? J Pediatr Surg 2008;43(12):2151–5.

31. Sarkar S, Hussain N, Herson V. Fibrin glue for persistent pneumothorax in neonates. J Perinatol 2003;23:82–4.

32. Canpolat FE, Yurdakok M, Yurttutan S. Fibrin glue for persistent pneumothorax in an extremely low birth weight infant. Indian Pediatr 2006;43:646–7.

33. Stringel G, Amin NS, Dozor AJ. Video-assisted thoracoscopy in the management of recurrent spontaneous pneumothorax in the pediatric population. JSLS 1999;3:113.

34. Inderbitzi RGC, Furrer M, Striffeler H, et al. Thoracoscopic pleurectomy for treatment of complicated spontaneous pneumothorax. J Thorac Cardiovasc Surg 1993;105:84.

35. Özcan C, McGahren ED, Rodgers BM. Thoracoscopic treatment of spontaneous pneumothorax in children. J Pediatr Surg 2003;38(10):1459–64.

36. Treasure T. Minimally invasive surgery for pneumothorax: the evidence, changing practice and current opinion. J R Soc Med 2007;100:419–22.

37. Sakatmoto K, Takei H, Nishii T, et al. Staple line coverage with absorbable mesh after thoracoscopic bullectomy for spontaneous pneumothorax. Surg Endosc 2004;18:478–81.

38. Cho S, Ryu KM, Jheon S, et al. Additional mechanical pleurodesis after thoracoscopic wedge resection and covering procedure for primary spontaneous pneumothorax. Surg Endosc 2009;23:986–90.

39. de Campos JR, Vargas FS, de Campos WE, et al. Thoracoscopy talc poudrage: a 15-year experience. Chest 2001;119:801–6.

40. Hunt I, Barber B, Southon R, et al. Is talc pleurodesis safe for young patients following primary spontaneous pneumothorax? Inter Cardiovasc Thor Surg 2007;6:117–20.

41. Gyorik S, Erni S, Studler U, et al. Long-term follow-up of thoracoscopic talc pleurodesis for primary spontaneous pneumothorax. Eur Respir J 2007;29:757–60.

42. Cardillo G, Carleo F, Giunti R, et al. Videothoracoscopic talc poudrage in primary spontaneous pneumothorax: a single institution experience in 861 cases. J Thorac Cardiovasc Surg 2006;131:322–8.

43. Plentinckx P, Muysoms F, De Decker C, et al. Thoracoscopic talc pleurodesis for the treatment of spontaneous pneumothorax. Acta Chir Belg 2005;105(5):504–7.

44. Tribble CG, Selden RF, Rodgers BM. Talc poudrage in the treatment of spontaneous pneumothoraces in patients with cystic fibrosis. Ann Surg 1986;204: 677–80.

45. Austin EH, Flye MW. The treatment of recurrent malignant pleural effusion. Ann Thorac Surg 1979;28:190–203.

46. Spector ML, Stern RC. Pneumothorax in cystic fibrosis: a 26-year experience. Ann Thorac Surg 1989;47:204–7.

47. Stephenson LW. Treatment of pneumothorax with intrapleural tetracycline. Chest 1985;88:803–4.

48. Chen JS, Tsai KT, Hsu HH, et al. Intrapleural minocycline following simple aspiration for initial treatment of primary spontaneous pneumothorax. Respir Med 2008;102:1004–10.

49. Chen JS, Hsu HH, Chen RJ, et al. Additional minocylcline pleurodesis after thoracoscopic surgery for primary spontaneous pneumothorax. Am J Respir Crit Care Med 2006;173:548–54.

50. Hazelrigg SR, Landreneau RJ, Mack M, et al. Thoracoscopic stapled resection for spontaneous pneumothorax. J Thorac Cardiovasc Surg 1993;105: 389–93.

51. Rodgers BM, McGahren ED. Endoscopy in children. Chest Surg Clin N Am 1993;3:405.

52. Kokoska ER, Chen MK. The New Technology Committee. Position paper on video-assisted thoracoscopic surgery as treatment of pediatric empyema. J Pediatr Surg 2009;44:289–93.

53. Fajardo JE, Chang MG. Pleural empyema in children: a nationwide retrospective study. South Med J 1987;80:593–6.

54. Bartlett JG, Gorbach SL, Thadepalli HT, et al. Bacteriology of empyema. Lancet 1974;1:338–40.

55. American Thoracic Society. Management of nontuberculous empyema. Am Rev Respir Dis 1962;85:935–6.

56. Chonmaitree T, Powell KR. Parapneumonic pleural effusion and empyema in children. Clin Pediatr 1983;22:414–9.

57. St. Peter SD, Tsao K, Harrison C, et al. Thoracoscopic decortication vs tube thoracoscopy with fibrinolysis for empyema in children: a prospective, randomized trial. J Pediatr Surg 2009;44:106–11.

58. Martinón-Torres F, Dosil-Gallardo S, Perez del Molino-Bernal ML, et al. Pleural antigen assay in the diagnosis of pediatric pneumococcal empyema. J Crit Care 2011. [Epub ahead of print].

59. Dass R, Deka NM, Barman H, et al. Empyema thoracis: analysis of 150 cases from a tertiary care center in North East India. Indian J Pediatr 2011;78(11):1371–7.

60. Picard E, Joseph L, Goldberg S, et al. Predictive factors of morbidity in childhood parapneumonic effusion-associated pneumonia: a prospective study. Pediatr Infect Dis J 2010;29:840–3.

61. Strachan RE, Cornelius A, Gilbert GL, et al. A bedside assay to detect streptococcus pneumoniae in children with empyema. Pediatr Pulmonol 2011;46: 179–83.

62. Li ST, Tancredi DJ. Empyema hospitalization increased in US children despite pneumococcal conjugate vaccine. Pediatrics 2010;125(1):26–33.

63. Lewis KT, Bukstein DA. Parapneumonic empyema in children: diagnosis and management. Am Fam Physician 1992;46:1443–55.

64. Gustafson RA, Murray GF, Warden HE, et al. Role of lung decortication in symptomatic empyemas in children. Ann Thorac Surg 1990;49:940–7.

65. Hoff SJ, Neblett WW, Heller RM, et al. Postpneumonic empyema in childhood: selecting appropriate therapy. J Pediatr Surg 1989;24:659–64.

66. Ramnath RR, Heller RM, Ben-Ami T, et al. Implications of early sonographic evaluation of parapneumonic effusions in children with pneumonia. Pediatrics 1998; 101:68–71.

67. Carter E, Waldhausen J, Zhang W, et al. Management of children with empyema: pleural drainage is not always necessary. Pediatr Pulmonol 2010; 45:475–80.

68. Kosloske AM, Carwright KC. The controversial role of decortication in the management of pediatric empyema. J Thorac Cardiovasc Surg 1988;96: 166–70.

69. Chan PW, Crawford O, Wallis C, et al. Treatment of pleural empyema. J Paediatr Child Health 2000;36:375–7.

70. Chan W, Keyser-Gauvin E, Davis GM, et al. Empyema thoracis in children: a 26-year review of the Montreal Children's Hospital experience. J Pediatr Surg 1997; 32:870–2.

71. Kern JA, Rodgers BD. Thoracoscopy in the management of empyema in children. J Pediatr Surg 1993;28:1128–32.

72. Cohen G, Hjortdal V, Ricci M, et al. Primary thoracoscopic treatment of empyema in children. J Thorac Cardiovasc Surg 2003;125:79–84.

73. Kercher KW, Attori RJ, Hoover JD, et al. Thoracoscopic decortication as first-line therapy for pediatric parapneumonic empyema. A case series. Chest 2000;118: 24–7.

74. Meier AH, Smith B, Raghavan A, et al. Rational treatment of empyema in children. Arch Surg 2000;135:907–12.

75. Chen LE, Langer JC, Dillon PA, et al. Management of late-stage parapneumonic empyema. J Pediatr Surg 2002;37:371–4.

76. Stovroff M, Teague G, Heiss KH, et al. Thoracoscopy in the management of pediatric empyema. J Pediatr Surg 1995;30:1211–5.

77. Schneider CR, Gauderer MW, Blackhurst D, et al. Video-assisted thoracoscopic surgery as a primary intervention in pediatric effusion and empyema. Am Surg 2010;76:957–61.

78. Aziz A, Healey JM, Qureshi F, et al. Comparative analysis of chest tube thoracostomy and video-assisted thoracoscopic surgery in empyema and parapneumonic effusion associated with pneumonia in children. Surg Infect 2008;9(3):317–23.

79. Menon P, Kanojia RP, Rao KL. Empyema thoracis: surgical management in children. J Indian Assoc Pediatr Surg 2009;14(3):85–93.

80. Cochran JB, Tecklenburg FW, Turner RB. Intrapleural instillation of fibrinolytic agents for treatment of pleural empyema. Pediatr Crit Care Med 2003;4:39–43.

81. Wells RG, Havens PL. Intrapleural fibrinolysis for parapnuemonic effusion and empyema in children. Radiology 2003;228:370–8.

82. Nagasawa KK, Johnson SM. Thoracoscopic treatment of pediatric lung abscesses. J Pediatr Surg 2010;45:574–8.

83. Kosloske AM, Ball WS, Butler C, et al. Drainage of pediatric lung abscess by cough, catheter, or complete resection. J Pediatr Surg 1986;21:596–600.

84. Lacey SR, Kosloske AM. Pneumonostomy in the management of pediatric lung abscess. J Pediatr Surg 1983;18:625–7.

85. Gocman A, Kiper N, Toppare M, et al. Conservative treatment of empyema in children. Respiration 1993;60:182–5.

86. Redding GJ, Walund L, Walund D, et al. Lung function in children following empyema. Am J Dis Child 1990;144:1337–42.
87. Helin RD, Angeles ST, Bhat R. Octreotide therapy for infants and children: a brief review. Pediatr Crit Care Med 2006;7:576–9.
88. Gallego C, Martin P, Moral MT, et al. Congenital chylothorax: from foetal life to adolescence. Acta Paediatr 2010;99:1571–7.
89. Dubin PJ, King IN, Gallagher PG. Congenital chylothorax. Curr Opin Pediatr 2000;12:505–9.
90. Al-Tawil K, Ahmed G, Al-Hathal M, et al. Congenital chylothorax. Am J Perinatol 2000;17(3):121–6.
91. Allen EM, Van Heeckeren DW, Spector ML, et al. Management of nutritional and infectious complications of postoperative chylothorax in children. J Pediatr Surg 1991;26:1169–74.
92. Chan EH, Russell JL, Williams WG, et al. Postoperative chylothorax after cardiothoracic surgery in children. Ann Thorac Surg 2005;80:1864–71.
93. Hanekamp MN, Tjin A, Djie GC, et al. Does V-A ECMO increase the likelihood of chylothorax after congenital diaphragmatic hernia repair? J Pediatr Surg 2003; 38:971–4.
94. Zavala A, Campos JM, Ruitort C, et al. Chylothorax in congenital diaphragmatic hernia. Pediatr Surg Int 2010;26:919–22.
95. Kamiyama M, Usui N, Tani G, et al. Postoperative chylothorax in congenital diaphragmatic hernia. Eur J Pediatr Surg 2010;20:391–4.
96. Gonzalez R, Bryner BS, Teitelbaum DH, et al. Chylothorax after congenital diaphragmatic hernia repair. J Pediatr Surg 2009;44:1181–5.
97. Easa D, Balaraman V, Ash K, et al. Congenital chylothorax and mediastinal neuroblastoma. J Pediatr Surg 1991;26:96–8.
98. McCulloch MA, Conaway MR, Haizlip JA, et al. Postoperative chylothorax development is associated with increased incidence and risk profile for central venous thromboses. Pediatr Cardiol 2008;29:556–61.
99. Geismer S, Tilelli JA, Campbell JB, et al. Chylothorax as a manifestation of child abuse. Pediatr Emerg Care 1997;13(6):386–9.
100. Gulesarian KJ, Gilchrist BF, Luks FI, et al. Child abuse as a cause of traumatic chylothorax. J Pediatr Surg 1996;31:1696–7.
101. Beghetti M, La Scala G, Belli D, et al. Etiology and management of pediatric chylothorax. J Pediatr 2000;136:653–8.
102. Paget-Brown A, Kattwinkel J, Rodgers BM, et al. The use of octreotide to treat congenital chylothorax. J Pediatr Surg 2006;41:845–7.
103. Biewer ES, Zürn C, Arnold R, et al. Chylothorax after surgery on congenital heart disease in newborns and infants–risk factors and efficacy of MCT-diet. J Cardiothorac Surg 2010;5:127–33.
104. Milonakis M, Chatzis AC, Giannopoulos NM, et al. Etiology and management of chylothorax following pediatric heart surgery. J Card Surg 2009;24:369–73.
105. Das A, Shah PS. Octreotide for the treatment of chylothorax in neonates (review). Cochrane Database Syst Rev 2010;(9):1–16.
106. Au M, Weber TR, Fleming RE. Successful use of somatostatin in a case of neonatal chylothorax. J Pediatr Surg 2003;38:1106–7.
107. Tauber MT, Harris AG, Rochicciol P. Clinical use of the long acting somatostatin analogue octreotide in pediatrics. Eur J Pediatr 1994;153:304–10.
108. Caverly L, Rausch CM, da Cruz E, et al. Octreotide treatment of chylothorax in pediatric patients following cardiothoracic surgery. Congenit Heart Dis 2010; 5(6):573–8.

109. Wright SB, Mainwaring RD. Octreotide management of chylothorax following bidirectional Glenn in a three-month old infant. J Card Surg 2009;24:216–8.

110. Rosti L, De Battisti F, Butera G, et al. Octreotide in the management of postoperative chylothorax. Pediatr Cardiol 2005;26:440–3.

111. Landvoight MT, Mullett CJ. Octreotide efficacy in the treatment of chylothoraces following cardiac surgery in infants and children. Pediatr Crit Care Med 2006; 7(3):245–8.

112. Murphy MC, Newman BM, Rodgers BM. Pleuro-peritoneal shunts in the management of persistent chylothorax. Ann Thorac Surg 1989;48:195–200.

113. Engum SA, Rescorla FJ, West KW, et al. The use of pleuroperitoneal shunts in the management of persistent chylothorax in infants. J Pediatr Surg 1999;34: 286–90.

114. Wolff AB, Silen ML, Kokoska ER, et al. Treatment of refractory chylothorax with externalized pleuroperitoneal shunts in children. Ann Thorac Surg 1999;65: 1053–7.

115. Rheuban KS, Kron IL, Carpenter MA. Pleuroperitoneal shunts for refractory chylothorax after operation for congenital heart disease. Ann Thorac Surg 1992;53: 85–7.

116. Itkin M, Krishnamurthy G, Naim MY, et al. Percutaneous thoracic duct embolization as a treatment for intrathoracic chyle leaks in infants. Pediatrics 2011;128: e237–41.

117. Le Nué R, Molinaro F, Gomes-Ferreira C, et al. Surgical management of congenital chylothorax in children. Eur J Pediatr Surg 2010;20:307–11.

118. Nath DS, Savla J, Robinder BS, et al. Thoracic duct ligation for persistent chylothorax after pediatric cardiothoracic surgery. Ann Thorac Surg 2009;88: 246–52.

119. Cleveland K, Zook D, Harvey K, et al. Massive chylothorax in small babies. J Pediatr Surg 2009;44:546–50.

120. Graham DD, McGahren ED, Tribble CG, et al. Use of video- assisted thoracic surgery in the treatment of chylothorax. Ann Thorac Surg 1994;57:1507–12.

121. Nagata K, Masumoto K, Tesiba R, et al. Outcome and treatment in an antenatally diagnosed congenital cystic adenomatoid malformation of the lung. Pediatr Surg Int 2009;25:753–7.

122. Wong A, Vieten D, Singh S, et al. Long-term outcome of asymptomatic patients with congenital cystic adenomatoid malformation. Pediatr Surg Int 2009;25: 479–85.

123. Adzick NS. Management of fetal lung lesions. Clin Perinatol 2009;39:363–6.

124. Rothenberg SS, Kuenzler KA, Middlesworth W, et al. Thoracoscopic lobectomy in infants less than 10 kg with prenatally diagnosed cystic lung disease. J Laparoendosc Adv Surg Tech A 2011;21(2):181–4.

125. Chen H, Hsu W, Lu FL, et al. Management of congenital cystic adenomatoid malformation and bronchopulmonary sequestration in newborns. Pediatric Neonatology 2010;51(3):172–7.

126. MacSweeney F, Papagiannopoulos K, Goldstraw P, et al. An assessment of the expanded classification of congenital cystic adenomatoid malformations and their relationship to malignant transformation. Am J Surg Pathol 2003;27(8): 1139–46.

127. Hammond PJ, Devdas JM, Ray B, et al. The outcome of expectant management of congenital cystic adenomatoid malformations (CCAM) of the lung. Eur J Pediatr Surg 2010;20:145–9.

128. Sauvat F, Michel J, Benachi A, et al. Management of asymptomatic neonatal cystic adenomatoid malformations. J Pediatr Surg 2003;38:548–52.

129. Raychaudhuri P, Pasupati A, James A, et al. Prospective study of antenatally diagnosed congenital cystic malformations. Pediatr Surg Int 2011;27(11): 1156–64.

130. Wilson RD, Hedrick HL, Liechty KW, et al. Cystic adenomatoid malformation of the lung: review of genetics, prenatal diagnosis, and in utero treatment. Am J Med Genet 2005;140:151–5.

131. Ozcan C, Celik A, Ural Z, et al. Primary pulmonary rhabdomyosarcoma arising within cystic adenomatoid malformation: a case report and review of the literature. J Pediatr Surg 2001;36(7):1062–5.

132. Nasr A, Himidan S, Pastor AC, et al. Is congenital cystic adenomatoid malformation a premalignant lesion for pleuropulmonary blastoma? J Pediatr Surg 2010; 45:1086–9.

133. West D, Nicholson AG, Colquhoun I, et al. Bronchioloalveolar carcinoma in congenital cystic adenomatoid malformation. Ann Thorac Surg 2007;83: 687–9.

134. Hill AD, Dehner LP. A cautionary note about congenital cystic adenomatoid malformation (CCAM) type 4. Am J Surg Pathol 2004;28(4):554–5.

135. Vu LT, Farmer DL, Nobuhara KK, et al. Thoracoscopic versus open resection for congenital cystic adenomatoid malformations of the lung. J Pediatr Surg 2008; 43:359.

136. Azizkhan RG, Crombleholme TM. Congenital cystic lung disease: contemporary antenatal and postnatal management. Pediatr Surg Int 2008;24:643–57.

137. Laberge J, Puligandla P, Flageole H. Asymptomatic congenital lung malformations. Semin Pediatr Surg 2005;14:16–33.

138. Taylor JA, Laor T, Warner BW. Extralobar pulmonary sequestration. Surgery 2008;143:833–4.

139. Laje P, Martinez-Ferro M, Grisoni E, et al. Intraabdominal pulmonary sequestration. a case series and review of the literature. J Pediatr Surg 2006;41: 1309–12.

140. Joyeux L, Mejean N, Rousseau T, et al. Ectopic extralobar pulmonary sequestrations in children: interest of the laparoscopic approach. J Pediatr Surg 2010;45: 2269–73.

141. Moore KL, Persaud TV. The developing human: clinically oriented embryology. 7th edition. Philadelphia: Elsevier; 2003. p. 242–52.

142. Lee BS, Kim JT, Kim EA, et al. Neonatal pulmonary sequestration: clinical experience with transumbilical arterial embolization. Pediatr Pulmonol 2008;43: 404–13.

143. Stern R, Berger S, Casaulta C, et al. Bilateral intralobar pulmonary sequestration in a newborn, case report and review of the literature on bilateral pulmonary sequestrations. J Pediatr Surg 2007;42:E19–23.

144. Pinkerton HJ, Oldham KT. Lung. In: Oldham KT, Colombani PM, Foglia RP, et al, editors. Principles and practice of pediatric surgery. Philadelphia: Lippincott Williams & Wilkins; 2005. p. 951–82.

145. Ulku R, Onat S, Ozçelik C. Congenital lobar emphysema: differential diagnosis and therapeutic approach. Pediatr Int 2008;50:658–61.

146. Robers PA, Holland AJ, Halliday RJ, et al. Congenital lobar emphysema: like father, like son. J Pediatr Surg 2002;37:799–801.

147. Thakral CL, Maji DC, Sajwani MJ. Congenital lobar emphysema: experience with 21 cases. Pediatr Surg Int 2001;17:88–91.

148. Mei-Zahav M, Konen O, Manson D, et al. Is congenital lobar emphysema a surgical disease? J Pediatr Surg 2006;41:1058–61.
149. Mendeloff EN. Sequestrations, congenital cystic adenomatoid malformations, and congenital lobar emphysema. Semin Thorac Cardiovasc Surg 2004;16: 209–14.
150. Seo T, Ando H, Kaneko K, et al. Two cases of prenatally diagnosed congenital lobar emphysema caused by lobar bronchial atresia. J Pediatr Surg 2006;41: E17–20.
151. Eber E. Antenatal diagnosis of congenital thoracic malformations. Early surgery, late surgery, or no surgery? Semin Respir Crit Care Med 2007;28:355–66.
152. Tapper D, Schuster S, McBride J, et al. Polyalveolar lobe: anatomic and physiologic parameters and their relationship to congenital lobar emphysema. J Pediatr Surg 1980;15:931–7.
153. Olutoye OO, Coleman BG, Hubbard AM, et al. Prenatal diagnosis and management of congenital lobar emphysema. J Pediatr Surg 2000;35:792–5.
154. Albanese CT, Rothenberg SS. Experience with 144 consecutive pediatric thoracoscopic lobectomies. J Laparoendosc Adv Surg Tech A 2007;17(3):339–41.
155. Rothenberg SS. First decade's experience with thoracoscopic lobectomy in infants and children. J Pediatr Surg 2008;43:40–5.
156. Man DW, Hamdy MH, Hendry GM, et al. Congenital lobar emphysema: problems in diagnosis and management. Arch Dis Child 1983;58:709–12.
157. Tander B, Yalçin M, Yilmax B, et al. Congenital lobar emphysema: a clinicopathologic evaluation of 14 cases. Eur J Pediatr Surg 2003;13:108–11.
158. Harmon CM, Coran AG. Congenital anomalies of the foregut. In: Grosfeld JL, O'Neill JA, Fonkalsrud EW, et al, editors. Pediatric surgery. 6th edition. Philadelphia: Mosby; 2006. p. 1051–81.
159. Beasley SW, Williams AK, Qi BQ, et al. The development of the proximal oesophageal pouch in the adriamycin rat model of oesophageal atresia with tracheoesophageal fistula. Pediatr Surg Int 2004;20(7):548–50.
160. Spilde T, Bhatia A, Ostlie D, et al. A role for sonic hedgehog signaling in the pathogenesis of human tracheoesophageal fistula. J Pediatr Surg 2003;38(3): 465–8.
161. Spilde TL, Bhatia AM, Miller KA, et al. Thyroid transcription factor-1 expression in the human neonatal tracheoesophageal fistula. J Pediatr Surg 2002;37(7):1065–7.
162. Quan L, Smith DW. The VATER association. Vertebral defects, anal atresia, T-E fistula with esophageal atresia, radial and renal dysplasia: a spectrum of associated defects. J Pediatr 1973;82(1):104–7.
163. Barry JE, Auldist AW. The Vater association; one end of a spectrum of anomalies. Am J Dis Child 1974;128(6):769–71.
164. Stringer MD, McKenna KM, Goldstein RB, et al. Prenatal diagnosis of esophageal atresia. J Pediatr Surg 1995;30:1258–63.
165. Langer JC, Hussain H, Khan A, et al. Prenatal diagnosis of esophageal atresia using sonography and magnetic resonance imaging. J Pediatr Surg 2001;36(5): 804–7.
166. Kluth D. Atlas of esophageal atresia. J Pediatr Surg 1976;11:901–19.
167. Johnson AM, Rodgers BM, Alford B, et al. Esophageal atresia with double fistula: the missed anomaly. Ann Thorac Surg 1984;38(3):195–200.
168. Rothenberg SS. Thoracoscopic repair of tracheoesophageal fistula in newborns. J Pediatr Surg 2002;37(6):869–72.
169. Babu R, Pierro A, Spitz L, et al. The management of oesophageal atresia in neonates with right-sided arch. J Pediatr Surg 2000;35(1):56–8.

170. Canty TG Jr, Boyle EM, Linden B, et al. Aortic arch anomalies associated with long gap esophageal atresia and tracheoesophageal fistula. J Pediatr Surg 1997;32(11):1587–91.

171. Puri P, Ninan GK, Blake NS, et al. Delayed primary anastomosis for esophageal atresia: 18 months' to 11 years' follow-up. J Pediatr Surg 1992;27(8):1127–30.

172. Davison P, Poenaru D, Kamal I. Esophageal atresia: primary repair of a rare long gap variant involving distal pouch mobilization. J Pediatr Surg 1999;34(2):1881–3.

173. Lopes MF, Reis A, Coutinho S, et al. Very long gap esophageal atresia successfully treated by esophageal lengthening using external traction suture. J Pediatr Surg 2004;39(8):1286–7.

174. Bagolan P, Iacobelli Bd B, De Angelis P, et al. Long gap esophageal atresia and esophageal replacement: moving toward a separation. J Pediatr Surg 2004; 39(7):1084–90.

175. Al-Qahtani AR, Yazbeck S, Rosen NG, et al. Lengthening technique for long gap esophageal atresia and early anastomosis. J Pediatr Surg 2003;38(5):737–9.

176. Farkash U, Lazar L, Erez I, et al. The distal pouch in esophageal atresia–to dissect or not to dissect, that is the question. Eur J Pediatr Surg 2002;12:19–23.

177. Varjavandi V, Shi E. Early primary repair of long gap esophageal atresia: the VA-TER operation. J Pediatr Surg 2000;35:1830–2.

178. Healey PJ, Sawin RS, Hall DG, et al. Delayed primary repair of esophageal atresia with tracheoesophageal fistula: is it worth the wait? Arch Surg 1998; 133(5):552–6.

179. Allal H, Montes-Tapia F, Andina G, et al. Thoracoscopic repair of H-type tracheoesophageal fistula in the newborn: a technical case report. J Pediatr Surg 2004;39(10):1568–70.

180. Schmittenbacher PP, Mantel K, Hofmann U, et al. Treatment of congenital tracheoesophageal fistula by endoscopic laser coagulation: preliminary report of three cases. J Pediatr Surg 1992;27(1):26–8.

181. Kovesi T, Rubin S. Long-term complications of congenital esophageal atresia and/or tracheoesophageal fistula. Chest 2004;126(3):915–25.

182. Little DC, Rescorla FJ, Grosfeld JL, et al. Long-term analysis of children with esophageal atresia and tracheoesophageal fistula. J Pediatr Surg 2000;38: 852–6.

183. Said M, Mekki M, Golli M, et al. Balloon dilatation of anastomotic strictures secondary to surgical repair of oesophageal atresia. Br J Radiol 2003; 76(901):26–31.

184. Lang T, Hümmer HP, Behrens R. Balloon dilation is preferable to bougienage in children with esophageal atresia. Endoscopy 2001;33(4):329–35.

185. Vos A, Ekkelkamp S. Congenital tracheoesophageal fistula: preventing recurrence. J Pediatr Surg 1996;31(7):936–8.

186. Wheatley MJ, Coran AG. Pericardial flap interposition for the definitive management of recurrent tracheoesophageal fistula. J Pediatr Surg 1992; 27(8):1122–6.

187. Ein SH, Stringer DA, Stephens CA, et al. Recurrent tracheoesophageal fistulas seventeen-year review. J Pediatr Surg 1983;18(4):436–41.

188. McGahren ED, Rodgers BM. Bronchoscopic obliteration of recurrent tracheoesophageal fistula in an infant. Pediatric Endosurgery and Innovative Techniques 2001;5(1):37–41.

189. Duerloo JA, Ekkelkamp S, Bartelsman JF, et al. Gastroesophageal reflux: prevalence in adults older than 28 years after correction of esophageal atresia. Ann Surg 2003;238(5):686–9.

190. Schalamon J, Lindahl H, Saarikoski H, et al. Endoscopic follow-up in esophageal atresia–for how long is it necessary? J Pediatr Surg 2003;38(5):702–4.
191. Montgomery M, Witt H, Kuylenstierna R, et al. Swallowing disorders after esophageal atresia evaluated with videomanometry. J Pediatr Surg 1998;33(8): 1219–23.

# Pediatric Chest II
## Benign Tumors and Cysts

Robin Petroze, MD[a], Eugene D. McGahren, MD[b],*

**KEYWORDS**

- Thoracic tumors • Mediastinal tumors • Benign thoracic tumors
- Pediatric thoracic tumors

**KEY POINTS**

- Thoracic tumors are rare in children, and metastatic or malignant conditions must be excluded during the diagnostic evaluation.
- Tumors of the mediastinum reflect the nature of the tissue in the particular section of the mediastinum in which they arise.
- Diagnostic evaluation usually begins with chest radiography. However, computed tomography and/or magnetic resonance imaging are typically needed.
- Patients may present with upper respiratory symptoms, pain, cough, a mass, and airway, esophageal, or vascular compression.

Thoracic tumors are rare in children, and metastatic or malignant conditions must be excluded during the diagnostic evaluation. The majority of primary pulmonary neoplasms in children are malignant.[1] A review of 383 children with primary pulmonary neoplasms in children found only 24% to be benign.[2] Tumors of the pediatric chest can originate from the lung parenchyma, pleura, chest wall, or mediastinum. Tumors of the chest wall are mostly commonly of the Ewing types (Askin or primitive neuroectodermal tumor [PNET]) or rhabdomyosarcoma. Others include lymphoma, fibrosarcoma, chondrosarcoma, and osteochondroma.[3–6] Tumors of the mediastinum reflect the nature of the tissue in the particular section of the mediastinum in which they arise. Most arise in the posterior compartment (51%), followed by the middle mediastinum and the anterior mediastinum.[5,7] Tumors of the thymus, germ cell tumors, lymphomas, and lymphangiomas occur in the anterior mediastinum. Bronchogenic cysts occur in the middle mediastinum. Neurogenic tumors, which are the most common mediastinal tumors, and esophageal duplication cysts arise in the posterior

a Department of General Surgery, University of Virginia Health System, Box 800709, Charlottesville, VA 22908, USA; b Division of Pediatric Surgery, University of Virginia Children's Hospital, University of Virginia Health System, Box 800709, Charlottesville, VA 22908, USA
* Corresponding author.
*E-mail address:* edm6k@virginia.edu

Surg Clin N Am 92 (2012) 645–658
doi:10.1016/j.suc.2012.03.014
0039-6109/12/$ – see front matter © 2012 Elsevier Inc. All rights reserved.

surgical.theclinics.com

mediastinum. About 75% of malignant mediastinal tumors are symptomatic, whereas only 32% of nonmalignant mediastinal masses are symptomatic.[5]

In general, thoracic tumors can present incidentally without symptoms, or with symptoms of fever, cough, pneumonitis, chest pain, a chest wall mass, or effects of compression of adjacent structures such as the airway, esophagus, or superior central venous system. Compression of airway or mediastinal vasculature can be life-threatening.[5,8–10]

Diagnostic evaluation usually begins with chest radiography. However, computed tomography (CT) and/or magnetic resonance imaging (MRI) are typically needed. CT is most useful for parenchymal lesions, whereas MRI provides better visualization of soft-tissue lesions, vascular anatomy, and tumors of the posterior mediastinum.[11,12] Surgical resection is the standard treatment for benign thoracic tumors in children. Thoracotomy is a traditional approach, but the thoracoscopic technique for diagnosis and treatment of thoracic tumors is well established, and may be particularly useful in the case of benign neurogenic tumors of the posterior mediastinum.[13,14] The term benign tumors can be a misnomer in that although their histology is not malignant, these tumors can be locally aggressive with significant associated morbidity and potential for mortality, because of the proximity to, and compromise of, intrathoracic and mediastinal structures.

The treatment of malignant tumors is predicated on the nature of the tumor. Most tumors such as neuroblastoma, rhabdomyosarcoma, Ewing tumors, fibrosarcoma, and osteosarcoma will ultimately need surgical resection. However, lymphomas are treated medically. Therefore, biopsy of large tumors is usually initially performed to determine the nature of the tumor and whether chemotherapy might reduce the size of the tumor for easier resection if indicated.[15] This article primarily addresses benign tumors; pediatric malignant conditions are more extensively addressed in another article elsewhere in this issue.

## NEUROFIBROMA

Neurogenic tumors are the most common benign tumor of the mediastinum in children. Such tumors are most frequently located in the posterior mediastinum and may extend along the nerves, making complete surgical resection difficult even in benign cases. Neurofibromas are nerve-sheath tumors that can arise from peripheral nerves, sympathetic ganglia, or mediastinal chemoreceptors of the paraganglion system.[10,15,16] Neurofibromas can present in isolation or as one of multiple tumors associated with neurofibromatosis type 1. Neurofibromatosis type 1 is an autosomal dominant disorder with an incidence of 1 in 3000 individuals and equal incidence in males and females. Plexiform neurofibromas (PNF) are considered pathognomonic for neurofibromatosis.[17]

Patients may present with upper respiratory symptoms, tracheal compression (more common in infants), or scoliosis. The tumor may be detected incidentally on chest radiograph. The diagnosis may be suggested by the radiographic presence of scoliosis, widened intervertebral foramina, or disruption of the costovertebral angle. MRI is useful in assessing extension of the tumor into the spinal canal. Surgical resection of these tumors is the standard treatment option. A thoracoscopic approach is increasingly used to access neurogenic tumors of the posterior mediastinum.[13,18,19] However, complete resection can pose a challenge because PNFs have a tendency toward large size, local invasiveness, involvement of critical nerves, and recurrence. Malignant degeneration is more common in older patients, but frequent monitoring is required in children with neurofibromatosis type 1.[20–22] Clinical trials of molecular drug targets for children with large PNFs are ongoing.[23]

## GERM CELL TUMORS

Pediatric germ cell tumors (GCTs) of the chest represent only 5% of all GCTs but are the third most common mediastinal tumor in children. Teratomas are the most common form of mediastinal GCT, comprising 80% of all such tumors, and 10% of all teratomas. GCTs are almost always located in the anterior mediastinum, although posterior mediastinal, pericardial, and intraparenchymal teratomas have been described.[24–26] As with extrathoracic teratomas, the tumors originate from primordial germ cells, contain elements of fetal endoderm, mesoderm, and ectoderm, and can be cystic, solid, or contain mixed cystic and solid elements. Hair, sebaceous glands, teeth, bone, and muscle, as well as well-differentiated thyroid, adrenal, or pancreatic tissue have been observed.[27]

Nearly 80% of teratomas of the chest are benign, and teratomas containing mature tissue elements are believed to have less malignant potential than immature teratomas.[16,25] Teratomas may be detected on prenatal ultrasonography and be associated with fetal hydrops and polyhydramnios.[28] However, if undetected prenatally, few of these lesions present in the neonatal period.[29] Benign teratomas are commonly asymptomatic and are discovered as anterior mediastinal calcifications on routine chest radiograph in older children. Large teratomas present with respiratory distress caused by compression of the trachea and/or adjoining parenchyma, or resulting from rupture. Imaging of a mediastinal teratoma may be accomplished by either CT or MRI. However, CT is particularly useful for identifying fatty and calcified tissue within the tumor.[30] Surgery is indicated to relieve symptoms and to rule out malignant elements. Resection is generally achieved via median sternotomy or thoracotomy as appropriate. Care must be taken during anesthesia induction, as loss of muscle tone can lead to life-threatening airway collapse resulting from tumor compression.[25,26] Even if the tumor is benign, any recurrence has a high risk of being malignant, so long-term follow-up is required.[26]

## OSTEOCHONDROMA

Osteochondromas are the most common of all benign bone tumors and account for half of all rib tumors. These tumors exhibit a 3:1 male predominance and usually present in the first to third decade of life, with growth beginning before puberty and continuing until bone maturation.[31,32] Tumors originate from the rib cortex and can present as a painless mass or with complications of hemothorax, pneumothorax, nerve or vascular impingement, or fracture.[9,33] Chest radiograph showing a pedunculated mass with a cartilaginous cap is highly suggestive of osteochondroma. Surgical resection is indicated, as only 10% of all rib tumors are benign and malignant transformation of osteochondromas can occur. Surgery should be delayed until after puberty except in cases of increasing size or symptoms.[9] Chest wall reconstruction may be indicated following removal of large tumors, but late complications such as restrictive lung disease or scoliosis are uncommon following resection of benign osteochondromas.[34]

## MYOFIBROMA

Myofibromas are the most common benign lung tumor in children, and the most common fibrous disorder of infancy and childhood. These tumors can present as parenchymal lesions or endobronchial masses causing obstruction. Tumors can be solitary or multicentric, and the literature reveals a variety of nomenclature: infantile myofibromatosis, inflammatory myofibroblastic tumor, inflammatory pseudotumor, plasma cell granuloma, histiocytoma, fibroxanthoma, fibrohistiocytoma, or solitary myofibroma.[1,3] Visceral and cutaneous involvement has been described in the multicentric form.[35,36]

Presenting symptoms include cough, chest pain, fever, hemoptysis, pneumonitis, dysphagia, and airway obstruction in the case of endobronchial lesions.[1] Histologically, tumors contain inflammatory cells and contractile myofibroblastic cells. An antecedent pulmonary infection is present in up to 30% of cases, with research suggesting possible associations with viral agents such as human herpesvirus 8 and Epstein-Barr virus.[37]

Spontaneous regression of myofibromas has been described and is more common in the solitary form. However, recurrence and aggressive local invasion, including malignant degeneration, can occur.[38,39] In cases where complete surgical resection cannot be achieved, nonsteroidal anti-inflammatory agents have shown efficacy in tumor regression.[40]

## LYMPHOMA

Lymphoma, both Hodgkin and non-Hodgkin, is the most common cause of anterior and middle mediastinal masses in children. Hodgkin disease has a predisposition to the cervical or mediastinal regions and may present as local or disseminated disease. Non-Hodgkin lymphomas in children fall into 3 categories: lymphoblastic, small noncleaved cell, and large cell. Non-Hodgkin lymphomas are assumed to be disseminated when first discovered. Most non-Hodgkin tumors found in the mediastinum are of a lymphoblastic T-cell origin because these cells arise from T-cell precursors. The thymus has a major role in producing these cells. About 70% of children with lymphoblastic lymphoma will have an anterior mediastinal mass.[41–43]

A mediastinal lymphoma may present as an incidental finding on a chest radiograph. However, if there is compression of the trachea or the upper central venous system, respiratory distress, cough, chest pain, neck swelling, or superior vena cava syndrome may be presenting symptoms.[42–46] Non-Hodgkin lymphomas grow quickly, and frequently cause notable, if not severe, respiratory compromise. Pleural effusions are present in 50% to 70% of these cases.[43,46] A chest CT scan can delineate the size and location of the tumor and the degree of airway compression.[47] Hodgkin lymphoma may present with fever or systemic symptoms in addition to cervical or mediastinal adenopathy.

The diagnosis of lymphoma is best established by tissue biopsy. Attempts should be made to establish the diagnosis of lymphoma in the least invasive way, especially if there is an anterior mediastinal mass that threatens the child's respiratory status. In many instances, diagnosis can be established from a blood sample, biopsy of a peripheral or cervical lymph node, or aspiration of pleural fluid or bone marrow.[41] However, when a mediastinal mass represents the only identifiable tissue or when symptomatology does not allow delay in diagnosis and treatment, direct biopsy of the mediastinal mass is necessary.[48,49] A fine-needle aspirate (FNA) may be considered, but this technique is unsuccessful in obtaining diagnostic material up to 50% of the time. Moreover, current biological studies for tumor subtyping often require an amount of tissue beyond that obtainable by FNA.[41,50] Therefore, more aggressive procedures are usually needed, such as percutaneous core-needle biopsies, thoracoscopic-assisted biopsy, or anterior thoracotomy.[46,51] Local anesthesia may be adequate for needle aspirations or for biopsies requiring limited incisions. If general anesthesia is needed, the patient is best positioned in a partial or total upright position, or other position that is determined to relieve pressure on the airway, with the patient breathing spontaneously. A rigid bronchoscope should be available to access and support the lower airway should any difficulties arise. Airway collapse may ensue with general anesthesia, and muscle relaxants are best avoided.[42,48] It is difficult to know ahead of time which patient will not tolerate anesthesia. Traditionally it has been thought that the more significant the respiratory symptoms, the greater the risk of anesthesia, although there is often not a direct correlation.[41] Shamberger and colleagues[47] attempted to quantify this risk by measuring the cross-sectional area of the compressed trachea by CT. If the cross-sectional area of the most compressed portion of the trachea is larger than 50% of the expected normal cross-sectional area, this study suggests that an uneventful anesthesia should ensue.

If respiratory symptoms truly prohibit manipulation of the patient, chemotherapy may be required without a tissue diagnosis. Radiation therapy is not commonly used in this setting as it was in the past. However, emergent use of chemotherapy to reduce tumor bulk may eliminate any opportunity of obtaining reliable tissue to provide a precise diagnosis of the type of lymphoma.[47–49,52] Therefore, it is desirable to obtain tissue before treatment if possible.

## ENLARGED BENIGN MEDIASTINAL LYMPH NODES

Several nonmalignant conditions may cause enlargement of mediastinal lymph nodes. Such ailments include sarcoidosis, Castleman disease, histoplasmosis, coccidiomycosis, tuberculosis and, rarely, bacterial and viral infections.[53–55] Enlarged lymph nodes may cause compression of the trachea or bronchi, the esophagus, or the central venous system, resulting in respiratory compromise, dysphagia, or superior vena cava syndrome. A chest CT or MRI may be required to delineate the extent of mediastinal nodal pathology. If diagnostic tests are inconclusive, nodal biopsy may be required; this can be accomplished by ultrasound- or CT-guided percutaneous needle biopsy, biopsy using the thoracoscopic technique or, rarely, open thoracotomy.

## THYMOMA

Thymomas are the most common neoplasms of the anterior mediastinum in adults, but they are rare in children,[56–59] and comprise only 1% to 4% of pediatric mediastinal tumors.[5,60] Thymomas are commonly associated with myasthenia gravis in adults, but this association is very rare in children.[61] Immunodeficiency and pure red cell aplasia may also be associated with thymoma in children. Thymomas represent neoplasms of epithelial or lymphocytic origin. On imaging they are typically soft-tissue masses, but may have cystic components and calcifications as well.[61–63] Malignant potential is determined by the presence and extent of microscopic or macroscopic invasion beyond the capsule of the gland.[57–60,64] Malignant thymomas occur as 1 of 3 histologic classes: lymphocytic, mixed lymphoepithelial, and predominantly epithelial. Moreover, differentiation between lymphocytic thymoma and lymphoblastic lymphoma can be difficult. However, the distinction is important, as the latter may have leukemogenic potential.[56,60,65] There are various staging classifications, with a recent one introduced by the World Health Organization.[60,61] More traditional stagings are described by Masaoka and colleagues and Bergh and colleagues.[66–68] Thymomas are best treated by total surgical excision. Radiation therapy and chemotherapy may be required for advanced stages of malignancy or partially resected or unresectable disease.[58,60,69,70]

## LYMPHANGIOMA

Lymphangiomas are congenital lesions that contain an abnormal proliferation of lymphatic and vascular tissue. These tumors can be composed principally of large lymphatic cysts or they can consist of denser tissue with more prominent vascular elements. The term cystic hygroma is often used to describe large cystic lymphangiomas. Lymphangiomatous tissue has a thin endothelial lining and may also contain smooth muscle. There are several theories regarding the formation of lymphangiomas, the most commonly accepted of which suggests that lymphangiomas represent the failure of embryonic lymph sacs to establish adequate drainage into the venous system.[65,71,72]

Lymphangiomas occur in about 1 in 6000 births, and only about 1% are confined to the thoracic cavity.[73–76] Large cervical lymphangiomas, however, may extend into the mediastinum in 2% to 10% of cases.[65,74] Isolated thoracic lymphangiomas are usually found in the anterior mediastinum, although they can be found in other compartments of the mediastinum and in the lung tissue as well.[65,73] Cervical lymphangiomas often extend into the posterior mediastinum. Prenatal ultrasonography may detect an intrathoracic lymphangioma.[76]

Thoracic lymphangiomas are often incidental findings on chest imaging. If symptoms are present, they are the result of impingement on the airway, lungs, or other mediastinal structures by the lymphangioma. Symptoms include cough, stridor, dyspnea, dysphagia, hemoptysis, superior vena cava syndrome, and Horner syndrome. Infection or collections of chyle in the pleura or pericardium may occur. Hemorrhage into a lymphangioma with rapid enlargement and sudden onset of symptoms has been described.[73,75–78] Thoracic lymphangiomas appear as homogeneous masses on a chest radiograph. Ultrasonography reveals a lesion that is primarily cystic in nature, sometimes containing debris. CT or MRI reveals the cystic nature of the lesion as well as the extent of its involvement with other mediastinal and thoracic structures. Calcifications may occasionally be present if there is a significant vascular component.[73,75,77]

There have been reports of spontaneous regression of lymphangiomas, but these are very rare and are not part of the natural course of this lesion. The optimal therapy for mediastinal lymphangiomas is total excision, but it is widely agreed that vital structures should not be sacrificed during attempts at total excision.[65,72,74] Because tissue must often be left behind and because some lesions are simply not resectable because of their extensive involvement of vital structures, alternative strategies for therapy have been advanced.[74] Intralesional injection of sclerosing agents is often used as a primary therapy. It may be definitive therapy in up to 80% of cases depending on reports, or may be a method of reducing a lymphangioma to a more easily resectable size. Injection of sclerosing agents has also been used to treat residual or recurrent tissue after resection. The more commonly used sclerosing agents have been bleomycin and OK-432. However, successful therapy has been reported with alcohol, alcoholic solution of zein (Ethibloc), dextrose, tetracycline, doxycycline, iodine, cyclophosphamide, and dexamethasone.[71,74,79–86] Irradiation of these lesions is discouraged.[72]

The most common postoperative complication after resection of a lymphangioma is lymph accumulation in the surgical area. Repeated aspiration of the fluid often resolves this difficulty. Use of fibrin glue as a sclerosant may be helpful if aspiration fails.[86] In some cases, resection of all or part of the residual tissue may be necessary. Lymphangiomas recur in at least 10% to 15% of cases if resection has not been complete. Therefore, close long-term follow-up of these children is necessary.

## BRONCHOGENIC CYSTS

Bronchogenic cysts result from abnormal budding of the tracheal diverticulum during formation of the foregut. These tumors tend to be more commonly found in the right chest and are more common in males.[87] A bronchogenic cyst may be one component of a constellation of anomalies that result from anomalous lung and foregut development and that sometimes have related characteristics and histologic findings, including congenital cystic adenomatous malformation (CCAM), bronchopulmonary sequestrations, congenital lobar emphysema, bronchogenic cysts, esophageal duplication cysts, and neurenteric cysts. For example, CCAM and pulmonary sequestration may manifest as hybrid lesions, and esophageal duplication and bronchogenic cysts have common elements of histology.[88–90] Gerle and colleagues[91] proposed the term bronchopulmonary-foregut malformations to encompass the anomalies of bronchogenic cysts, pulmonary sequestrations, and abnormalities of tracheal budding. Most bronchogenic cysts are located in the middle mediastinum in paratracheal, carinal, hilar, or paraesophageal positions,[88] and may also be located within the lung parenchyma itself.[92] Bronchogenic cysts are typically lined with ciliated columnar epithelium and contain thick mucus. The walls of the cysts usually contain hyaline cartilage, smooth muscle, mucus glands, and nerve fibers.[87,88,93–95] Bronchogenic cysts rarely communicate with the airway, but they may densely adhere to it.[87,92] There may be associated vertebral anomalies.[96]

Bronchogenic cysts become symptomatic as a result of compromise of the airway or infection (**Fig. 1**). Airway compromise is more typically seen in infants, whereas infection tends to present in older children. Symptoms related to airway compromise include stridor, wheezing, cough, nasal flaring, retractions, and intermittent cyanotic spells. Symptoms related to infection include fever, cough, hemoptysis, sputum production, and recurrent pneumonia.[87] In many cases, however, bronchogenic cysts are asymptomatic and are discovered as incidental findings on chest radiography as either a space-occupying lesion or a cyst with an air-fluid level.[89] If a bronchogenic cyst is suspected, a contrast-enhanced CT or MRI will best delineate the anatomy.[97,98]

Once detected, bronchogenic cysts should be excised, and this may be done either via thoracotomy or thoracoscopic technique.[99–103] Cysts that are asymptomatic at the time of diagnosis should still be removed because they are prone to causing airway compromise and infection. In rare instances, malignancy, including adenocarcinoma and rhabdomyosarcoma, has been reported to be associated with bronchogenic cysts.[92,97,99,104,105] If a bronchogenic cyst cannot be completely excised, the

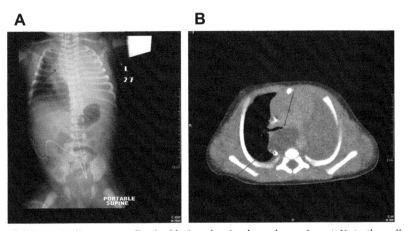

**Fig. 1.** (*A*) Arrow indicates a mediastinal lesion that is a bronchogenic cyst. Note the collapse of the left lung. (*B*) CT image of the bronchogenic cyst shown in the radiograph in *A* reveals how it compresses the left main stem bronchus, resulting in the collapse of the left lung.

remaining epithelium should be fulgurated. These children must be monitored for recurrence.[106]

## ESOPHAGEAL DUPLICATION CYSTS

Esophageal duplication cysts result from a failure of appropriate vacuolization of the esophagus during embryologic development. Embryologic development may also be related to the development of other congenital anomalies, particularly broncho-genic cysts.[88–90,107] Esophageal duplication cysts may be associated with other anomalies including intestinal duplications, esophageal atresia and fistula, and spinal anomalies. These cysts are more common in males than in females, and are more frequently found in the right side of the chest and toward the lower esophagus. Esoph-ageal duplication cysts are typically attached to, or within, the esophageal wall, are covered by a smooth muscle, and may be lined by squamous, columnar, cuboidal, pseudostratified, or ciliated epithelium, or some combination of these types.[107–109] It is estimated that 10% of esophageal duplication cysts communicate with the lumen of the esophagus.[107]

Many esophageal duplication cysts are asymptomatic, and are discovered inciden-tally in late childhood or adulthood. If these cysts become symptomatic in infants, it is usually because they are higher in the mediastinum and are causing respiratory compromise resulting from compression of the trachea and mediastinum. Dysphagia and neck swelling may also be noted. In older children and adults, typical symptoms are dysphagia, epigastric discomfort, and retrosternal pain. Other reported symptoms and complications of esophageal duplication cysts have included anorexia, regurgita-tion, empyema, pyopericardium, mediastinitis, cardiac arrhythmias, and erosion and bleeding from ectopic gastric mucosa within the cyst.[107,108,110,111]

An esophageal duplication cyst may be suspected by mediastinal widening and/or tracheal deviation or compression on chest radiography. Barium swallow may show a mass effect on the esophagus. The best imaging tools are CT and MRI.[108] Therapy is surgical excision of the cyst, which may be accomplished by thoracotomy or thor-acoscopic technique. If the entire cyst cannot be removed, the mucosa of the remain-ing cyst should be fulgurated. If an opening is made into the esophagus, this can be primarily repaired.[99,107,110]

## THYMIC CYSTS

Thymic cysts are uncommon lesions and may present as either mediastinal and/or neck masses in children.[65,112–116] Mediastinal thymic cysts are typically asymptomatic and are found incidentally as a widening of the mediastinum on chest radiography, or as a cystic structure in the anterior mediastinum on CT or MRI. If symptoms are present they may include wheezing, cough, upper respiratory infection, fever, or airway obstruction.[117] Thymic cysts may be congenital or acquired. Congenital cysts are characterized as unilocular with a thin translucent wall. Acquired cysts are thought to be the result of inflammation, and are multilocular with thick walls.[118] However, they are uniformly benign in children. Thymic cysts are lined by ciliated epithelium with components of lymphocytes, thymic tissue, cholesterol crystals, and Hassall corpus-cles within the wall.[113] When a thymic cyst is suspected, ultrasonography, CT, and MRI are useful imaging modalities. Needle aspiration has been suggested as helpful in making the diagnosis as well, but examination of surgically resected specimens is ultimately optimal for diagnosis.[114,119] Cystic thymomas that can mimic the appear-ance of thymic cysts on imaging have been reported.[63] Thymic cysts rarely involve adjacent structures and can typically be easily resected. Resection of a thymic cyst can be accomplished thoracoscopically (the author's unpublished experience).[120]

## PERICARDIAL CYSTS

Pericardial cysts form when the mesodermal lacunae fail to coalesce during development of the pericardium.[55,112] These cysts are typically found at the cardiophrenic angle in the middle mediastinum, and are thin-walled with a flat mesothelial lining. Histology is uniformly benign.[65,113] Pericardial cysts are usually found incidentally on chest images. Because the histology is benign and most cysts are asymptomatic at presentation, some investigators believe that observation of pericardial cysts is appropriate. However, others cite their potential for symptomatology, such as inflammation, as justification for their removal.[112,121] Cardiac tamponade, attributable to hemorrhage or effusion, has been reported.[122,123] Ultrasonography and CT usually confirm the diagnosis. Surgical excision is usually uncomplicated and can be accomplished by thoracotomy or a thoracoscopic technique (the author's unpublished experience).[124,125]

## REFERENCES

1. Shochat SJ. Tumors of the lung. In: Grosfeld JL, O'Neill JA, Fonkalsrud EW, et al, editors. Pediatric surgery. 6th edition. Philadelphia: Mosby; 2006. p. 640–8.
2. Hancock BJ, Di Lorenzo M, Youssef S, et al. Childhood primary pulmonary neoplasms. J Pediatr Surg 1993;28(9):1133–6.
3. Hartman GE, Shochat SJ. Primary pulmonary neoplasms of childhood: a review. Ann Thorac Surg 1983;36(1):108–19.
4. Rich BS, McEvoy MP, honeyman JN, et al. Hodgkin disease presenting with chest wall involvement: a case series. J Pediatr Surg 2011;46:1835–7.
5. Takeda S, Miyoshi S, Akashi A, et al. Clinical spectrum of primary mediastinal tumors: a comparison of adult and pediatric populations at a single Japanese institution. J Surg Oncol 2003;83(1):24–30.
6. van den Berg H, van Rijn RR, Merks JH. Management of tumors of the chest wall in childhood: a review. J Pediatr Hematol Oncol 2008;30(3):214–21.
7. Azizkhan RG, Dudgeon DL, Buck JR. Life-threatening airway obstruction as a complication to the management of mediastinal masses in children. J Pediatr Surg 1985;20:816–22.
8. Newman B. Thoracic neoplasms in children. Radiol Clin North Am 2011;49(4): 633–64.
9. Shah AA, D'Amico TA. Primary chest wall tumors. J Am Coll Surg 2010;210(3): 360–6.
10. Jaggers J, Balsara K. Mediastinal masses in children. Semin Thorac Cardiovasc Surg 2004;16(3):201–8.
11. Wyttenbach R, Vock P, Tschappeler H. Cross-sectional imaging with CT and/or MRI of pediatric chest tumors. Eur Radiol 1998;8(6):1040–6.
12. Anthony E. Imaging of pediatric chest masses. Paediatr Respir Rev 2006; 7(Suppl 1):S39–40.
13. Lacreuse I, Valla JS, de Lagausie P, et al. Thoracoscopic resection of neurogenic tumors in children. J Pediatr Surg 2007;42(10):1725–8.
14. Petty JK, Bensard DD, Partrick DA, et al. Resection of neurogenic tumors in children: is thoracoscopy superior to thoracotomy? J Am Coll Surg 2006;203(5): 699–703.

15. Azarow KS, Pearl RH, Zurcher R, et al. Primary mediastinal masses. A comparison of adult and pediatric populations. J Thorac Cardiovasc Surg 1993;106(1): 67–72.

16. Grosfeld JL, Weinberger M, Kilman JW, et al. Primary mediastinal neoplasms in infants and children. Ann Thorac Surg 1971;12(2):179–90.

17. Ardern-Holmes SL, North KN. Therapeutics for childhood neurofibromatosis type 1 and type 2. Curr Treat Options Neurol 2011;13(6):529–43.

18. Fraga JC, Aydogdu B, Aufieri R, et al. Surgical treatment for pediatric mediastinal neurogenic tumors. Ann Thorac Surg 2010;90(2):413–8.

19. Nio M, Nakamura M, Yoshida S, et al. Thoracoscopic removal of neurogenic mediastinal tumors in children. J Laparoendosc Adv Surg Tech A 2005;15(1):80–3.

20. Prada CE, Rangwala FA, Martin LJ, et al. Pediatric plexiform neurofibromas: impact on morbidity and mortality in neurofibromatosis type 1. J Pediatr 2012; 160(3):461–7.

21. Campione A, Di Bisceglie M, Lonzi M, et al. Sudden onset of thoracic pain: neurofibroma with intracystic haemorrhage. Interact Cardiovasc Thorac Surg 2004;3(3):533–4.

22. Cebesoy O, Tutar E, Isik M, et al. A case of isolated giant plexiform neurofibroma involving all branches of the common peroneal nerve. Arch Orthop Trauma Surg 2007;127(8):709–12.

23. Kim A, Gillespie A, Dombi E, et al. Characteristics of children enrolled in treatment trials for NF1-related plexiform neurofibromas. Neurology 2009;73(16): 1273–9.

24. Grosfeld JL, Skinner MA, Rescorla FJ, et al. Mediastinal tumors in children: experience with 196 cases. Ann Surg Oncol 1994;1:121.

25. Horton Z, Schlatter M, Schultz S. Pediatric germ cell tumors. Surg Oncol 2007; 16(3):205–13.

26. Lakhoo K, Boyle M, Drake DP. Mediastinal teratomas: review of 15 pediatric cases. J Pediatr Surg 1993;28(9):1161–4.

27. Azizkhan RG. Teratomas and other germ cell tumors. In: Grosfeld JL, O'Neill JA, Fonkalsrud EW, et al, editors. Pediatric surgery. 6th edition. Philadelphia: Mosby; 2006. p. 554–74.

28. Kuller JA, Laifer SA, Martin JG, et al. Unusual presentations of fetal teratoma. J Perinatol 1991;40:294–6.

29. Seibert J, Marvin WJ, Rose EF, et al. Mediastinal teratoma: a rare cause of severe respiratory distress in the newborn. J Pediatr Surg 1976;11:253–5.

30. Link KM, Samuels LJ, Reed JC, et al. Magnetic resonance imaging of the mediastinum. J Thorac Imaging 1993;8:34–53.

31. Marino-Nieto J, Lugo-Vicente H. Rib osteochondroma in a child: case report and review of literature. Bol Asoc Med P R 2011;103(1):47–50.

32. Smith SE, Keshavjee S. Primary chest wall tumors. Thorac Surg Clin 2010;20(4): 495–507.

33. O'Brien PJ, Ramasunder S, Cox MW. Venous thoracic outlet syndrome secondary to first rib osteochondroma in a pediatric patient. J Vasc Surg 2011;53(3):811–3.

34. Soyer T, Karnak I, Ciftci AO, et al. The results of surgical treatment of chest wall tumors in childhood. Pediatr Surg Int 2006;22(2):135–9.

35. Behar PM, Albritton FD, Muller S, et al. Multicentric infantile myofibromatosis. Int J Pediatr Otorhinolaryngol 1998;45(3):249–54.

36. Pelluard-Nehme F, Coatleven F, Carles D, et al. Multicentric infantile myofibromatosis: two perinatal cases. Eur J Pediatr 2007;166(10):997–1001.

37. Mergan F, Jaubert F, Sauvat F, et al. Inflammatory myofibroblastic tumor in children: clinical review with anaplastic lymphoma kinase, Epstein-Barr virus, and human herpesvirus 8 detection analysis. J Pediatr Surg 2005;40(10):1581–6.
38. Haspel AC, Coviello VF, Stevens M, et al. Myofibroma of the mandible in an infant: case report, review of the literature, and discussion. J Oral Maxillofac Surg 2011. [Epub ahead of print].
39. Karnak I, Senocak ME, Ciftci AO, et al. Inflammatory myofibroblastic tumor in children: diagnosis and treatment. J Pediatr Surg 2001;36(6):908–12.
40. Su W, Ko A, O'Connell T, et al. Treatment of pseudotumors with nonsteroidal anti-inflammatory drugs. J Pediatr Surg 2000;35(11):1635–7.
41. White KS. Thoracic imaging of pediatric lymphomas. J Thorac Imaging 2001; 16(4):224–37.
42. Garey CL, Laituri CA, Valusek PA, et al. Management of anterior mediastinal masses in children. Eur J Pediatr Surg 2011;21:310–3.
43. Mauch PM, Kalish LA, Kadin M, et al. Patterns of presentation of Hodgkin disease: implication for etiology and pathogenesis. Cancer 1993;71:2062–71.
44. Ingram L, Rivera GK, Shapiro DN. Superior vena cava syndrome associated with childhood malignancy: analysis of 24 cases. Med Pediatr Oncol 1990;18: 476–81.
45. Yellin A, Mandel M, Rechavi G, et al. Superior vena cava syndrome associated with lymphoma. Am J Dis Child 1992;146(9):1060–3.
46. Shorter NA, Fiston HC. Lymphomas. In: Ashcraft KW, Holder TM, editors. Pediatric surgery. 2nd edition. Philadelphia: WB Saunders; 1993. p. 863.
47. Shamberger RC, Holyman RS, Griscom NT, et al. CT quantitation of tracheal cross-section area as a guide to the surgical and anesthetic management of children with anterior mediastinal masses. J Pediatr Surg 1991;26:138–42.
48. Ferrari LR, Bedford RF. General anesthesia prior to treatment of anterior mediastinal masses in pediatric cancer patients. Anesthesiology 1990;72:991–5.
49. Halpern S, Chatten J, Meadows AT, et al. Anterior mediastinal masses: anesthesia hazards and other problems. J Pediatr 1983;102:407–10.
50. King MR, Telander RL, Smithson WA, et al. Primary mediastinal tumors in children. J Pediatr Surg 1982;17:512–20.
51. Carr TF, Lockwood L, Stevens RF, et al. Childhood B cell lymphomas arising in the mediastinum. J Clin Pathol 1993;46:513–6.
52. Loeffler JS, Leopold KA, Recht A, et al. Emergency prebiopsy radiation for mediastinal masses: impact on subsequent pathologic diagnosis and outcome. J Clin Oncol 1986;4:716–21.
53. Lemonine G, Montupet P. Mediastinal tumors in infancy and childhood. In: Fallis JC, Filler RM, Lemoina G, editors. Pediatric thoracic surgery. New York: Elsevier; 1991. p. 258.
54. Sills RH. The spleen and lymph nodes. In: Oski FA, editor. Principles and practice of pediatrics. Philadelphia: JB Lippincott; 1990. p. 1540.
55. McGahren ED, Rodgers BM. Mediastinum and pleura. In: Oldham KT, Colombani PM, Foglia RP, et al, editors. Principles and practice of pediatric surgery. Philadelphia: Lippincott Williams & Wilkins; 2005. p. 929–49.
56. Copper JD. Current therapy for thymoma. Chest 1993;103(Suppl 4):334S–6S.
57. Couture MM, Mountain CP. Thymoma. Semin Surg Oncol 1990;6:110–4.
58. Pokorny WJ. Thymomas. In: Oski FA, editor. Principles and practice of pediatrics. 1st edition. Philadelphia: JB Lippincott; 1990. p. 1613.
59. Spigland N, Di Lorenzo M, Youssef S, et al. Malignant thymoma in children: a 20-year review. J Pediatr Surg 1990;25:1143–6.

60. Rothstein DH, Voss SD, Isakoff M, et al. Thymoma in a child: case report and review of the literature. Pediatr Surg Int 2005;21:548–51.
61. Dhall G, Ginsburg H, Bodenstein L, et al. Thymoma in children: report of two cases and review of literature. J Pediatr Hematol Oncol 2004;26:681–5.
62. Bikchandani J, Valusek PA, Juang D, et al. Giant ossifying malignant thymoma in a child. J Pediatr Surg 2010;45:E31–4.
63. Honda S, Morikawa T, Sasaki F, et al. Cystic thymoma in a child: a rare case and review of the literature. Pediatr Surg Int 2007;23:1015–7.
64. Sicherer SH, Cabana MD, Perlman EJ, et al. Thymoma and cellular immune deficiency in an adolescent. Pediatr Allergy Immunol 1998;9:49–52.
65. Tova JA. Mediastinal tumors. In: Holcomb GW III, Murphy JP, editors. Ashcraft's pediatric surgery. 5th edition. Philadelphia: Saunders; 2010. p. 345–61.
66. Masaoka A, Monden Y, Nakahara K, et al. Following study of thymoma with special reference to their clinical stages. Cancer 1981;48:2485–92.
67. Masaoka A, Yamakawa Y, Niwa H, et al. Thymectomy and malignancy. Eur J Cardiothorac Surg 1994;8:251–3.
68. Bergh NP, Gatzinsky P, Larsson S, et al. Tumors of the thymus and thymic region: I. clinicopathological studies on thymomas. Ann Thorac Surg 1978;25: 91–8.
69. Pollack A, Komaki R, Cox JD, et al. Thymoma: treatment and prognosis. Int J Radiat Oncol Biol Phys 1992;23:1037–43.
70. Niehues T, Harms D, Jurgens H, et al. Treatment of pediatric malignant thymoma: long-term remission in a 14-year-old boy with EBV-associated thymic carcinoma by aggressive, combined modality treatment. Med Pediatr Oncol 1996; 26:419–24.
71. Emran MA, Dubois J, Laberge L, et al. Alcoholic solution of zein (Ethibloc) sclerotherapy for treatment of lymphangiomas in children. J Pediatr Surg 2006;41: 975–9.
72. Glasson MJ, Taylor SF. Cervical cervico-mediastinal and intrathoracic lymphangioma. Prog Pediatr Surg 1991;27:62–83.
73. Green NA, Diaz MC. Pulmonary lymphangioma in a 14-month old. Pediatr Emerg Care 2011;27(1):52–4.
74. Hancock BJ, St-Vil D, Luks FL, et al. Complications of lymphangiomas in children. J Pediatr Surg 1992;27:220–6.
75. Kostopoulos GK, Fessatidis JT, Hevas AL, et al. Mediastinal cystic hygroma: report of a case with review of the literature. Eur J Cardiothorac Surg 1993;7: 166–7.
76. Zalel Y, Shalev E, Ben-Ami M, et al. Ultrasonic diagnosis of mediastinal cystic hygroma. Prenat Diagn 1992;12:541–4.
77. Gupta AK, Bery M, Raghav B, et al. Mediastinal and skeletal lymphangiomas in a child. Pediatr Radiol 1991;21:129.
78. Ağartan C, Olguner M, Akgur FM, et al. A case of mediastinal hygroma whose only symptom was hoarseness. J Pediatr Surg 1998;33:642–3.
79. Okazaki T, Iwatani S, Yanai T, et al. Treatment of lymphangioma in children: our experience of 128 cases. J Pediatr Surg 2007;42:386–9.
80. Degenhardt P, Dieckow B, Mau H, et al. Huge intra- and extrathoracic lymphangioma in a baby successfully treated by sclerotherapy with OK-432. Eur J Pediatr Surg 2006;16:197–200.
81. Pokorny WJ. Congenital malformations of the lymphatic system. In: Oski FA, editor. Principles and practice of pediatrics. 1st edition. Philadelphia: JB Lippincott; 1990. p. 1612.

82. Ogita S, Tsuto T, Deguchi E, et al. OK-432 therapy for unresectable lymphangiomas in children. J Pediatr Surg 1991;26:263–70.
83. Okada A, Kubota A, Fukuzawa M, et al. Injection of bleomycin as a primary therapy of cystic lymphangioma. J Pediatr Surg 1992;27:440–3.
84. Ogita S, Tsuto T, Nakamura K, et al. OK-432 therapy for lymphangioma in children: why and how does it work? J Pediatr Surg 1996;31:477–80.
85. Orford J, Barker A, Thonell S, et al. Bleomycin therapy for cystic hygroma. J Pediatr Surg 1995;30:1282–7.
86. Castañón M, Margarit J, Carrasco R, et al. Long-term follow-up of nineteen cystic lymphangiomas treated with fibrin sealant. J Pediatr Surg 1999;34:1276–9.
87. Stewart B, Cochran A, Iglesia K, et al. Unusual case of stridor and wheeze in an infant. Pediatr Pulmonol 2002;34:320–3.
88. Tomita SS, Wojtczak H, Pickard R, et al. Congenital cystic adenomatoid malformation and bronchogenic cyst in a 4-month-old infant. Ann Thorac Cardiovasc Surg 2009;15:394–6.
89. Mampilly T, Kurian R, Shenai A. Bronchogenic cyst-cause of refractory wheezing in infancy. Indian J Pediatr 2005;72(4):363–4.
90. Nobuhara KK, Gorski YC, La Quaglia MP, et al. Bronchogenic cysts and esophageal duplications: common origins and treatment. J Pediatr Surg 1997;32(10):1408–13.
91. Gerle RD, Jaretzki A, Ashley CA, et al. Congenital bronchopulmonary-foregut malformation: pulmonary sequestration communicating with the gastrointestinal tract. N Engl J Med 1968;278:1413–9.
92. St Georges R, Deslauriers J, Duranceau A, et al. Clinical spectrum of bronchogenic cysts of the mediastinum and lung in the adult. Ann Thorac Surg 1991;52(1):6–13.
93. Hausen T, Corbet A, Avery ME. Malformations of the mediastinum and lung parenchyma. In: Taeusch WH, Ballard RA, editors. Avery's disease of the newborn. 7th edition. Philadelphia: W.B. Saunders; 1998. p. 672–3, 1991;52:6–13.
94. Stern RC. Lower respiratory tract—congenital abnormalities. In: . In: Nelson WE, Behrman RE, Kliegman RM, et al, editors. Nelson's textbook of pediatrics, vol. 2, 16th edition. Saunders WB; 1996. p. 331–5, 1200.
95. Ahrens B, Wit J, Schmitt M, et al. Symptomatic bronchogenic cyst in a six-month-old infant: case report and review of the literature. J Thorac Cardiovasc Surg 2001;122:1021–3.
96. Lazar RH, Younis BT, Bassila MN. Bronchogenic cysts: a cause of stridor in the neonate. Am J Otolaryngol 1991;12:117–21.
97. Suen GC, Mathisen DJ, Grillo HC, et al. Surgical management and radiological characteristics of bronchogenic cysts. Ann Thorac Surg 1993;55:476–81.
98. McAdams HP, Kirejczyk WM, Rosado-de-Christenson ML, et al. Bronchogenic cyst: imaging features with clinical and histopathological correlation. Radiology 2000;217:441–6.
99. Bratu I, Laberge JM, Flageole H, et al. Foregut duplications: is there an advantage to thoracoscopic resection? J Pediatr Surg 2005;40:138–41.
100. Tolg C, Abelin K, Laudenbach V, et al. Open vs thoracoscopic surgical management of bronchogenic cysts. Surg Endosc 2005;19:77–80.
101. Kern JA, Daniel TM, Tribble CO, et al. Thoracoscopic diagnosis and treatment of mediastinal masses. Ann Thorac Surg 1993;56:92–6.
102. Dillon PW, Cilley RE, Krummel TM. Video-assisted thoracoscopic excision of intrathoracic masses in children: report of two cases. Surg Laparosc Endosc 1993;3:433–6.

103. Lobe TE. Pediatric thoracoscopy. Semin Thorac Cardiovasc Surg 1993;5: 298–302.
104. Olsen JB, Clemmensen O, Andersen K. Adenocarcinoma arising in a foregut cyst of the mediastinum. Ann Thorac Surg 1991;51:497–9.
105. de Perrot M, Pache JC, Spiliopoulos A. Carcinoma arising in congenital lung cysts. Thorac Cardiovasc Surg 2001;49:184–5.
106. Read CA, Moront M, Carangelo R. Recurrent bronchogenic cyst: an argument for complete surgical excision. Arch Surg 1991;126:1306–8.
107. Gupta B, Meher R, Raj A, et al. Duplication cyst of oesophagus: a case report. J Paediatr Child Health 2010;46:134–5.
108. Sodhi KS, Saxena AK, Narashimha Rao KL, et al. Esophageal duplication cyst, an unusual cause of respiratory distress in infants. Pediatr Emerg Care 2005; 21(12):854–6.
109. Snyder CL, Bickler SW, Gittes GK, et al. Esophageal duplication cyst with esophageal web and tracheoesophageal fistula. J Pediatr Surg 1996;31(7): 968–9.
110. Hirose S, Clifton MS, Bratton B, et al. Thoracoscopic resection of foregut duplication cysts. J Laparoendosc Adv Surg Tech A 2006;16:526–9.
111. Overhaus M, Decker P, Zhou H, et al. The congenital duplication cyst: a rare differential diagnosis of retrosternal pain and dysphagia in a young patient. Scand J Gastroenterol 2003;38:337–40.
112. Rice TW. Benign neoplasms and cysts of the mediastinum. Semin Thorac Cardiovasc Surg 1992;4:25–33.
113. Wick MR. Mediastinal cysts and intrathoracic thyroid tumors. Semin Diagn Pathol 1990;7:285–94.
114. Komura M, Kanamori Y, Sugiyama M, et al. A pediatric care of life-threatening airway obstruction caused by a cervicomediastinal thymic cyst. Pediatr Radiol 2010;40:1569–71.
115. Amanatidou V, Mavrokosta M, Koutesis A, et al. Cervicomediastinal thymic cyst-report of a case. Thorac Cardiovasc Surg 2008;56:177–8.
116. Cigliano B, Baltogiannis N, De Marco M, et al. Cervical thymic cysts. Pediatr Surg Int 2007;23:1219–25.
117. Hendrickson M, Azarow K, Eon S, et al. Congenital thymic cysts in children— mostly misdiagnosed. J Pediatr Surg 1998;33:821–5.
118. Bouziri A, Khaldi A, Louati H, et al. Respiratory failure revealing a multilocular thymic cyst in an infant. Ann Thorac Surg 2010;90:305–8.
119. Tollefsen I, Yoo M, Bland JD, et al. Thymic cyst: is a correct pre-operative diagnosis possible? Report of a case and review of the literature. Eur J Pediatr 2001; 160:620–2.
120. Hazelrigg SR, Landreneau RI, Mack MJ, et al. Thoracoscopic resection of mediastinal cysts. Ann Thorac Surg 1993;56:659–60.
121. Noyes BC, Weber T, Vogler C. Pericardial cysts in children: surgical or conservative approach? J Pediatr Surg 2003;38:1263–5.
122. Shiraishi I, Yamagishi M, Kawakita A, et al. Acute cardiac tamponade caused by massive hemorrhage from pericardial cyst. Circulation 2000;101:E196–7.
123. Bava GL, Magliani L, Bertoli D, et al. Complicated pericardial cyst: atypical anatomy and clinical course. Clin Cardiol 1998;21:862–4.
124. Szinicz G, Taxer F, Riedlinger J, et al. Thoracoscopic resection of a pericardial cyst. Thorac Cardiovasc Surg 1992;40:190–1.
125. Eto A, Arima T, Nagashima A. Pericardial cyst in a child treated with video-assisted thoracoscopic surgery. Eur J Pediatr 2000;159:889–91.

# Congenital Diaphragmatic Hernia and Protective Ventilation Strategies in Pediatric Surgery

Alejandro Garcia, MD, Charles J.H. Stolar, MD*

## KEYWORDS

- Congenital diaphragmatic hernia • Lung protective ventilation • Neonate • ECMO

## KEY POINTS

- All infants affected with congenital diaphragmatic hernias (CDH) suffer from some degree of respiratory insufficiency arising from a combination of pulmonary hypoplasia and pulmonary hypertension.
- Respiratory care strategies using high peak airway pressures, muscle paralysis or excessive sedation, hyperventilation, and induced alkalosis to optimize blood gasses lead to significant barotrauma, increased morbidity, and overuse of extracorporeal membrane oxygenation (ECMO).
- Newer permissive hypercapnia/spontaneous ventilation protocols geared to accept moderate hypercapnia at lower peak airway pressures, allowing for spontaneous ventilation, and minimizing sedation have led to improved outcomes.
- High-frequency oscillatory ventilation can be used in infants with CDH who continue to have persistent respiratory distress despite conventional ventilation. It may also be effective as an initial approach as opposed to rescue therapy.
- ECMO can be used successfully in infants with CDH as a resuscitative strategy to minimize further barotrauma in carefully selected patients.

Congenital diaphragmatic hernia (CDH) is an uncommon entity with an estimated annual incidence of about 1 in 3000 live births. CDH results from a defect in the diaphragm that allows evisceration of the abdominal contents into the thorax, most commonly on the left, resulting in maldevelopment of the bronchioles and intra-acinar arterioles. Despite advances in neonatal intensive care, CDH is associated with a high morbidity and mortality stemming from the degree of pulmonary hypoplasia present. This pulmonary hypoplasia is associated with a variable amount of potentially reversible persistent pulmonary hypertension of the newborn (PPHN).

The authors have nothing to disclose.
Division of Pediatric Surgery, Columbia University College of Physicians and Surgeons, 3959 Broadway, CHN 214, New York, NY 10032, USA
* Corresponding author.
E-mail address: cjs3@columbia.edu

This PPHN is the result of a reduced number and generations of airways, increased muscularization of the intra-acinar pulmonary arteries, a small cross-sectional area of the pulmonary vascular bed, and abnormal pulmonary vasoconstriction. Most infants with CDH have some degree of respiratory distress in the perinatal period and require mechanical ventilator support. This can lead to a vicious cycle of pulmonary vasospasm, pulmonary hypertension, right-to-left shunting at the ductal and foramen levels, progressive hypoxemia, hypercarbia, and acidosis.

It is imperative to use ventilator strategies that optimize ventilation and minimize barotrauma and oxygen toxicity, while maintaining adequate oxygen delivery. Some modalities that have been used to minimize ventilator-induced injury include pressure controlled ventilation and high-frequency oscillatory ventilation. Extracorporeal membrane oxygenation (ECMO) has been used as a salvage strategy to prevent further mechanical pulmonary injury. Currently, infants with CDH are initially managed with lung protective ventilation with subsequent surgical repair after a period of stabilization. Definitive treatment involves reduction of the abdominal viscera to close the defect without undue tension on the abdominal wall and repair of the diaphragmatic defect. Appropriate ventilator management is crucial for successful outcomes in these infants.

## NEONATAL PULMONARY DEVELOPMENT IN CDH

Fetal pulmonary development is divided into different stages. Most of the major airways have formed by 16 weeks and canalization of the major airways with formation of the air-blood barrier occurs by 24 weeks of gestation. This is followed by a period of differentiation and further growth of the air spaces. At 36 weeks of gestation, much of the lung growth is completed, along with the continued production of surfactant. The mechanism by which the diaphragm fails to form in infants with CDH is not well understood. The diaphragmatic defect allows the abdominal organs to develop in the thorax, leading to mediastinal shift and abnormal lung growth.

Pulmonary hypoplasia, elevated pulmonary vascular resistance, and subsequent right heart failure are the main contributors of mortality in infants with CDH. Traditionally, infants with a right-sided CDH have an overall worse prognosis and have a higher requirement for ECMO than those with left-sided hernias.[1] Lung hypoplasia in CDH is associated with a variable reduction in lung tissue that is characterized by a decrease in airway number, smaller airspaces, and a decrease in vascular branches with increased adventitia and medial thickness.[2] Airway smooth muscle dysregulation may also contribute to airway obstruction and respiratory distress in these infants.[3] In addition, lung volumes of both the ipsilateral and contralateral lungs are decreased in infants with CDH.[4] It is important to consider that in infants with CDH, pulmonary airway and vascular development may continue after birth.[5] To preserve viable lung parenchyma and allow further development, it is important to minimize injury from overly aggressive ventilation strategies.

## MECHANICAL VENTILATION IN CHILDREN

After the birth of an infant with CDH, all efforts should be made to stabilize the cardiopulmonary system while inducing minimal iatrogenic injury from therapeutic interventions. The diagnosis of CDH is no longer considered a surgical emergency and attention should be made to address the physiologic distress that may be present at birth. Immediate intubation and mechanical ventilation is important in nearly all cases of CDH to minimize respiratory distress. Bag masking may lead to gastrointestinal distension with further compression of the hypoplastic lungs and should therefore be avoided. Nasogastric decompression should be implemented in all patients to minimize gastric and abdominal distention. Preductal and postductal oxygen saturations should be monitored to assess degree of ductal shunting present owing to pulmonary hypertension. A transthoracic echocardiogram should be obtained to assess overall cardiac function and severity of pulmonary hypertension. Arterial and venous access should be acquired through the umbilicus for monitoring of hemodynamics.

Ventilator management in preterm infants and adults is extensively described; however, few prospective studies exist that provide a clinically validated approach to ventilator management in neonates and children. Current ventilator strategies in children are largely extrapolated from data obtained from adult series. There are important differences to consider between adult and neonatal lung physiology. The maturation of the human lung and alveolization continues beyond infancy. At birth, a term infant has about 50 million alveoli and this number increases to about 300 million by age 2. The lung parenchyma of a neonate is relatively devoid of collagen. The elastin-to-collagen ratio changes over the first few years of life and this affects the stiffness and the potential for overdistention and recoil of the infant lung. The ratio of lung volume, including total lung capacity and functional residual capacity, to body weight continues to change throughout development.[6] Ventilator protocols that calculate tidal volumes based on body weight may have different effects in neonates than adults. The changes to the structure of the chest wall during development may also affect ventilation strategies. The orientation of the ribs is horizontal during infancy but becomes oriented downward by age 10. Ossification of the rib cage, calcification of the costal cartilage, and development of muscular mass progressively changes during childhood and adolescence. These important physiologic changes must be considered when determining appropriate ventilation strategies in children.

## VENTILATOR-INDUCED LUNG INJURY

Much of the information that is known on ventilator-induced lung injury (VILI) arises from the adult management of acute respiratory distress syndrome (ARDS). VILI results from high peak airway pressures leading to a high transpulmonary pressure gradient with excessive distending pressures and subsequent lung overdistension (volutrauma). VILI can lead to systemic effects by initiating an inflammatory cascade within the lungs. Mechanical ventilation can also lead to shear stress and injure the alveolar-capillary barrier, which allows fluid extravasation and the efflux of inflammatory mediators from the alveolar space into the general circulation. Studies have shown that ventilator strategies can have an impact in pulmonary and systemic cytokine release and these changes are associated with multisystem organ failure.[7] This mechanical injury also leads to dysfunction of the type II pneumocyte and a concomitant reduction in surfactant production. The resulting pulmonary edema and loss of surfactant can lead to whole alveoli collapse and subsequent right-to-left shunting that is typically seen in ARDS. The inflammation caused by lung overdistention and oxygen toxicity is also thought to be important in the development of bronchopulmonary dysplasia and chronic lung disease in infants.

In adults, a lung protective strategy focused on low tidal volume, high positive end-expiratory pressure (PEEP), and recruitment maneuvers was found to be beneficial in patients with ARDS.[8] Studies from the ARDS Network demonstrated that ventilation with lower tidal volumes resulted in an overall lower mortality.[9] In a large series of nonsurvivors of CDH, autopsy and clinical data revealed that the predominant strategy among nonsurvivors were high peak airway pressures, which were associated with diffuse alveolar damage, evidence of air leak, and pulmonary hemorrhage.[10] This has led to a paradigm shift in the management of ventilation in neonates with CDH.

## EARLY VENTILATION STRATEGIES: INDUCED ALKALOSIS

In the early 1980s, management of pulmonary hypertension in infants with CDH involved treatment with chemical-induced and ventilator-induced alkalosis. Early attempts at using the ventilator to optimize blood gases led to significant morbidity from barotrauma and exacerbation of pulmonary hypertension. Alkalosis was used to significantly attenuate right-to-left ductal and atrial shunting by decreasing pulmonary vascular resistance.[11] Higher peak inspiratory pressures and mean airway pressures were used to achieve adequate alkalosis. These high airway pressures exacerbated lung injury to the abnormal lung parenchyma and led to an increase in morbidity.[10,12] Studies suggest that chemical-induced alkalosis may also be associated with an increased risk of neurologic injury[13] and the need for ECMO.[14]

## A RADICAL APPROACH: PERMISSIVE HYPERCAPNIA

In approaching ventilation management in infants with CDH, it is important to minimize ventilator-induced lung injury from overdistention of the terminal lung units. In 1985, Wung and colleagues[15] introduced the concept of permissive hypercapnia with "gentle ventilation." Infants were intubated nasotracheally and were initially ventilated with intermittent mandatory ventilation. Peak inspiratory pressures were determined by clinical assessment of chest excursion. Ventilator settings and fractional inspiratory oxygen ($FiO_2$) were selected to maintain a arterial partial pressure of oxygen ($PaO_2$) between 50 and 70 mm Hg. Arterial partial pressure of carbon dioxide ($PaCO_2$) was not a controlling parameter and was allowed to increase as high as 60 mm Hg. By tolerating a higher level of $PaCO_2$, lower levels of mean airway pressures could be achieved. Muscle relaxants were avoided. This was considered a radical approach, as prior studies described improved outcomes with maintenance of $PaCO_2$ within the normal range.[11] Permissive hypercapnia eventually became part of a coordinated approach in the care of patients with CDH, including delayed surgery, spontaneous ventilation, and minimizing sedation.[15–17]

Most infants can be managed successfully with a simple pressure-cycle ventilation using a rate of 20 to 40 breaths per minute and moderate peak airway pressures (22–35 cm H2O). If adequate gas exchange is not achieved using conventional ventilator settings, high-rate ventilation should be considered. Discontinuously, increasing the rate of ventilation while decreasing PEEP can lead to improved gas exchange while minimizing high mean airway pressures (MAPs). Initial settings of a rate of 100, peak inspiratory pressure of 18–22 cm H2O, PEEP of 0 to 1, and $FiO_2$ as needed are adequate and can be adjusted as necessary to provide adequate oxygenation and ventilation. Peak airway pressures should be minimized, preferably below 25 cm H2O.

There remain no clear guidelines for acceptable blood gas ranges for infants with CDH. Given the large variations from multiple studies, it is clear that markers of adequate oxygen delivery must be used to determine the adequacy of ventilation. Preductal oxygen saturations offer an estimate of brain and coronary oxygen delivery and the oxygenation of blood entering the circulation. Preductal saturations between 85% and 95% are generally acceptable. Other markers of systemic perfusion that can be used include serum lactate, urine output, pH, mixed venous oxygen saturations, and clinical features of distal perfusion. These markers can assist the clinician in determining the need for increases in ventilation or pharmacologic support.

## HIGH-FREQUENCY OSCILLATORY VENTILATION

High airway pressures and subsequent barotrauma to the hypoplastic lungs limit the utility of conventional ventilation in critically ill infants with CDH. This led to the consideration of high-frequency oscillatory ventilation (HFOV) in infants with CDH with respiratory failure. HFOV combines very high respiratory rates with low tidal volumes. HFOV minimizes alveolar overdistention and injury at end-inspiration by preserving uniform lung inflation. Studies have shown improved outcomes and less barotrauma in neonates with respiratory distress using HFOV compared with conventional ventilation as front-end, not rescue therapy; however, the literature is mixed. Early use of HFOV in patients with CDH aids in the stabilization before operative repair.[18] HFOV has also been successfully applied during operative repair of the diaphragmatic defect.[19] In a large 2-center study comparing ventilator strategies in infants with CDH, early use of HFOV did not improve outcomes over conventional ventilation.[20,21] The use of HFOV may be beneficial to those patients who have failed an initial trial of conventional ventilation.

Management of HFOV can be technically challenging, especially in infants with CDH, given the abnormal lung volumes that are present. Eight-rib expansion on the contralateral side to the defect, as seen on chest radiograph, is an adequate starting point for ventilation.[22] Adjustments to tidal volume must be made by changes to amplitude and frequency, which are inversely related. Changes in settings must be monitored closely to prevent lung hyperinflation and minimize the effects of high airway pressures on lung hyperinflation, venous return, pulmonary vascular resistance, and cardiac output.[23] Frequent assessment of adequate tissue perfusion is imperative when high airway pressures are required on HFOV.

Pressure-limited HFOV can be effectively applied as rescue therapy to infants with CDH to minimize the effects of barotrauma (MAP <18). An initial strategy using an $FiO_2$ as needed and a MAP of 12 cm H2O is a reasonable starting point for infants with CDH. We advocate starting with a fixed frequency (10 Hz) and making adjustments to amplitude as needed to maintain adequate ventilation while minimizing MAPs. Preoperative stabilization of an infant with CDH using pressure-limited HFOV and delayed surgery has resulted in a decreased need for ECMO and improved survival.[16,18,21]

## INHALED NITRIC OXIDE

Regulation of the vascular smooth muscle tone is significantly influenced by nitric oxide. Nitric oxide exists not only as an endogenous molecule but also as a gas that can be inhaled. When administered as a gas, it is delivered directly to ventilated areas of the lung and acts as a selective pulmonary vasodilator. Since 1992, inhaled nitric oxide (iNO) has been used as a treatment modality for patients with pulmonary hypertension. Inhaled nitric oxide interferes with the cGMP pathway and results in vasodilation by reducing intracellular calcium levels. It functions to improve oxygenation, decrease pulmonary vascular resistance, and decrease right ventricle afterload without producing a concomitant decrease in systemic vascular resistance. Inhaled nitric oxide is generally safe, well tolerated, and easy to administer.

In the Neonatal Inhaled Nitric Oxide Study (NINOS), term or near-term infants with hypoxic respiratory failure treated with iNO had an acute improvement in oxygenation and a significant reduction in the need for ECMO compared with the placebo-treated group but with no difference in mortality.[24] In a separate parallel study focusing on patients with CDH, iNO led to temporary stabilization, but treated patients trended toward a higher likelihood of ECMO or death.[25] Rebound pulmonary hypertension may occur as iNO is being weaned and about 30% of newborns with CDH may not respond to iNO treatment.[26] The exact role of iNO in infants with CDH is unclear, further prospective studies are needed.

## EXTRACORPOREAL MEMBRANE OXYGENATION

ECMO is a life-saving technology that uses partial heart/lung bypass to support a patient in cardiopulmonary failure. It is supportive and therapeutic for infants with an acute but reversible respiratory or cardiac condition. Since 1974, the Extracorporeal Life Support Organization (ELSO) has recorded approximately 28,000 newborns who have been supported with ECMO for a variety of cardiopulmonary disorders. To date, more than 6200 infants with CDH have been supported on ECMO with an overall survival of 51%. For infants who exceed maximal medical management, ECMO may provide an opportunity to allow cardiopulmonary rest and protect the lungs from further injury.

For the past few decades, numerous studies in infants with CDH have sought to elucidate which factors could determine which infants would fail medical management and require ECMO. Infants with an intra-abdominal liver position, as determined by prenatal magnetic resonance imaging, had a greater chance of survival using high-frequency oscillatory ventilation without ECMO in a few studies. Prenatal lung-to-head ratios (LHR) have also been used to prognosticate the need for ECMO and overall survival in patients with CDH. LHR values, when measured at 24 to 26 weeks' gestation, less than 0.85 had poor survival despite ECMO and those with values greater than 1.4 survived with few requiring ECMO.[27] No prenatal test perfectly predicts survival or need for ECMO in patients with CDH so careful prenatal counseling is necessary.

Patient selection of newborns with CDH for ECMO support is controversial. Neonates with CDH who present with severe pulmonary hypoplasia that precludes adequate gas exchange should not be offered ECMO. Patients who are unable to achieve a preductal oxygen saturation greater than 90% on an FiO2 of 1.0 and then go on to deteriorate generally have inadequate lung volume for survival and ECMO should not be considered. Typically, ECMO candidates will maintain adequate oxygenation within the first few hours of life during the "honeymoon" period, but then subsequently deteriorate owing to the effects of pulmonary hypertension that are generally reversible. Patients who maintain a preductal arterial oxygen saturation (SaO2) of greater than 90% on FiO2 of 1.0 or a PaCO2 less than 50 for a period of time but subsequently develop sustained hypoxia (SaO2 <60%), acidosis (pH <7.2), or an alveolar arterial oxygen gradient greater than 600 for 10 hours, then ECMO should be initiated. This can also be manifest by mixed venous desaturations and multiple end organ failure. Following these criteria, patients with CDH supported on ECMO had an 86% percent overall survival.[28]

Once the desired oxygen delivery is obtained, the ventilator should be promptly weaned to avoid further oxygen toxicity and barotrauma. The optimal rest settings are patient dependent but generally consist of an FiO2 of 0.21, PEEP of 5 cm H2O, peak inspiratory pressure of 20 to 25 cm H2O, a rate of 12 breaths/minute and an inspiratory time of 0.5 seconds once adequate perfusion and oxygenation on ECMO are obtained.[29] On weaning off ECMO, or after surgical repair on ECMO, ventilator settings can be increased as necessary to obtain successful decannulation hemodynamics. Occasionally, infants may develop airway reactivity and exacerbation of pulmonary hypertension after surgical repair, which may require increased ventilator support or ECMO in the postoperative period.[30]

## LIQUID VENTILATION

Numerous groups have studied perfluorocarbons as a medium for respiration for the past 4 decades. Perflubrons are a group of chemicals that are liquid at room temperature, heavier but less viscous than water, have surfactant properties, and can carry large amounts of respiratory gases. Previous studies have demonstrated the ability of perfluorocarbon-filled lungs to improve gas exchange and pulmonary compliance in both full-term and premature neonatal animal models of respiratory failure. After the lungs are filled with perfluorocarbons, there are 2 modes of ventilation: (1) total liquid ventilation, in which the lungs are ventilated with tidal volumes of perfluorocarbon using a liquid ventilator, or (2) partial liquid ventilation, in which the lungs are ventilated with gas tidal volumes using a standard gas mechanical ventilator. Some of the limitations of partial liquid ventilator include lack of precise measurements of perfluorocarbon dose, pressure and volume changes in alveoli, oxygenation at alveoli, and clearance of debris.[31] Partial liquid ventilation has been applied to infants with CDH on ECMO support as a means to improve gas exchange.[32] Currently approved by the Food and Drug Administration for clinical trials only, future large prospective trials are needed to determine the true efficacy of liquid ventilation in patients with CDH.

## SURFACTANT ADMINISTRATION

Patients with congenital diaphragmatic hernias not only have pulmonary hypertension but also suffer from an acquired surfactant inactivation. Postmortem examinations of the lung in infants with CDH demonstrate lower phospholipid and surface active lecithin concentrations. Surfactant deficiency in CDH is usually acquired secondary to ventilator-induced damage to type II pneumocytes or from the severity of the disease itself. The risk of administration of surfactant is that routine dosages of surfactant may exceed the normal tidal volumes of many infants with CDH. Surfactant therapy also carries adverse side effects, such as severe hypotension and acute respiratory distress. Despite its widespread use in many centers, its safety in patients with CDH is currently unknown. Small studies evaluating the efficacy of exogenous surfactant administration in patients with CDH on ECMO have failed to show a significant long-term improvement in respiratory function. Some studies indicate that surfactant therapy is associated with a higher mortality rate, greater use of ECMO, and more chronic lung disease in infants with CDH.[33,34] In preterm infants with CDH, surfactant administration was also associated with lower survival rate. Based on the limited available evidence, the routine use of surfactant replacement in infants with CDH should be avoided.

## SUMMARY

The main goal of ventilator management in neonates with congenital diaphragmatic hernias is to provide adequate gas exchange while minimizing barotrauma before surgical repair. This can be achieved by implementing a lung protective strategy where permissive hypercapnea is used and adequate tidal volumes are achieved at lower airway pressures. In infants with CDH, hypercapnea and preductal saturations as low as 85% can be accepted to minimize the hazardous effects of ventilator-induced lung injury. Markers of systemic perfusion should be used to guide the effectiveness of ventilation and oxygenation.

Various ventilation strategies have been used to prevent ventilator-induced lung injury. An initial trial of ventilation with permissive hypercapnea and spontaneous respirations can be initiated in all patients with CDH. If oxygenation or ventilation is inadequate, a trial of high-rate/low-pressure ventilation should be used. Once high mean airway pressures are required using conventional ventilation, then conversion to pressure-limited high-frequency oscillatory ventilation should be considered. ECMO is appropriate for subsequent failures if there is adequate lung parenchyma to support life. Additional modalities, such as surfactant administration and inhaled nitric oxide, have not shown consistent benefits in infants with CDH, and their routine use should be with caution. Future research with liquid ventilation may provide an attractive alternative option for infants with CDH requiring increased ventilator support. It is important for centers to adapt an algorithm with defined decision points to allow consistent ventilation strategies for infants with CDH.

Any fetus diagnosed with CDH should be born in close proximity to a full-service neonatal intensive care unit. It is important to consider early coordinated transfer, given the inability of transporting patients on portable HFOV in many areas. The perinatal care of infants with CDH is complex and requires a multidisciplinary group of pediatric neonatologists, surgeons, cardiologists, and social workers. Early lung protective ventilation is critical for successful outcomes in infants with CDH.

## REFERENCES

1. Fisher JC, Jefferson RA, Arkovitz MS, et al. Redefining outcomes in right congenital diaphragmatic hernia. J Pediatr Surg 2008;43(2):373–9.
2. Levin DL. Morphologic analysis of the pulmonary vascular bed in congenital left-sided diaphragmatic hernia. J Pediatr 1978;92(5):805–9.
3. Jesudason EC. Small lungs and suspect smooth muscle: congenital diaphragmatic hernia and the smooth muscle hypothesis. J Pediatr Surg 2006;41(2): 431–5.
4. Jani J, Peralta CF, Benachi A, et al. Assessment of lung area in fetuses with congenital diaphragmatic hernia. Ultrasound Obstet Gynecol 2007;30(1):72–6.
5. Beals DA, Schloo BL, Vacanti JP, et al. Pulmonary growth and remodeling in infants with high-risk congenital diaphragmatic hernia. J Pediatr Surg 1992;27(8):997–1001 [discussion: 1001–2].
6. Thorsteinsson A, Larsson A, Jonmarker C, et al. Pressure-volume relations of the respiratory system in healthy children. Am J Respir Crit Care Med 1994;150(2): 421–30.
7. Logan JW, Cotten CM, Goldberg RN, et al. Mechanical ventilation strategies in the management of congenital diaphragmatic hernia. Semin Pediatr Surg 2007; 16(2):115–25.
8. Amato MB, Barbas CS, Medeiros DM, et al. Effect of a protective-ventilation strategy on mortality in the acute respiratory distress syndrome. N Engl J Med 1998;338(6):347–54.
9. Ventilation with lower tidal volumes as compared with traditional tidal volumes for acute lung injury and the acute respiratory distress syndrome. The Acute Respiratory Distress Syndrome Network. N Engl J Med 2000;342(18):1301–8.
10. Sakurai Y, Azarow K, Cutz E, et al. Pulmonary barotrauma in congenital diaphragmatic hernia: a clinicopathological correlation. J Pediatr Surg 1999;34(12):1813–7.
11. Drummond WH, Gregory GA, Heymann MA, et al. The independent effects of hyperventilation, tolazoline, and dopamine on infants with persistent pulmonary hypertension. J Pediatr 1981;98(4):603–11.
12. Thibeault DW, Haney B. Lung volume, pulmonary vasculature, and factors affecting survival in congenital diaphragmatic hernia. Pediatrics 1998;101(2): 289–95.

13. Murase M, Ishida A. Early hypocarbia of preterm infants: its relationship to periventricular leukomalacia and cerebral palsy, and its perinatal risk factors. Acta Paediatr 2005;94(1):85–91.

14. Walsh MC, Stork EK. Persistent pulmonary hypertension of the newborn. Rational therapy based on pathophysiology. Clin Perinatol 2001;28(3):609–27, vii.

15. Wung JT, James LS, Kilchevsky E, et al. Management of infants with severe respiratory failure and persistence of the fetal circulation, without hyperventilation. Pediatrics 1985;76(4):488–94.

16. Wung JT, Sahni R, Moffitt ST, et al. Congenital diaphragmatic hernia: survival treated with very delayed surgery, spontaneous respiration, and no chest tube. J Pediatr Surg 1995;30(3):406–9.

17. Boloker J, Bateman DA, Wung JT, et al. Congenital diaphragmatic hernia in 120 infants treated consecutively with permissive hypercapnea/spontaneous respiration/elective repair. J Pediatr Surg 2002;37(3):357–66.

18. Reyes C, Chang LK, Waffarn F, et al. Delayed repair of congenital diaphragmatic hernia with early high-frequency oscillatory ventilation during preoperative stabilization. J Pediatr Surg 1998;33(7):1010–4 [discussion: 1014–6].

19. Bouchut JC, Dubois R, Moussa M, et al. High frequency oscillatory ventilation during repair of neonatal congenital diaphragmatic hernia. Paediatr Anaesth 2000;10(4): 377–9.

20. Azarow K, Messineo A, Pearl R, et al. Congenital diaphragmatic hernia—a tale of two cities: the Toronto experience. J Pediatr Surg 1997;32(3):395–400.

21. Wilson JM, Lund DP, Lillehei CW, et al. Congenital diaphragmatic hernia—a tale of two cities: the Boston experience. J Pediatr Surg 1997;32(3):401–5.

22. Cotten M, Clark RH. The science of neonatal high-frequency ventilation. Respir Care Clin N Am 2001;7(4):611–31.

23. Traverse JH, Korvenranta H, Adams EM, et al. Impairment of hemodynamics with increasing mean airway pressure during high-frequency oscillatory ventilation. Pediatr Res 1988;23(6):628–31.

24. Inhaled nitric oxide in full-term and nearly full-term infants with hypoxic respiratory failure. The Neonatal Inhaled Nitric Oxide Study Group. N Engl J Med 1997; 336(9):597–604.

25. Inhaled nitric oxide and hypoxic respiratory failure in infants with congenital diaphragmatic hernia. The Neonatal Inhaled Nitric Oxide Study Group (NINOS). Pediatrics 1997;99(6):838–45.

26. Goldman AP, Tasker RC, Hosiasson S, et al. Early response to inhaled nitric oxide and its relationship to outcome in children with severe hypoxemic respiratory failure. Chest 1997;112(3):752–8.

27. Aspelund G, Fisher JC, Simpson LL, et al. Prenatal lung-head ratio: threshold to predict outcome for congenital diaphragmatic hernia. J Matern Fetal Neonatal Med 2011. [Epub ahead of print].

28. Stolar C, Dillon P, Reyes C. Selective use of extracorporeal membrane oxygenation in the management of congenital diaphragmatic hernia. J Pediatr Surg 1988; 23(3):207–11.

29. Keszler M, Subramanian KN, Smith YA, et al. Pulmonary management during extracorporeal membrane oxygenation. Crit Care Med 1989;17(6):495–500.

30. Nakayama DK, Motoyama EK, Mutich RL, et al. Pulmonary function in newborns after repair of congenital diaphragmatic hernia. Pediatr Pulmonol 1991;11(1): 49–55.

31. Wolfson MR, Shaffer TH. Pulmonary applications of perfluorochemical liquids: ventilation and beyond. Paediatr Respir Rev 2005;6(2):117–27.

32. Pranikoff T, Gauger PG, Hirschl RB. Partial liquid ventilation in newborn patients with congenital diaphragmatic hernia. J Pediatr Surg 1996;31(5):613–8.
33. Van Meurs K. Is surfactant therapy beneficial in the treatment of the term newborn infant with congenital diaphragmatic hernia? J Pediatr 2004;145(3):312–6.
34. Lally KP, Lally PA, Langham MR, et al. Surfactant does not improve survival rate in preterm infants with congenital diaphragmatic hernia. J Pediatr Surg 2004;39(6): 829–33.

# Chest Wall Deformities in Pediatric Surgery

Robert J. Obermeyer, MD[a,b,*], Michael J. Goretsky, MD[a,b]

## KEYWORDS

- Pectus excavatum • Pectus carinatum • Nuss procedure • Chest wall deformities

## KEY POINTS

- The most common chest wall deformities are congenital pectus excavatum and pectus carinatum.
- Most young children with pectus excavatum are asymptomatic, but as they become more active in their pre- and early teenage years the most common complaints are exercise intolerance, lack of endurance, and shortness of breath on exertion.
- Despite the varied results of studies designed to evaluate the pulmonary and cardiac pathophysiologic effects of pectus excavatum, the majority of patients indicate improved exercise tolerance after surgery.
- Patients with pectus carinatum also may present with similar symptoms, although they are much less likely to do so than patients with pectus excavatum.
- The primary therapy for pectus carinatum is orthotic bracing. Failing this, both the open and minimally invasive techniques are good alternatives.

Chest wall deformities can be divided into 2 main categories, congenital and acquired. Congenital chest wall deformities may present any time between birth and early adolescence. Acquired chest wall deformities typically follow prior chest surgery or a posterolateral diaphragmatic hernia repair (Bochdalek). Congenital chest wall deformities fall within 2 main groups, those with either a depression or protrusion of the sternum and those with varying degrees of aplasia or dysplasia (thoracic ectopia cordis, sternal clefts, Poland syndrome, Jeune asphyxiating thoracic dystrophy). The most common chest wall deformities are congenital pectus excavatum (88%) and pectus carinatum (5%).

## PECTUS EXCAVATUM

Depression of the anterior chest wall is known as pectus excavatum (PE), but has also been termed funnel chest and trichterbrust.[1] PE is the most common chest wall

The authors have nothing to disclose.
[a] Eastern Virginia Medical School, 700 West Olney Road, Norfolk, VA 23507, USA; [b] Pediatric Surgery, Children's Hospital of The King's Daughters, 601 Children's Lane, Norfolk, VA 23507, USA
* Pediatric Surgery, Children's Hospital of The King's Daughters, 601 Children's Lane, Norfolk, VA 23507.
E-mail address: Robert.Obermeyer@chkd.org

Surg Clin N Am 92 (2012) 669–684
doi:10.1016/j.suc.2012.03.001
0039-6109/12/$ – see front matter © 2012 Elsevier Inc. All rights reserved.

deformity and has an incidence of 1 in 400 births (0.25%). It occurs more frequently in boys than girls by a 5:1 ratio. About 95% of cases occur in Caucasian patients whereas Asian, African American, and Hispanic patients each only present about 1% to 2% of the time.[2,3] PE is most often noted in the first year of life (86%), and in the remaining cases will present sometime before or during the early teenage years.[4] Cases of spontaneous resolution during this time frame are very uncommon, and the more typical course is worsening of the depression during phases of rapid vertical growth and puberty.[5]

### Etiology

The mechanism and cause of PE has not been established. One physical mechanism commonly described is a disproportionate overgrowth of the costal cartilages that pushes the sternum posteriorly,[6] but more recent computed tomography (CT) studies have cast doubt on this theory. Nakaoka and colleagues[7] demonstrated that in PE patients the costal cartilage lengths relative to the adjacent rib were not longer than in healthy control patients. Another mechanism proposed is an abnormal tethering of the sternum to the diaphragm posteriorly. This theory is supported by a 33% incidence of acquired PE in patients after repair of posterolateral congenital diaphragmatic hernias (Bochdalek).[8] Alternatively, a relative weakening of the costal cartilages could be the culprit, which would align mechanistically with the association of PE with other musculoskeletal abnormalities such as scoliosis, Marfan syndrome, Ehlers-Danlos syndrome, and osteogenesis imperfecta.[9–11]

The cause of this mechanistic aberration is also unclear, but histopathologic (disorderly arrangement and distribution of collagen, perichondritis, areas of aseptic necrosis) and mineral (decreased zinc and elevated magnesium and calcium) eccentricities have been identified that may be responsible for the weakening of the costal cartilages relative to the posterior sternal attachments, resulting in posterior migration of the sternum.[12]

Although there is no confirmed chromosomal abnormality, there is a genetic predisposition supported by roughly 40% of patients having a family member with a chest wall deformity. Evaluation of 34 families with a 4-generation pedigree analysis suggested 4 different possible patterns of inheritance: autosomal dominant, autosomal recessive, X-linked recessive, and complex.[3,13]

### Pathophysiology

#### Pulmonary

In 1992, Kaguraoka and colleagues[14] had one of the largest series evaluating pulmonary function, in 138 PE patients before and after open repair. Although vital capacity (VC) decreased within 2 months after surgery, it was noted to recover to preoperative levels within 1 year after surgery and remain at baseline for up to 42 months without improvement, despite significant morphologic improvement. In 2000, Haller and Loughlin[15] evaluated pulmonary function in 36 PE patients and 10 normal controls, and demonstrated a decrease in forced VC (FVC) in the PE cohort. Six months after open surgical repair, the studies were repeated on 15 PE patients and 6 normal controls. Although surgical repair did not improve FVC in the PE group, patients did show increased exercise tolerance and a higher oxygen pulse, which is a surrogate for cardiac output.

The largest study by 2005 was performed by Lawson and colleagues,[16] and evaluated 408 PE patients as well as 45 patients following minimally invasive repair of pectus excavatum (MIRPE) with subsequent bar removal. With normal average values defined as 100% of predicted for FVC, forced expired volume in 1 second (FEV$_1$), and forced expiratory flow ($FEF_{25\%-75\%}$), the uncorrected PE patients demonstrated a statistically significant decrease in these pulmonary function testing values by an average of 13% to 20%. Only patients 11 years and older at the time of surgery appreciated a significant 6% to 15% improvement in mean PFT after bar removal. Patients with surgical correction before 11 years of age did not have significant improvement in PFT values. More recently Lawson and colleagues[17] demonstrated, in a multicenter study of 310 subjects, more data supporting these PFT derangements in PE patients. Patients with a median Haller index greater than 4.3 were found to have a significant decrease in these PFT values by an average of 14% to 20%, which is similar to their findings in 2005. Of further interest in this study was the finding that for each unit increase in the Haller index, patients were 1.4 times more likely to show a restrictive pattern. Postoperative PFT values from the multicenter study by Kelly and colleagues[3] are pending, and will help elucidate the effects of surgical correction of PE on PFT values.

Another possible explanation for ease of fatigability in PE patients is a less efficient mechanism of breathing. In 2011, Redlinger and colleagues[18] demonstrated focal chest wall motion abnormalities in 64 PE patients versus 55 controls. Using motion analysis technology, PE patients were determined to have significantly decreased chest wall motion at the area of the pectus defect and increased abdominal contributions to respiration. This phenomenon in PE patients may result in a less efficient mechanism of breathing and thus help explain symptoms such as ease of fatigability (**Fig. 1**).

### Cardiac

Thoracic CT and magnetic resonance imaging (MRI) scans often demonstrate that the right ventricle is deformed by the posterior displacement of the sternum in PE patients. The degree of deformity is variable, depending on the severity and asymmetry of the PE as well as the occasional repositioning of the heart into the left thoracic cavity. Pectus carinatum (PC) patients do not have cardiac compression, so these patients should be spared any adverse cardiac effects. To that effect, in 1984 Cahill and colleagues[19] evaluated 14 PE and 5 PC patients for progressive work exercise performance. Exercise performance was improved for PE patients when assessed by effort-related total exercise time and the maximal oxygen consumption, but more compelling was the lower pulse at 3 given workloads. There was a consistent decrease in heart rate at each given power output ($P<.02$; paired $t$-test) for the PE

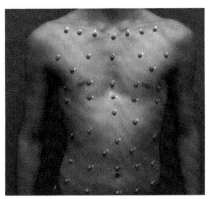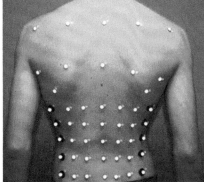

**Fig. 1.** Markers used to track motion of the chest wall during deep breathing in patients with pectus excavatum.

patients, but no decrease was observed in PC patients. These findings support the hypothesis that cardiac stroke volume in PE is impaired and may be improved by surgical correction.

Later, Kowalewski and colleagues[20] addressed the effects of surgical correction in 1999 using digital subtraction echocardiographic evaluation of right ventricular structure and function in 42 patients, before and 6 months after repair of PE. Statistically significant increases were seen in the right ventricular volume indices (systolic, diastolic, and stroke volume) after surgery, but the amount of improvement did not have a direct correlation to the degree of sternocostal elevation.

In 2000, Zhao and colleagues[21] compared the effects of position in 13 PE patients versus 20 control subjects. Peak oxygen uptake ($Vo_2$max) and Doppler stroke volume (SV) were assessed while cycling in the sitting and supine positions. PE patients exercising in the sitting position demonstrated decreased $Vo_2$max and SV, but during supine exercise they approached the same values as the control subjects. These findings support the theory that exercise capacity is limited as a result of reduced filling of the right heart by the compressive effects of PE.

In addition to the compressive effects of PE on filling and emptying of the right heart, there is also thought to be deformation of the mitral valve annulus, producing mitral valve prolapse (MVP) and mitral valve regurgitation (MVR). To support this theory, in 2006 Coln and colleagues,[22] using echocardiography, evaluated 123 patients who had undergone repair of PE by the Nuss procedure. Preoperative echocardiography revealed cardiac compression in 95% (117 of 123) and mitral valve abnormalities in 44% (25 MVP and 29 MVR of 123) of patients. Postoperative echocardiography revealed resolution of compression in all cases, and only mild persistent MVP in 7 patients and asymptomatic MVR in 1 patient. The interplay between impaired right heart filling, impaired right ventricular SV, and valvular dysfunction may help explain why the symptoms related to exertion, present in 86% (106 of 123) of the PE patients preoperatively, resolved in all patients postoperatively.

### Clinical Evaluation

#### Signs

Initial consultation should include a complete history and physical examination, which includes questions regarding onset, duration, and progression of chest wall deformity. The morphology of the PE should be described in detail. The degree of depression of the body of the sternum and the lower costal cartilages should be noted. The deformity may be described as symmetric or asymmetric with a deeper depression on one side of the sternum. Asymmetry is often associated with sternal rotation, and this should be identified too. The deepest point of the PE should be noted, and is often below the sternum. The deformity may be localized (cup-shaped), diffuse (saucer-shaped), or long and unilateral (grand-canyon type). A mixed deformity with protrusion of the upper sternum and depression of the lower sternum has been termed Currarino-Silverman deformity, also known as horns-of-steer deformity (**Fig. 2**).[23] This type of PE defect is the only one that the authors have found not to be amenable to the Nuss procedure. Photographic documentation with a minimum of 6 angles (face shot, frontal, left and right lateral, left and right oblique) is very helpful in following these patients before and after repair.

#### Symptoms

Symptom assessment should be thorough, with focused questioning regarding the pulmonary and cardiac systems. Most young children with PE are asymptomatic, but as they become more active in their pre- and early teenage years the most

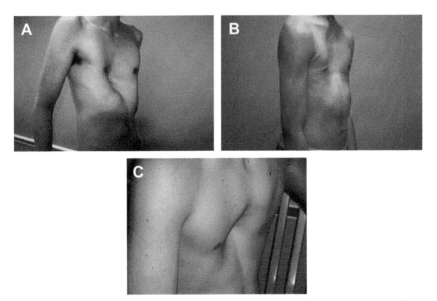

**Fig. 2.** (*A*) Cup-shaped deformity. (*B*) Saucer-shaped deformity. (*C*) Horns-of-steer deformity.

common complaints are exercise intolerance, lack of endurance, and shortness of breath on exertion. Body image is also an important part of the history because these patients may be at risk for poor body image, social withdrawal, and even suicidal tendencies. PE has been determined to have lower HRQL (Health-Related Quality-of-Life) scores than age-matched population norms.[24] In a multicenter study by Kelly and colleagues[25] using previously validated psychometric assessments, 264 patients (age 8–21 years) were found to have a statistically significant improvement in body image when assessed after their surgical repair. Emotional difficulties and social self-consciousness were also statistically significantly improved when judged by the parents.

### Objective Evaluation

Pulmonary function testing, CT or MRI of the chest, and a cardiac evaluation to include electrocardiogram and echocardiogram are a routine part of the evaluation for a patient with PE. More recently, MRI of the chest with cardiac function assessment has been used to avoid radiation exposure and replace the echocardiogram. Radiographic evaluation with a thoracic CT scan or MRI allows the physician to grade the severity of the PE by calculating the Haller index that uses the internal measurements of the transverse and anteroposterior dimension at the deepest point of the deformity (**Fig. 3**).[26] Thin-layer rapid-use epicutaneous (TRUE) patch testing (**Fig. 4**) can be useful in all patients to identify metal allergies. This test must be performed if a history of metal allergy or atopy (eczema, allergic rhinitis, or asthma) is identified. If the patient is found to be allergic to nickel or chromium, a custom titanium bar must be used. Only about 2% to 3% of patients have been identified as having metal allergies, but if this is not detected preoperatively, bar removal may be required.[27]

### Management

Asymptomatic patients with mild PE (ie, Haller index <3.25) are encouraged to perform deep breathing with 5- to 10-second breath-holding as tolerated, and to continue

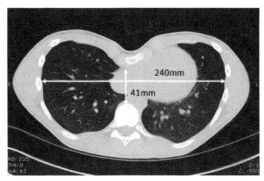

**Fig. 3.** Haller index = 240/41 = 5.85.

aerobic activities. Surgical correction of PE is offered to those patients who are interested in attempting to improve their exercise tolerance. Most surgeons agree that surgical correction is recommended if the patient has 2 or more of the following[28]:

1. Compression abnormalities: chest CT or MRI showing cardiac or pulmonary compression with a Haller index of 3.25 or greater
2. Pulmonary abnormalities: restrictive lung disease by PFT evaluation
3. Cardiac abnormalities: cardiac compression, MVP, or conduction abnormalities
4. Performance abnormalities: exercise intolerance, lack of endurance, and shortness of breath on exertion
5. Recurrence: following an open or MIRPE procedure.

The optimal age for repair is 10 to 14 years old because at this time the thoracic rib cage is more malleable, thus allowing for rapid recovery, better results, and a lower recurrence rate as the bar remains in place during musculoskeletal maturation. However, the authors have had equally good results in patients older than 18 years.

### Vacuum bell

Although not a surgical technique for correction of PE, the vacuum bell may represent a future method of treating selected PE patients noninvasively. At the time of writing, the vacuum bell is not approved by the Food and Drug Administration nor is it readily available in the United States. The concept of applying vacuum to the chest wall to correct deformities was initially described more than 100 years ago.[29] Modernization and refinement of a vacuum bell was performed by an engineer, who himself suffered from PE (Klobe, http://www.trichterbrust.de) (**Fig. 5**). In 2005, Schier and colleagues[30] introduced the use of this device with 60 patients (age 6.1–34.9 years, median

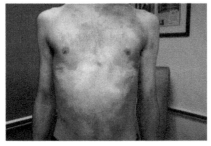
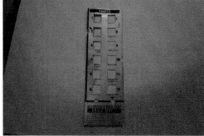

**Fig. 4.** A patient with allergy and TRUE patch.

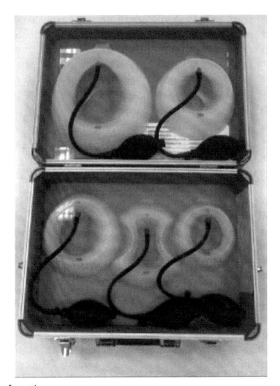

**Fig. 5.** A variety of suction cups.

14.8 years). After 1 month 85% achieved 1 cm of sternal elevation, but only 20% had complete correction after 5 months. Longer-term results that included 133 patients (age 3–61 years, median 16.2 years) were published by Haecker[31] in 2011. Overall the results were similar, with 79% having 1-cm lift after 3 months and complete correction in only 13.5% after 18 months. One conclusion by Haecker was that results were better for patients with mild and symmetric PE.[31] The vacuum bell was also described in both of these studies as a way to temporarily elevate the sternum intraoperatively while using the introducer to dissect under the sternum during the MIRPE procedure. The authors have had a positive experience with this technique, and a video presentation is available with detailed descriptions.[32] Future uses for the vacuum bell may include the use of the suction cup for young patients, under-correction, recurrences, and more liberal use in the operating room.

### Minimally invasive repair of pectus excavatum (nuss repair)
The Nuss repair is performed with the arms abducted approximately 70° from the thorax and 90° at the elbow to prevent excess traction on the brachial plexus. The chest is measured transversely with a paper ruler from bilateral points located slightly medial to the anterior axillary line. The bar length selected is 1 inch less than this measurement to account for the shorter course the bar takes as it traverses the chest wall. The optimal shape is different for each patient, but a slight bend on the ends of the bar with an approximately 2-cm flat section in the middle to support the sternum is recommended.

Lateral incisions are made and tunnels are created to the planned entrance and exit sites, which are medial to the greatest apex. All this is done under direct thoracoscopic visualization. Using an umbilical tape, the bar that has previously been measured and bent is then passed and flipped. In older patients or those with stiff, asymmetric, or saucer-shaped defects, 2 bars are frequently required. The bar is then secured with a stabilizer and pericostal sutures. The incisions are closed in 3 layers, air is evacuated, and an intraoperative chest radiograph is acquired to ensure there is not an unrecognized pneumothorax or bar shift. The bar is maintained for 2 to 3 years to decrease recurrence rates.

### Open repair (Ravitch procedure)

An open method to repair PE is used in some centers. Repair in young children is discouraged because of the risk of interference with the growth plates and subsequent development of acquired thoracic chondrodystrophy. The surgical repair involves various modifications of the original procedure described by Brown and modified by Ravitch.[33,34]

A transverse thoracic incision is made in the inframammary crease. Electrocautery is used to create cutaneous flaps, and the pectoralis muscle is elevated to expose the depressed sternum and costal cartilages from at least T3 to T7. The perichondrium is scored longitudinally, and the deformed cartilages are resected either partially or completely with preservation of the perichondrial sheaths. The xiphoid may require division from the sternum if it is expected to protrude after correction. An anterior table, wedge-shaped, sternal osteotomy is performed at the cephalad transition from the normal to the depressed sternum near the level of the insertion of the second or third costal cartilages. For an optimal cosmetic result, the osteotomy may need to be at an angle if the sternum is rotated. The posterior aspect of the sternum is dissected free, elevated, and fractured by upward traction. The osteotomy is closed with nonabsorbable sutures. A drain is positioned below the muscle flaps. The muscle flaps are sutured back into position and the incisions are closed.

### Postoperative care

While hospitalized and until 2 weeks postoperatively, incentive spirometry is recommended 10 times per hour while awake to minimize respiratory complications. A patient-controlled analgesia pump is used for pain control up to the second postoperative day, at which time the patients are transitioned to oral pain medication. Hospital stays range from 3 to 6 days. On discharge patients are given copies of their chest radiograph, a Medic alert application ("metal bars in chest, press harder for CPR, apply defibrillation pads on the front and back of the chest"), and routine discharge instructions (**Box 1**). After discharge, deep-breathing exercises are also strongly recommended as described previously.

### Outcomes

Complications for both surgical techniques are low and of similar frequency.[4,10] The most recent data from the last 21 years including 1123 primary and 92 redo repairs performed using the Nuss procedure at the Children's Hospital of the King's Daughters, Norfolk, Virginia was recently published.[35] Of the 790 patients who have had their bar removed, a good or excellent result was obtained in 96%, fair in 1.4%, and poor in 0.8%. Chest tube drainage to correct the inability to evacuate air from the thoracic space is recommended, and was required in about 4% of cases. Postoperative chest tubes to treat hemothorax or effusions were required in 0.9%. Pneumonia occurred in 0.5% and pericarditis requiring indomethacin was required in 0.4%. Superficial wound infections (1%) were twice as common as deep infections involving the bar (0.5%). Only 3 patients (0.2%) required early bar removal because of infection. Before modifications in bar fixation the bar-displacement rate was 12% to 13%, but it

---

**Box 1**
**Discharge instructions for PE repair patients**

Week 4:

    You may sleep on your side

    You may twist at the waist

Week 6:

    You may drive

    We highly recommend that you begin cardiovascular conditioning such as running, swimming, biking (only if you are skilled), pilates, yoga, and so forth

Week 8:

    We highly recommend that you begin light upper body weight training (no more than 2–5 lbs)

3 Months:

    You may carry a back pack

    You may return to noncontact sports such as basketball, soccer, baseball, and so forth

    You can ride a rollercoaster

6 Months:

    You are restriction free except for the following activities: football, sparring with martial arts, wrestling/boxing, hockey

We do not recommend that you participate in any activity that you are likely to receive a forcible blow to the chest while the bar is in place, in order to decrease the possibility of the bar from shifting.

---

is now less than 2%.[35] Overcorrection occurred in 2% of primary repairs and only 0.4% developed a PC. Despite the varied results of studies designed to evaluate the pulmonary and cardiac pathophysiologic effects of PE, the majority of patients indicate subjectively improved exercise tolerance after surgery. Recurrences requiring redo operation should be low, and occurred in only 11 of the authors' patients (1.4%).

## PECTUS CARINATUM

PC is the second most common congenital chest wall deformity. It is also frequently referred to as pigeon chest, chicken breast, and pyramidal chest. It is 5 times less common than PE in North America.[36] However, in other countries it is much more common. In Argentina it has been reported to comprise 55% of chest wall deformities,[37] and in Brazil it has a frequency of half that of PE.[38] Similarly to PE, it is more common in boys than in girls, with a ratio of 4:1.[39] Most children present as teenagers because the deformity usually is not appreciated until after 11 years of age, and then worsens with puberty.

### Pathophysiology and Clinical Evaluation

The origin of PC is similar to that of PE. Although there is no clear etiology, there is some genetic predisposition because 26% of patients have a family history of chest wall deformities.[36] In addition, there is an abnormality of connective tissue development because 12% of patients also have scoliosis.[36]

    A complete history and physical examination is warranted. There is always a prominent protrusion of the sternum, with several patterns that may be present. The most common deformity is the chondrogladiolar protrusion, which is a symmetric protrusion of the sternum (gladiolus) and coastal cartilages (**Fig. 6**); this is also called keel chest. Lateral depression of the ribs accentuates the protrusion and can be asymmetric. Mixed deformities occur that involve components of both protrusion and depression. The sternum is rotated posteriorly toward the depressed side. Imaging can be helpful in determining the degree of compression, which may be falsely accentuated by the protrusion defect. Poland syndrome is commonly associated with mixed defects. There is an increased incidence of congenital heart disease in these children.[40] Chondromanubrial defects are much less common and are referred to as pouter pigeon deformities. This condition has a protrusion of the manubrium and superior costal cartilages, with a relative depression of the body of the sternum. Premature fusion and synostosis of the sternum creates this deformity.

Most children will not have significant symptoms with PC. Tenderness when lying prone is a common complaint, and musculoskeletal pain of the chest and epigastrium may also be present. Psychological distress and negative body image can be identified, and in severe cases patients may complain of physiologic deficits such as shortness of breath. Supplements to the physical examination include posteroanterior and lateral chest radiographs, and in certain cases chest imaging with either a CT or MRI may be helpful. A Haller index of 1.2 to 2 is often found in those patients who will benefit from therapy.[39]

### Management

Orthotic bracing is the first line therapy recommended for most patients, especially those who are motivated, have a malleable chest wall, and are younger than 18 years. Success rates of 65% to 80% have been reported with orthotic bracing alone, with good long-term results. Success is strongly dependent on the patient's motivation and chest wall flexibility. By making the brace comfortable to wear, easy to conceal, with incremental corrections over time, there has been a higher rate of success. Recently, Martinez-Ferro and colleagues[37] have reported the use of a dynamic compression system for the correction of PC (**Fig. 7**). This device uses a custom-made aluminum brace with an electronic pressure-measuring device. By using this system investigators have reported an 88% good to excellent result, and avoidance of skin complications, suboptimal results, and patient noncompliance[41] Regardless of which brace is used, the use in conjunction with physical therapists and/or physical

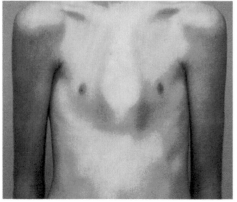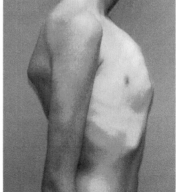

**Fig. 6.** Pectus carinatum (chondrogladiolar type).

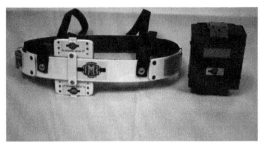

**Fig. 7.** Dynamic compression system that is custom fit to the patient. An electronic pressure measuring device is placed in the docking stating of the brace, and the brace is adjusted to a pressure of treatment of 2.5 psi.

medicine and rehabilitation physicians is advantageous.[42,43] In addition, the peer-pressure effect of having a bracing clinic helps with noncompliance in teenagers.

The surgical management of PC is also presently in evolution, with newer minimally invasive techniques being evaluated. The time-honored open approach is most often used, and is similar to that used for open repairs of PE. This approach was first promoted by Ravitch[44] in 1952 for the surgical correction of PC. A transverse incision is usually made, followed by skin and pectoralis muscle flaps. It is recommended that all and partially deformed cartilages are removed, because with continued growth they can worsen and become apparent.[36,45,46] It is important to leave the perichondrium behind. The type of deformity of the carinatum defect will dictate subsequent steps in the procedure. For chondrogladiolar defects, double osteotomies are often needed to allow the posterior plate of the sternum to be fractured and return to a more normal position. For mixed defects and asymmetric defects, it is important to resect cartilages on both sides of the sternum to allow it to flatten. A transverse offset wedge-shaped osteotomy is used. Closure of this defect then allows anterior displacement and rotation of the sternum. Closed suction drains are placed and are usually removed before discharge.

In 2009, Abramson and colleagues[41,47] from Buenos Aires reported a 5-year experience with a minimally invasive technique for PC repair. With this technique a Nuss bar is tunneled subcutaneously via lateral thoracic incisions and placed anterior to the sternum. Stabilizers are attached to the ribs on both sides with subperiosteally placed wires. The bar is then attached to the stabilizers and secured, once the desired configuration of the chest is obtained, with manual pressure. A modification of thoracoscopic cartilage resection for stiff chests has been reported by Kim and Idowu.[48] The use of these 2 modifications are still in evolution in the United States, and initial anecdotal reports have been promising. Issues with securing the stabilizers to the ribs and securing the bar to the stabilizer have been some of the areas of concern that are undergoing further modifications.

### Outcomes

Some form of orthotic bracing is the first-line therapy for PC. With essentially no morbidity except minor skin irritation, there is no reason not to try bracing for at least 12 to 24 months. In compliant patients who have not finished puberty, success rates approaching 80% have been reported.[42,43,49] In older patients with stiff chests, bypassing bracing and going straight to surgery is reasonable.

Overall success from the surgical techniques is high, with minimal complications. Most complications are minor and consist of wound infections, pneumothorax, pneumonia, wound separation, and minor cosmetic issues. Recurrence is rare and is usually associated with incomplete initial repair and repair at an early age.[36,45,50] Patients have reported a subjective improvement in chest discomfort, dyspnea, and stamina after repair, but any objective reports are limited.

## STERNAL DEFECTS

Sternal defects are extremely rare and, except for sternal clefts, have a high mortality. The types of sternal defects are based on the tissue coverage of the heart. Thoracic ectopia cordis is the "naked heart" with no somatic overlying structures. Intrinsic cardiac defects are common and survival is rare. Successful repairs usually require the absence of intrinsic cardiac anomalies and require some form of grafting (autologous vs synthetic materials) that avoids posterior compression of the heart into a limited thoracic space.[51–53] Cervical ectopia cordis is based on the extent of superior displacement of the heart. There is fusion between the apex of the heart and the mouth, with severe craniofacial anomalies. No survivors have been reported.[54] Thoracoabdominal ectopia cordis consists of a heart covered by a thin membrane with a cleft sternum. It is frequently associated with Cantrell pentalogy, which includes a bifid sternum, diaphragmatic defect, pericardial defect, omphalocele, and intracardiac lesions. Pulmonary hypoplasia can occur with this anomaly and is usually fatal.[55] Successful surgical repair is possible, but mortality is usually the final outcome resulting from the intracardiac lesion or pulmonary hypoplasia. Initial surgical intervention has to address the skin defect over the abdomen and heart. Topical astringents to allow secondary epithelialization have been used to allow time for definitive repair of the cardiac lesion, which should be completed before any placement of a prosthetic material if needed.

### Sternal Cleft (Bifid Sternum)

Congenital sternal cleft or bifid sternum is the least severe anomaly of the sternum. There is a gap in the midline of the anterior chest between the two halves of the sternum. Newborns have an orthotopic heart with normal skin coverage and an intact pericardium. The cleft in the sternum can be partial or complete; however, most are partial, with an intact lower sternum and xiphoid. The most common cleft is an incomplete one with a bridge of bony tissue inferiorly joining the 2 edges, creating a U- or V-shaped defect (**Fig. 8**). The incomplete superior cleft sternum (bony connection inferiorly) may also be associated with a midline raphe or bandlike scar that extends to the umbilicus.[56] This sternal defect is the only one in which intracardiac defects are rare, thus rendering low mortality. Craniofacial defects and, rarely, vascular malformations can be associated with sternal clefts.[57]

Most newborns are asymptomatic, and occasionally presentation may be delayed. On examination the heart can be seen beating directly under the skin. Paradoxic motion of the defect can be seen, which may cause compromise of respiratory mechanics in the newborn. There also may be ulcerated skin over the defect or a draining sinus tract that originates from the pericardium.[58]

Sternal clefts should be repaired to provide bony protection of the heart and great vessels, to improve respiratory dynamics, and to improve the appearance of the chest wall.[59] This repair should ideally be done in the neonatal period when the chest wall is compliant, and at this stage the clefts can usually be repaired primarily. A midline incision is made, and the sternal edges are dissected free with a usually intact pericardium and diaphragm. In an incomplete cleft, a wedge of cartilage is resected to make it complete and the edges are freshened sharply with a scalpel. The edges can then

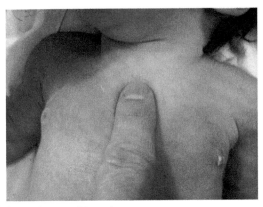

**Fig. 8.** Sternal cleft (superior U or V type).

usually be reapproximated primarily with interrupted sutures. It is important to assess the hemodynamic status after approximation of the sternal plates before completing closure.[59] The pectoralis muscles are closed in the midline.

Patients who present later require more complex repairs. It is almost impossible to repair primarily, and these patients require some form of grafting. A variety of techniques have been described,[60–63] all of which use some form of chondrotomy and division of the abnormal cartilages. Usually costal cartilage or rib grafts are then placed on the vascularized periosteal bed to bridge the gap between the edges of the sternal defect. If muscle cannot be placed on top of this in some fashion, a prosthetic material, such as Marlex, is then used.[56] Outcomes are very good in patients of all ages, assuming no other comorbidities are present.

## REFERENCES

1. Nowak H. Die erbliche trichterbrust. Dtsch med Wochenschr 1936;62(49):2003–4 [in German].
2. Fonkalsrud EW. Current management of pectus excavatum. World J Surg 2003; 27(5):502–8.
3. Kelly RE, Shamberger RC, Mellins RB, et al. Prospective multicenter study of surgical correction of pectus excavatum, 2007 correction of pectus excavatum: design, perioperative complications, pain, and baseline pulmonary function facilitated by internet-based data collection. J Am Coll Surg 2007;205(2):205–16.
4. Shamberger RC, Welch KJ. Surgical repair of pectus excavatum. J Pediatr Surg 1988;23(7):615–22.
5. Ohno K, Nakahira M, Takeuchi S, et al. Indications for surgical treatment of funnel chest by chest radiograph. Pediatr Surg Int 2001;17(8):591–5.
6. Sweet RH. Pectus excavatum. Ann Surg 1944;119:922–34.
7. Nakaoka T, Uemura S, Yoshida T, et al. Overgrowth of costal cartilage is not the etiology of pectus excavatum. J Pediatr Surg 2010;45(10):2015–8.
8. Nobuhara KK, Lund DP, Mitchell J, et al. Long-term outlook for survivors of congenital diaphragmatic hernia. Clin Perinatol 1996;23:873–87.
9. Waters P, Welch K, Micheli LJ, et al. Scoliosis in children with pectus excavatum and pectus carinatum. J Pediatr Orthop 1989;9(5):551–6.
10. Kelly RE, Lawson ML, Paidas CN, et al. Pectus excavatum in a 112-year autopsy series: anatomic findings and the effect on survival. J Pediatr Surg 2005;40(8): 1275–8.

11. Kotzot D, Schwabegger AH. Etiology of chest wall deformities—a genetic review for the treating physician. J Pediatr Surg 2009;44(10):2004–11.

12. Feng J, Hu T, Liu W, et al. The biomechanical, morphologic, and histochemical properties of the costal cartilages in children with pectus excavatum. J Pediatr Surg 2001;36(12):1770–6.

13. Creswick HA, Stacey MW, Kelly RE, et al. Family study of the inheritance of pectus excavatum. J Pediatr Surg 2006;41(10):1699–703.

14. Kaguraoka H, Ohnuki T, Itaoka T, et al. Degree of severity of pectus excavatum and pulmonary function in preoperative and postoperative periods. J Thorac Cardiovasc Surg 1992;104(5):1483–8.

15. Haller JA Jr, Loughlin GM. Cardiorespiratory function is significantly improved following corrective surgery for severe pectus excavatum. Proposed treatment guidelines. J Cardiovasc Surg (Torino) 2000;41(1):125–30.

16. Lawson ML, Mellins R, Tabangin M, et al. Impact of pectus excavatum on pulmonary function before and after repair with the Nuss procedure. J Pediatr Surg 2005;40(1):174–80.

17. Lawson ML, Mellins RB, Paulson JF, et al. Increasing severity of pectus excavatum is associated with reduced pulmonary function. J Pediatr 2011;159(2):256–61.

18. Redlinger RE, Kelly RE, Nuss D, et al. Regional chest wall motion dysfunction in patients with pectus excavatum demonstrated via optoelectronic plethysmography. J Pediatr Surg 2011;46(6):1172–6.

19. Cahill JL, Lees GM, Robertson HT. A summary of preoperative and postoperative cardiorespiratory performance in patients undergoing pectus excavatum and carinatum repair. J Pediatr Surg 1984;19(4):430–3.

20. Kowalewski J, Brocki M, Dryjanski T, et al. Pectus excavatum: increase of right ventricular systolic, diastolic, and stroke volumes after surgical repair. J Thorac Cardiovasc Surg 1999;118(1):87–92.

21. Zhao L, Feinberg MS, Gaides M, et al. Why is exercise capacity reduced in subjects with pectus excavatum? J Pediatr 2000;136(2):163–7.

22. Coln E, Carrasco J, Coln D. Demonstrating relief of cardiac compression with the Nuss minimally invasive repair for pectus excavatum. J Pediatr Surg 2006;41: 683–6.

23. Cartoski MJ, Nuss D, Goretsky MJ, et al. Classification of the dysmorphology of pectus excavatum. J Pediatr Surg 2006;41:1573–81.

24. Lam MW, Klassen AF, Montgomery CJ, et al. Quality-of-life outcomes after surgical correction of pectus excavatum: a comparison of the Ravitch and Nuss procedures. J Pediatr Surg 2008;43(5):819–25.

25. Kelly RE, Cash TF, Shamberger RC, et al. Surgical repair of pectus excavatum markedly improves body image and perceived ability for physical activity: multicenter study. Pediatrics 2008;122(6):1218–22.

26. Haller JA Jr, Kramer SS, Lietman SA. Use of CT scans in selection of patients for pectus excavatum surgery: a preliminary report. J Pediatr Surg 1987;22(10):904–6.

27. Rushing GD, Goretsky MJ, Gustin T, et al. When it is not an infection: metal allergy after the Nuss procedure for repair of pectus excavatum. J Pediatr Surg 2007; 42(1):93–7.

28. Croitoru DP, Kelly RE, Goretsky MJ, et al. Experience and modification update for the minimally invasive Nuss technique for pectus excavatum repair in 303 patients. J Pediatr Surg 2002;37(3):437–45.

29. Lange F. Thoraxdeformitäten. In: Pfaundler M, Schlossmann A, editors. Handbuch der kinderheilkunde, vol V. chirugie und orthopädie im kindersalter, vol. 5. Leipzig (Germany): FCW Vogel; 1910. p. 157.

30. Schier F, Bahr M, Klobe E. The vacuum chest wall lifter: an innovative, nonsurgical addition to the management of pectus excavatum. J Pediatr Surg 2005;40: 496–500.

31. Haecker FM. The vacuum bell for conservative treatment of pectus excavatum: the Basle experience. Pediatr Surg Int 2011;27:623–7.

32. Obermeyer RJ, Nuss D, Redlinger RE. Suction cup lift for severe pectus excavatum. Video presentation. Chicago: American College of Surgeons; 2009.

33. Brown AL. Pectus excavatum (funnel chest): anatomic basis, surgical treatment of the incipient stage in infancy, and correction of the deformity in the fully developed stage. J Thorac Surg 1939;9:164–84.

34. Ravitch M. The operative treatment of pectus excavatum. Ann Surg 1949;129(4): 429–44.

35. Kelly RE, Goretsky MJ, Obermeyer R, et al. Twenty-one years of experience with minimally invasive repair of pectus excavatum by the Nuss procedure in 1215 patients. Ann Surg 2010;252(6):1072–81.

36. Shamberger RC, Welch KJ. Surgical correction of pectus carinatum. J Pediatr Surg 1987;22:48–53.

37. Martinez-Ferro M, Fraire C, Bernard S. Dynamic compression system for the correction of pectus carinatum. Semin Pediatr Surg 2008;17(3):194–200.

38. Westphal FL, Lima LC, Lima Neto JC, et al. Prevalence of pectus carinatum and pectus excavatum in students in the city of Manaus, Brazil. J Bras Pneumol 2009; 35(3):221–6.

39. Fonkalsrud EW, Anselmo DM. Less extensive techniques for repair of pectus carinatum: the undertreated chest deformity. J Am Coll Surg 2004;198(6):898–905.

40. Currarino G, Silverman FN. Premature obliteration of the sternal sutures and pigeon-breast Deformity. Radiology 1958;70:532–40.

41. Abramson H, D'Agostino J, Wuscovi S. A 5-year experience with a minimally invasive technique for pectus carinatum repair. J Pediatr Surg 2009;44:118–24.

42. Egan JC, DuBois JJ, Morphy M, et al. Compressive orthotics in the treatment of asymmetric pectus carinatum: a preliminary report with an objective radiographic marker. J Pediatr Surg 2000;3:1183–6.

43. Haje SA, Bowen JR. Preliminary results of orthotic treatment of pectus deformities in children and adolescents. J Pediatr Orthop 1992;12:795–800.

44. Ravitch MM. Unusual sternal deformity with cardiac symptoms operative correction. J Thorac Surg 1952;23(2):138–44.

45. Sanger PW, Taylor FH, Robicsek F. Deformities of the anterior wall of the chest. Surg Gynecol Obstet 1963;116:515–22.

46. Fonkalsrud EW, Beanes S. Surgical management of pectus carinatum: 30 years' experience. World J Surg 2001;25(7):898–903.

47. Abramson H. A minimally invasive technique to repair pectus carinatum. Preliminary report. Arch Bronconeumol 2005;41(6):349–51.

48. Kim S, Idowu O. Minimally invasive thoracoscopic repair of unilateral pectus carinatum. J Pediatr Surg 2009;44:471–4.

49. Mielke CH, Winter RB. Pectus carinatum successfully treated with bracing: A case report. Int Orthop 1993;17:350–2.

50. Robicsek F, Cook JW, Daugherty HK, et al. Pectus carinatum. J Thorac Cardiovasc Surg 1979;78(1):52–61.

51. Haynor DR, Shuman WP, Brewers DK, et al. Imaging of fetal ectopia cordis: roles of sonography and computed tomography. J Ultrasound Med 1984;3:25–7.

52. Cutler GD, Wilens G. Ectopia cordis: report of a case. Am J Dis Child 1925;30: 76–81.

53. Dobell AR, Williams H, Long R. Staged repair of ectopia cordis. J Pediatr Surg 1982;17:353–8.
54. Shao-tsu L. Ectopia cordis congenital. Thoraxchirurgie 1957;5:197–212.
55. Shamberger R, Welch KJ. Sternal defects. Pediatr Surg Int 1990;5:156–64.
56. Acastello E, Majluf R, Garrido P, et al. Sternal cleft: a surgical opportunity. J Pediatr Surg 2003;38(2):178–83.
57. Pasic M, Carrel T, Tonz M, et al. Sternal cleft associated with vascular anomalies and micro-Gnathia. Ann Thorac Surg 1993;56(1):165–8.
58. Verska JJ. Surgical repair of total cleft sternum. J Thorac Cardiovasc Surg 1975; 69(2):301–5.
59. Domini M, Cupaioli M, Rossi F, et al. Bifid sternum: neonatal surgical treatment. Ann Thorac Surg 2000;69(1):267–9.
60. Maier HC, Bortone F. Complete failure of sternal fusion with herniation of pericardium. J Thorac Surg 1949;18:851–9.
61. Sabiston DC Jr. The surgical management of congenital bifid sternum with partial ectopia cordis. J Thorac Surg 1958;35:118–22.
62. Meissner F. Fissura sterni congenita. Zentralbl Chir 1964;89:1832–9.
63. Milanez de Campos JR, Das-Neves-Pereira JC, Lopes KM, et al. Technical modifications in stabilisers and in bar removal in the Nuss procedure. Eur J Cardiothorac Surg 2009;36(2):410–2.

# Neonatal Bowel Obstruction

David Juang, MD*, Charles L. Snyder, MD

## KEYWORDS

- Neonatal bowel obstruction • Intestinal atresia • Malrotation • Hirschsprung disease
- Meconium ileus • Anorectal malformations

## KEY POINTS

- There are 4 cardinal signs of intestinal obstruction in newborns: (1) maternal polyhydramnios, defined as amniotic fluid index more than the 95th percentile for the corresponding gestational age (or if the deepest vertical pool on ultrasound [US] is more than 8 cm)—it is more commonly associated with more proximal obstructions; (2) bilious emesis (again, more common in proximal obstructions); (3) failure to pass meconium in the first day of life; and (4) abdominal distention (more common in lower obstructions).
- Obstructions of the pylorus, duodenum, jejunum, ileum, and colon collectively are the most common causes of neonatal bowel obstruction.
- Many disease processes cause proximal intestinal obstruction and bilious emesis. The consequences of missing a diagnosis of malrotation and volvulus, however, are so devastating that it should be assumed present until proved otherwise. Radiologic studies can establish a definitive diagnosis but should not delay treatment if clinical suspicion is strong. Patients with suspected or confirmed midgut volvulus should be aggressively resuscitated, given intravenous broad-spectrum antibiotics, and taken to an operating room for immediate exploration.
- Key elements for the Ladd procedure for intestinal malrotation include evisceration of bowel, counterclockwise detorsion, division of bands, broadening of small bowel mesentery, appendectomy, and reorientation and placement of bowel.
- The intestinal lumen is intact in meconium disease but functionally obstructed by the thick, viscid protein-rich meconium, which adheres to the wall of the bowel, causing a blockage. A water-soluble hyperosmolar contrast enema may be diagnostic and therapeutic.
- Definitive diagnosis of Hirschsprung disease (HD) requires tissue. Absent ganglion cells in the submucosal and myenteric plexus, increased acetylcholinesterase in parasympathetic nerve fibers in the lamina propria, and muscularis mucosa are seen; abnormal nerve cells are identified.
- The incidence of anorectal malformations (ARMs) is approximately 1 in 5000 live births, with a slight male predominance. ARMs have a heterogeneous etiology, probably as a result of both genetic and environmental factors, although precise causation remains unknown. Evaluation of patients with an ARM should include echocardiogram, renal and bladder US, spinal US, voiding cystourethrogram, and plain radiographs of the abdomen and lower spine.

---

The authors have nothing to disclose, and no funding support.
Department of Surgery, Children's Mercy Hospital, University of Missouri–Kansas City, 2401 Gillham Road, Kansas City, MO 64108, USA
* Corresponding author.
E-mail address: djuang@cmh.edu

Surg Clin N Am 92 (2012) 685–711
doi:10.1016/j.suc.2012.03.008
0039-6109/12/$ – see front matter © 2012 Elsevier Inc. All rights reserved.

**surgical.theclinics.com**

Newborn intestinal obstructions are a common reason for admission to neonatal ICUs. The incidence is not precisely known but is estimated to be approximately 1 in 2000 live births.[1]

There are 4 cardinal signs of intestinal obstruction in newborns: (1) maternal polyhydramnios, defined as amniotic fluid index more than the 95th percentile for the corresponding gestational age (or if the deepest vertical pool on US is more than 8 cm)—it is more commonly associated with proximal obstructions; (2) bilious emesis (again, more common in proximal obstructions); (3) failure to pass meconium in the first day of life; and (4) abdominal distention (more common in lower obstructions).

The presentation may vary from subtle and easily overlooked findings on physical examination to massive abdominal distention with respiratory distress and cardiovascular collapse. A careful history (including maternal and prenatal) and physical examination often identify the diagnosis. Concomitant resuscitation (volume, gastric decompression, and ventilatory support) may be necessary.

## INTESTINAL ATRESIAS

Obstructions of the pylorus, duodenum, jejunum, ileum, and colon collectively are the most common causes of neonatal bowel obstruction. Approximately greater than 1:4000 live births are affected.

### Pyloric Atresia

Pyloric atresia is rare, with an incidence varying from 1 in 100,000 to 1 in 1,000,000 live births; it constitutes less than 1% of all gastrointestinal (GI) atresias.[2] There are several anatomic variants of pyloric atresia. One classification system consists of type I, pyloric membrane or web (57%); type II, pyloric canal replaced by solid tissue (34%); and type III, atretic pylorus with a gap between stomach and duodenum (9%).[3]

The cause is unknown but presumably is the result of a developmental problem during the first 1 to 2 months of gestation. An autosomal recessive genetic defect is suggested by familial cases.[4]

Approximately half the cases are associated with other anomalies, most commonly epidermolysis bullosa.[5] This association is highly lethal and is inherited in an autosomal recessive fashion. Genetic defects from mutations in the ITGA6, ITGB4, and PLEC genes areareare implicated.[6,7] Pyloric atresia may be also part of an extremely rare heritable syndrome of multiple intestinal atresias involving the stomach, duodenum, jejunum, ileum, colon, and rectum.[8]

Important differential diagnoses include malrotation with midgut volvulus, proximal duodenal atresia, and gastric volvulus.

### Clinical presentation
Polyhydramnios is identified prenatally in slightly more than half the cases. A single bubble rather than a double bubble is seen on prenatal US and plain abdominal films in the newborn (**Fig. 1**). The usual newborn presentation is that of a proximal obstruction with nonbilious emesis and a scaphoid abdomen. Epigastric distention and respiratory distress may be present.

Plain films often establish the diagnosis of gastric obstruction. Air may be insufflated into the stomach to assist in the diagnosis. Contrast is rarely needed.

### Treatment
Type I atresias are treated with web excision and a Heineke-Mikulicz pyloroplasty. Type II or III atresias may be managed with a pyloroplasty, if the gap is short. Longer

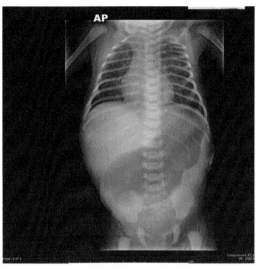

**Fig. 1.** Abdominal radiograph of newborn with pyloric atresia. The diagnosis is confirmed by the single large gastric bubble without distal intestinal air and maternal history of polyhydraminios.

gaps may require a Billroth I gastroduodenostomy.[9] Outcomes are variable and depend primarily on the presence or absence of associated anomalies.

### Duodenal Atresia

Congenital duodenal atresia or stenosis is the most common of the intestinal atresias, ranging from 1 in 5000 to 1 in 10,000 live births.[10,11]

Obstruction of the duodenum is postulated to result from a lack of revacuolization of the solid cord stage of intestinal development of the fetal duodenum by the 10th week of gestation.[12] Additionally, the pancreatic dorsal and ventral buds fuse near the 8th week of fetal development, and failure of the ventral bud to rotate completely may result in an annular pancreas.

More than half of patients have associated congenital anomalies.[13] Trisomy 21 is seen in approximately one-third of patients.[14] Congenital cardiac defects are found in another 30%, and 25% have other GI anomalies. Renal, skeletal, and central nervous system anomalies are less common associations.[15,16] Malrotation is found in up to 30% of patients with congenital duodenal obstruction.[10,17]

Prematurity is present in 45% of patients, and many are small for gestational age.[18,19] The incidence of polyhydramnios ranges from 32% to 81% in complete obstructions.[13,17,20]

### Pathology

Duodenal obstructions are classified as the more common atresia (including 3 subtypes) or as stenosis (extrinsic or intrinsic); 85% of duodenal obstructions occur distal to the ampulla of Vater in the second portion of the duodenum.[10,21] Bilious emesis with a relatively scaphoid abdomen is, therefore, a common presentation and may be difficult to discern from acute midgut volvulus secondary to malrotation.

**Fig. 2** depicts the various forms of duodenal atresia and stenosis. Type I atresias consist of an obstructing web and are the most common variant (**Fig. 3**). The web or diaphragm often balloons distally to create a windsock,[22] which leads to dilation

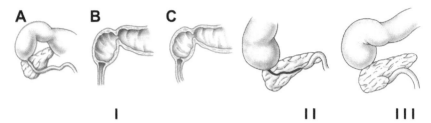

**Fig. 2.** Schematic of type *I* duodenal atresia (and stenosis) (*A, B, C*). Either a membrane (*B*) or web (*C*) causes the intrinsic duodenal obstruction. With a type *I* anomaly, there is no fibrous cord and the duodenum remains in continuity in a type *I* duodenal atresia. A type *II* duodenal atresia is characterized by complete obliteration of a segment of the duodenum with the proximal and distal portions attached via a fibrous cord (*II*). A type *III* duodenal atresia is associated with complete separation of the dilated proximal duodenum from the collapsed distal duodenum (*III*). (*From* Aguayo P, Ostlie D. Duodenal and intestinal atresia and stenosis. In: Holcomb III GW, Murphy JP, editors. Ashcraft's pediatric surgery. 5th edition. Philadelphia: WB Saunders; 2010. p. 400–15; with permission.)

of bowel distal to the origin of the obstruction (usually at or near the ampulla) and may mislead an inexperienced surgeon. Passage of a nasogastric catheter and manipulation of it into the distal duodenum demonstrate the site of origin of the web. Type II atresias (fibrous cord) are the least common, usually less than 10% of cases.[10]

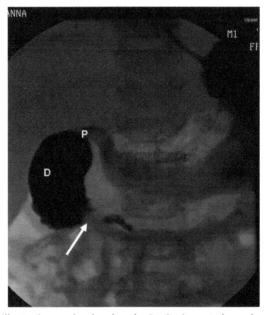

**Fig. 3.** UGI study illustrating a duodenal web. Beginning at the pylorus (P) the contrast outlines the markedly dilated proximal duodenum (D) with a collapsed distal segment. Note the absence of contrast at the location of the tiny web (*arrow*). (*From* Aguayo P, Ostlie D. Duodenal and intestinal atresia and stenosis. In: Holcomb III GW, Murphy JP, editors. Ashcraft's pediatric surgery. 5th edition. Philadelphia: WB Saunders; 2010. p. 400–15; with permission.)

Type III is complete separation of the atretic segments and also typically constitutes 10% or less of the total.

### Clinical presentation

US diagnosis of duodenal atresia can now be made in the late second or early third trimester. Approximately half of cases demonstrate a double bubble in fetuses of mothers with polyhydramnios.[23] Increased peristaltic activity of the stomach may also be noted.[24] Because approximately one-third of patients with duodenal atresia have trisomy 21, US characteristics of the disease should be sought.[25]

Classically, these otherwise stable patients present with bilious emesis within a few hours of life. However, 10% to 15% of patients with preampullary lesions have nonbilious emesis. Orogastric aspiration of more than 20 mL to 25 mL of fluid is suggestive of intestinal obstruction (normal aspirate volume in a neonate is <5 mL).[26] Abdominal radiographs reveal the characteristic double bubble with a paucity of distal bowel gas (**Fig. 4**). Neonates with bilious emesis and decompressed stomachs on abdominal radiographs may require an upper GI (UGI) contrast study to exclude malrotation with volvulus. Additionally, the double bubble may not be seen in duodenal stenosis, and a limited UGI study may be required to delineate this diagnosis.

Once a diagnosis of duodenal obstruction is made and malrotation with volvulus is excluded, the neonate should undergo resuscitation and gastric decompression.

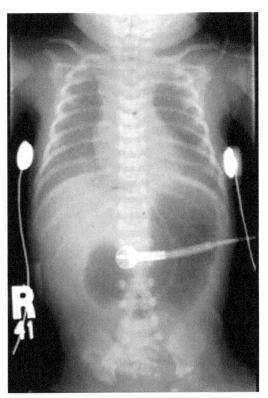

**Fig. 4.** Abdominal radiograph of neonate with the classic double bubble. Note the lack of distal intestinal air.

Imaging studies should be completed to evaluate for any skeletal, spinal, or cardiac abnormalities before operative intervention.

### Treatment

Laparoscopic or open duodenoduodenostomy is the procedure of choice.[16,27,28] A right supraumbilical transverse incision is used for exposure in the open approach. The right colon and hepatic flexure are reflected medially to visualize the duodenum. The position of the ligament of Treitz (if present) is identified, and the duodenum is inspected. Passage of a nasogastric tube and manual manipulation into the area of the obstruction may help identify a membrane or web. An annular pancreas, present in one-third of cases, may be found. Webs can be excised, but they are usually at or near the ampulla of Vater and may be fairly thick. Bypass via duodenoduodenostomy, with a proximal transverse to distal longitudinal (diamond-shaped) anastomosis (**Fig. 5**), is preferred in most cases, regardless of anatomic type.[11,18,29] Rarely, duodenojejunostomy is necessary due to anatomic considerations and the site of the obstruction. Although passage of a tube distally to rule out jejunoileal atresia (JIA) has been recommended historically, in a series of more than 400 patients, one study found such an association is less than 1%.[30]

The laparoscopic approach was first described by Rothenberg in 2002.[27] The standard laparoscopic approach begins with the patient supine. Once insufflation is established through the umbilical port, instruments are introduced through stab incisions in the right lower quadrant and one in the right midepigastric region. A liver retractor can be placed in the right or left upper quadrant if necessary. Alternatively, the liver can be elevated by placing a transabdominal wall suture around the falciform ligament and tying it outside the abdomen (**Fig. 6**). The duodenum is mobilized and the location of obstruction is identified. A standard diamond-shaped anastomosis is created with interrupted sutures. Our department has previously reported results using Nitinol U-Clips (Medtronic, Minneapolis, MN, USA) to create the duodenoduodenostomy with no leaks and more rapid initiation of feeds when compared with the traditional open

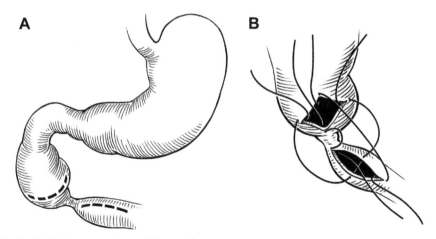

**Fig. 5.** (*A, B*) Representation of diamond anastomosis technique. A diamond-shaped anastomosis is created via the proximal transversely oriented and distal vertically oriented duodenotomies. (*From* Aguayo P, Ostlie D. Duodenal and intestinal atresia and stenosis. In: Holcomb III GW, Murphy JP, editors. Ashcraft's pediatric surgery. 5th edition. Philadelphia: WB Saunders; 2010. p. 400–15; with permission.)

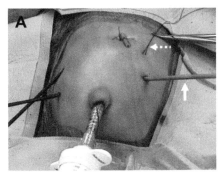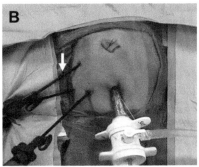

**Fig. 6.** Two approaches to placement of the instruments for a laparoscopic duodenal atresia repair are seen. On the left (*A*), the 2 right-sided instruments are the primary working sites for the surgeon. The liver retractor (*solid arrow*) has been placed in the left midepigastric region. The falciform ligament has been elevated by a suture placed under it and tied over the red rubber catheter, which is used as a bolster. The suture (*dotted arrow*) exteriorized in the baby's left upper abdomen was placed in the dilated proximal duodenum so that it could be easily manipulated. On the right (*B*), this is a similar configuration except the instrument elevating the liver (*arrow*) is placed in the baby's right upper abdomen rather than the left upper abdomen. The suture, which was placed through the proximal dilated duodenum in (*A*), was not needed in this particular case. (*From* Aguayo P, Ostlie D. Duodenal and intestinal atresia and stenosis. In: Holcomb III GW, Murphy JP, editors. Ashcraft's pediatric surgery. 5th edition. Philadelphia: WB Saunders; 2010. p. 400–15; with permission.)

approach.[28] The main advantage is a reduction in the time to complete the anastomosis.

Nasogastric decompression postoperatively is discontinued when bowel function returns. Delayed gastric emptying and slow return to feedings are the most common complications, usually as a result of dilation and poor motility. Late stenosis can occur but is infrequent. Other complications include gastroesophageal or duodenogastric reflux, gastritis or peptic ulcer, megaduodenum, blind-loop syndrome, and intestinal obstruction related to adhesions.[16]

Early postoperative mortality has been reported as low as 3% to 5%. Mortality is almost exclusively related to concurrent disease associated with related congenital abnormalities, especially cardiac anomalies and prematurity.[10,31] Long-term survival approaches 90%.[18,32,33]

### Jejunoileal Atresia

JIA occurs in approximately 1 in 5000 live births and affects male and female infants equally. Approximately 1 in 3 infants is premature.[10] Familial cases of intestinal atresias are rarely reported; most cases are sporadic.[34]

The hypothesis that most cases of JIA occur secondary to vascular disruption during fetal life is derived from experimental and clinical evidence. The ischemic insult to the midgut can affect single or multiple segments of the already developed intestine and the resulting ischemic necrosis of the bowel can lead to subsequent resorption of the affected segment.[10,35–37] The use of maternal vasoconstrictive medications as well as maternal cigarette smoking in the first trimester of pregnancy has been shown to increase the risk of small bowel atresia.[38] No correlations have been found between JIA and parental or maternal disease. There is no known genetic defect in most cases, except in rare heritable subgroups (discussed later) and in children with cystic fibrosis (CF).[39]

The presence of associated extraintestinal abnormalities in JIA is low (<10%) due to its occurrence late in fetal development.[40,41] Common associations include malrotation (10%–15%), gastroschisis (10%–15% of these infants have intestinal atresia), and CF (10%).[10,40–42] Rare associations with HD, trisomy 21, anorectal and vertebral anomalies, neural tube defects, congenital heart disease, and other GI atresias are reported.[37]

Atresia of the jejunum and ileum are approximately equally distributed between the 2 anatomic regions. JIA and stenosis are categorized into 4 distinct groups and with an additional consideration for type IIIb atresias (apple peel or Christmas tree appearance) (**Fig. 7**).[43] The latter group (type IIIb) accounts for 11% to 22% of JIA and consists of a proximal jejunal atresia with foreshortened small bowel. The distal small bowel receives its blood supply from a single ileocolic or right colic artery. Prematurity and low birth weight are more common in type IIIb JIA, and the incidence of malrotation and other anomalies is increased, as is familial tendency. Consequently, morbidity and mortality are increased.

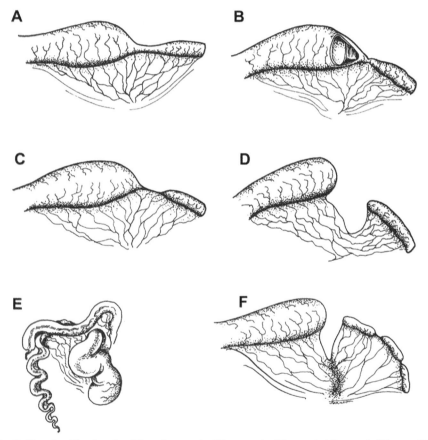

**Fig. 7.** The classification for JIA and stenosis: (A) stenosis, (B) type I, (C) type II, (D) type IIIa, (E) type IIIb, and (F) type IV. (*From* Aguayo P, Ostlie D. Duodenal and intestinal atresia and stenosis. In: Holcomb III GW, Murphy JP, editors. Ashcraft's pediatric surgery. 5th edition. Philadelphia: WB Saunders; 2010. p. 400–15; with permission.)

The most proximal atresia determines whether the atresia is classified as jejunal or ileal. Overall, type IIIa JIA is the most common variant. Multiple atresias are found in up to 25% of patients.[10,44] An extremely rare variant of JIA seen in scattered kindreds involves multiple atresias of the stomach, pylorus, duodenum, small bowel, and colon and is almost uniformly fatal.[45]

The differential diagnosis is wide, and includes malrotation, HD (specifically, total colonic aganglionosis), meconium ileus (MI), and sepsis (and other medical caused of ileus). Less commonly, internal hernias, intestinal duplications, or compressing mass lesions may be causative.

### Clinical presentation

Clinical presentation of JIA is variable, depending primarily on the anatomic location of the obstruction. A very proximal obstruction results in a scaphoid abdomen and bilious emesis, whereas a more distal ileal atresia can lead to massive abdominal distention and visible intestinal patterning. Distention may be progressive in the first hours or days of life, and most babies with JIA have significant distention. Polyhydramnios is seen in approximately one-quarter of cases and jaundice in a similar proportion. Failure to pass meconium is common.

Occasionally, the heavy dilated proximal blind end of the atretic bowel twists (volvulizes). If this occurs early in development, in utero perforation can result. Volvulus can occur postnatally and may require prompt intervention.

JIA usually is identified by flat and decubitus radiographic examination of the abdomen with only swallowed air as contrast. Swallowed air reaches the proximal bowel by 1 hour and the distal small bowel by 3 hours in a normal vigorous infant. Dilated loops of bowel with air-fluid levels are seen, with a paucity of gas distal to the obstruction. Newborn plain abdominal radiographs cannot usually differentiate colon from small bowel. The more distal the blockage, the more the dilation. Calcification may be the result of in utero perforation. A limited contrast UGI is not routinely necessary but may be useful if intestinal stenosis is suspected or if there is concern for malrotation (seen in approximately 10% to 15% of infants with JIA) with associated volvulus.[10] A contrast enema should be obtained and typically reveals a small unused colon (microcolon).

### Treatment

Initial treatment consists of nasogastric decompression, fluid resuscitation, and broad-spectrum antibiotics. Operative repair is usually not emergent (in uncomplicated cases) but should proceed expeditiously.

Surgical management of JIA is based on the location of the lesion, anatomic findings, associated conditions (malrotation, volvulus, or multiple atresias) noted at operation and the length of the remaining intestine. Resection of the dilated and hypertrophied proximal bowel with primary end-to-end anastomosis is the most common surgical approach.[46–48] Multiple atretic segments often require several anastomoses.

Repair of small intestinal atresia can be accomplished laparoscopically but markedly dilated bowel and the small confines of the neonatal abdomen make this difficult. The authors, therefore, have begun explorations through the umbilicus with a vertical incision of the fascia to the extent allowed by the umbilical incision. Transverse supraumbilical incisions also provide excellent exposure. Once the abdominal cavity is entered, careful inspection of the entire bowel is performed and the site and type of obstruction should be noted as well as any other abnormalities. The most distal limb of the atretic bowel should then be cannulated with a red rubber catheter and irrigated with warm saline to evaluate for distal obstruction. As described previously, the continuity of the colon can be established preoperatively by a contrast enema or with a prepositioned transrectal catheter placed before prepping. The length of bowel should then be carefully assessed. If the length of functional bowel is adequate, the bulbous hypertrophied proximal bowel should be resected (antimesenteric tapering jejunoplasty) to obviate more extensive resection. Intestinal imbrication is also used to reduce the caliber of the distended bowel while maintaining mucosal absorptive surface. The longevity of the imbrication is often limited, however, with breakdown of the suture plication over time.

Distally, a short segment (4–5 cm) of the bowel is removed obliquely leaving the mesenteric side longer than the antimesenteric aspect to create a fish mouth, which may be needed to create an adequate distal enterotomy for the anastomosis. The authors prefer a single-layer triangulated anastomosis. The suture line is tested for leaks and reinforcing sutures are placed as needed. A temporary enterostomy should be performed in cases of perforation with significant contamination or meconium peritonitis or if there is a question of bowel viability.

Postoperatively, supportive care consists of gastric decompression and parenteral nutrition. Total parenteral nutrition is mandatory and should begin as soon as possible. The time for return of bowel function varies. Prolonged dysmotility is seen in some infants, perhaps as a result of ischemic bowel and neuronal injury at the time of the initial atresia insult. Total parenteral nutrition should continue until infants are tolerating full enteral feeding. Enteral feedings are initiated when the gastric aspirate is clear, output is minimal, and the infant is stooling. All children with JIA should have a sweat chloride test and a genetic screen for CF.

The current survival rate is greater than 90%.[10] Intestinal obstruction and anastomotic complications are infrequent, but short gut syndrome may be a long-term sequela, particularly in type IIIb cases. Most children with JIA reach enteral intestinal autonomy.

### Colonic Atresia

Colonic atresia (CA) is a rare cause of intestinal obstruction, comprising 1.8% to 15% of all intestinal atresias.[49–51] The reported incidence varies but is approximately 1 in 20,000 live births.[52,53]

The colon forms at approximately 4 to 5 weeks of fetal life, and intestinal rotation takes place during weeks 4 to 12. The classically accepted explanation for JIA is a vascular insult to the fetal intestine, and this is still thought to be the primary cause for CA as well.[36] Recent studies have implicated the fibroblast growth factor (FGF) signaling process, however, because CA is observed in a mice model with a deficiency of expression of FGF10 and FGFR2b.[54,55] No genetic associations or defects have yet been identified, however, in humans with CA.

Associated anomalies are uncommon, and the defect is usually an isolated occurrence. CA has been found in approximately 2.5% of neonates with gastroschisis[56,57]; in some cases, compression of the intestine by the abdominal wall defect is a potential causative factor.

There are fewer than 25 published cases of CA and HD, but the association is real and a suction rectal biopsy should be obtained routinely.[58] Complex urologic abnormalities, multiple small intestinal atresias, an unfixed mesentery, and skeletal anomalies also are reported to occur with CA.[52,59–61]

CA is classified into 3 types: type I consists of mucosal atresia with an intact bowel wall and mesentery (web); type II consists of atretic ends separated by a fibrous cord; and type III, consists of atretic ends separated by a V-shaped mesenteric gap.[51] In the ascending and transverse colon, type III CAs predominate. Types I and II are seen more commonly distal to the splenic flexure.[52,59] Type III lesions are easily the most common variant overall.

In one review of 118 cases, approximately one-fourth occurred in each of these locations: ascending, transverse, splenic flexure, and descending/sigmoid colon. The hepatic flexure was an uncommon site.[53]

### Clinical presentation

The diagnosis may be suspected prenatally[62] but the US findings cannot usually be distinguished from other forms of intestinal atresia. Polyhydramnios is uncommon due to the distal nature of the obstruction. Most infants are born at term.

The primary items in the differential diagnosis are distal JIA or obstruction, rectal atresia, meconium disease, and HD.

The characteristic clinical features of CA are abdominal distention, bilious emesis, and failure to pass meconium. Plain abdominal films demonstrate a distal bowel obstruction (multiple dilated bowel loops with air-fluid levels). Occasionally, the dilation can be so massive that it mimics pneumoperitoneum. A microcolon distal to the atresia site and abrupt cutoff of retrograde contrast in found on a barium or water-soluble enema.

### Treatment

Diagnosis of CA is an indication for urgent surgical intervention because this anomaly has a higher risk of perforation (10% incidence) than seen in other intestinal atresias, presumably as a result of a closed loop obstruction from the intact ileocecal valve.

Initial management consists of bowel decompression, fluid resuscitation, and broad-spectrum antibiotics. Operative management should be prompt due the increased risk of perforation and volvulus. Surgical options are primary repair (resection and reanastomosis) versus a staged operative approach with an initial colostomy. The proximal and distal ends adjacent to the atresia are abnormal in both innervation and vascularity. Resection of the bulbous proximal colon and a portion of the distal microcolon is suggested.[63–65] Intraoperative exclusion of other intestinal atresias and stenoses is important because these may be coexistent.[15,46] A diagnosis of associated HD, although rare, must be made by frozen section analysis of rectal biopsies during initial surgery, because unrecognized HD may lead to anastomotic leak or functional obstruction.

In the absence of other serious comorbidities, the prognosis in CA is excellent. Survival should approach 100% in isolated CA. Complications (stomal prolapse, prolonged ileus, and adhesive obstruction) are seen in 25% to 50% of patients.[10,52] Familial recurrence is rare, and only one familial instance has been reported.[66]

## MALROTATION

The incidence of malrotation is estimated at approximately 1 in 6000 live births. Autopsy studies suggest that the true incidence may be as high as 1% of the total population.[67]

Intestinal rotation and fixation is normally an orderly sequence of embryologic events in early fetal development. Rapid intestinal growth after the fifth week of gestation results in herniation of the growing midgut through the umbilical ring. The superior mesenteric artery (SMA) functions as the central axis of an eventual counterclockwise 270° intestinal rotation. The duodenojejunal junction passes posterior to the SMA to its position to the left of the SMA whereas the cecocolic limb is on the right. The retroperitoneal fixation of the ascending and descending colon occurs subsequently, leaving a broad mesenteric base. The entire process is normally completed by the 12th week of gestation.[68] Disruption of any of these steps leads to rotational anomalies. A deficiency in duodenal growth, thus failing to drive the elongation and positioning of the intestine (rather than a true staged rotation), is also hypothesized as the primary cause.[68,69]

Associations are common in abnormal intestinal rotation, occurring in 30% to 60%.[70] Extraintestinal associations include congenital heart disease (specifically heterotaxia). Mutations in genes with a role in specifying left-right asymmetry in the early embryo are suggested by the former association.[71] Duodenal atresia is a well-recognized association, but JIA and CA as well as imperforate anus and HD may also coexist with the rotational anomalies.[70] Any abdominal wall malformation (gastroschisis, omphalocele, or a congenital diaphragmatic hernia) has varying degrees of abnormal intestinal rotation.

Rotational anomalies are classified as nonrotation, incomplete rotation, and reversed rotation. Nonrotation occurs when the intestine fails to rotate around the SMA in its usual 270° counterclockwise fashion. The duodenojejunal limb lies in the right abdomen with the cecocolic limb in the left abdomen, often close to each other. This creates a narrow mesenteric base through which the SMA passes. The mesenteric base are easily twisted (midgut volvulus), resulting initially in intestinal obstruction and then vascular compromise and eventual intestinal loss. In cases of incomplete rotation, normal rotation is arrested at or near 180°. The cecum usually resides in the right upper abdomen and obstructing peritoneal bands are present. Reversed rotation occurs when an errant clockwise rotation occurs, which leaves a tortuous transverse colon to the right of the SMA, passing through a retroduodenal tunnel behind the artery and in the small bowel mesentery. Reversed rotation with volvulus may occur with obstruction of the transverse colon. It almost never presents in the newborn period, however. Other rotational anomalies include the rare mesocolic hernias (paraduodenal) resulting from failure of the left or right mesocolon to become fully fixated to the posterior abdominal wall.

Many disease processes cause proximal intestinal obstruction and bilious emesis. The consequences of missing a diagnosis of malrotation and volvulus are so devastating, however, that it should be assumed present until proved otherwise.

### Clinical Presentation

Abnormal intestinal rotation presents in a chronic or acute manner, with or without volvulus, or even remains asymptomatic. The incidence of volvulus secondary to abnormal rotation is inversely proportional to age. Malrotation with midgut volvulus presents during the first week of life in 50% of children and within the first month of life in 75% of children; another 15% of children present within the first year.[72–74] Symptoms vary with progression of the volvulus, with acute onset of bilious emesis, irritability, an initially scaphoid abdomen with increasing distention, and tenderness. Delays in diagnosis can be devastating. Late signs include abdominal wall erythema and hematemesis or melena from progressive mucosal ischemia. Mesenteric vascular compromise rapidly leads to peritonitis, sepsis, shock, and death. Laboratory investigation may reveal leukocytosis or leukopenia, hyperkalemia, and thrombocytopenia. A metabolic acidosis occurs in the presence of ischemia.

Radiologic studies can establish a definitive diagnosis but should not delay treatment if clinical suspicion is strong. Patients with suspected or confirmed midgut volvulus should be aggressively resuscitated, given intravenous broad-spectrum antibiotics, and taken to an operating room for immediate exploration. In clinically stable patients, initial evaluation begins with a plain abdominal radiograph with a lateral decubitus view. Findings are nonspecific but may help differentiate other forms of neonatal obstruction. There are no plain film findings that rule out malrotation/volvulus. The gold standard for diagnosis is an upper GI (UGI) contrast study to evaluate the position of the duodenojejunal junction and rule out obstruction. UGI is preferred to the less accurate barium enema. The normal ligament of Treitz is to the left of the midline and above the gastric outlet. US is sometimes obtained (particularly if pyloric stenosis is suspected) and shows a superior mesenteric vein, which lies to the left of, or posterior to, the SMA. With volvulus, a swirl or whirlpool sign is seen on color Doppler US.[75] CT also can be diagnostic. The UGI series, however, remains the most accurate and preferred imaging study, demonstrating abnormal position of the duodenojejunal junction and/or volvulus (delayed or obstructed passage of contrast from the duodenum, often with a corkscrew appearance).

## Treatment

The key elements of the Ladd procedure are summarized in **Box 1**. With the exception of the laparoscopic approach, the original operation has remained unchanged.

The open technique typically begins through a right upper quadrant transverse incision. The entire bowel and mesentery should be eviscerated and a detorsed counterclockwise. Ischemic bowel should be warmed for 20 to 30 minutes and re-examined. The mesentery must be widened by excision of cecal peritoneal bands traversing the duodenum (Ladd bands) and mobilization of the duodenum. The dissection then continues to the base of the SMA and vein by incising the anterior mesenteric leaflet. Intrinsic duodenal obstruction should always be ruled out by catheter passage. An appendectomy is then completed and the small intestine returned to the right abdomen and colon to the left abdomen.

Necrotic or ischemic bowel may involve isolated segments or the entire midgut and is a devastating finding in a previously healthy newborn. A limited resection of clearly necrotic bowel can be performed if the remaining intestine is not threatened. A second-look operation is planned in 24 to 48 hours. Abdominal compartment syndrome is a possibility and may necessitate a temporary patch closure. Unfortunately, occasionally patients have complete infarction of the midgut. Previously, such infants were treated with abdominal closure and comfort care. Advances in intestinal and multivisceral transplantation have made the situation more complex, allowing limited survival for some infants. This ethical issue remains controversial and its discussion is beyond the scope of this article and alloted length.

Laparoscopy has been widely used in management of malrotation.[76] Diagnostic laparoscopy to confirm the diagnosis[77] has also been used in patients with atypical or marginal abnormal intestinal rotation without volvulus, followed by an open or

---

**Box 1**
**Key elements for operative correction of malrotation**

1. Evisceration of bowel

2. Counterclockwise detorsion of bowel

3. Division of Ladd cecal bands

4. Broadening of the small bowel mesentary

5. Appendectomy

6. Placement of small bowel along right lateral gutter and large colon along the left lateral gutter

laparoscopic Ladd procedure. Further studies with long-term follow-up are needed to confirm the advantages and disadvantages of the laparoscopic approach—the primary concern is that one of the major benefits of laparoscopy (diminished adhesion formation) may predispose to an increased risk of future volvulus.

Laparoscopic repair of malrotation with acute volvulus has also been reported[72,77–79] with favorable results despite the technical challenges. Most minimally invasive surgeons prefer an open approach in these infants/children.[76,77,79]

It is important to counsel families that no operation is 100% successful in preventing recurrent volvulus and that prompt evaluation of any future bilious emesis is mandatory. The incidence of recurrent volvulus after Ladd procedure is low, however—under 2% to 3% in most reports.[70]

Postoperative intussusception is reportedly increased after a Ladd procedure; Kidd and colleagues noted a 3% incidence (a more than 50-fold increase compared with laparotomy for other indications).[80] Adhesive small bowel obstruction requiring laparotomy occurs in approximately 10% of patients after open procedures.[81,82]

## MECONIUM DISEASE

MI is estimated to account for 10% to 30% of neonatal ICU bowel obstructions.[83,84] The incidence in the United States is approximately 1 in 3000 live births per year. The intestinal lumen is intact in MI but functionally obstructed by the thick, viscid protein-rich meconium, which adheres to the wall of the bowel causing a blockage.

Approximately 15% of patients with CF develop MI. Conversely, greater than 95% of patients with simple MI have CF.[85,86] Extremely low-birth-weight infants may also present with meconium obstruction in the absence of CF.[87,88]

There is some controversy regarding whether or not the development of MI in CF patients predicts poorer long-term outcome: a recent study of more than 27,000 patients indicated that this was the case.[89–92]

The carrier rate for CF in the US population is approximately 4% to 5%. There is variation in the incidence of CF: it is rare in Asians and much less common in African Americans than in white or Latin Americans.[84]

The genetic locus for the CF gene is chromosome 7q31. The primary defect is in the CFTR gene, a CF transmembrane (conductance) receptor gene that codes for a protein that is a chloride channel cyclic AMP mediator. The most common genetic defect is the delta-F508 abnormality, seen in approximately 70% of patients. There are more than 1000 genetic mutations, however, identified in the CFTR gene.[93,94]

CF results in mucoviscidosis in exocrine secretions throughout the body. This results in elevated levels of the chloride in the sweat. Historically, the diagnosis was sometimes suggested when kissing an affected baby resulted in a salty taste. There is also pancreatic exocrine insufficiency.

The abnormal meconium in MI contains decreased amounts of: water, pancreatic enzymes, lactase and sucrase, carbohydrates, sodium, potassium, and magnesium. Protein and albumin are increased. The result is thicker and stickier meconium.[95] MI itself is thought due more to intraluminal intestinal factors than the absence of pancreatic secretions.

The differential diagnosis usually includes JIA, HD, meconium plug syndrome, and neonatal small left colon syndrome.

### Clinical Presentation

Prenatal diagnosis of MI may be suspected as a result of US findings. Fetuses are classified as low risk or high risk: the low-risk group is those who have abnormal

US findings (discussed later). The high-risk group is those who have a family history of CF.

Abnormal US findings include hyperechoic intra-abdominal masses (due to the inspissated meconium). This has a low sensitivity, however, for MI (30%–70%). The positive predictive value of these findings is increased in high-risk patients (50% vs 6%). Other US findings include dilated bowel and inability to visualize the gallbladder.[25]

MI is often described as either simple (SMI) or complex (CMI). In SMI, diagnosis is often made within 1 or 2 days after birth. Patients usually do not pass meconium and have a somewhat distended abdomen due to the distal obstruction. The abdomen may feel doughy from the meconium. There is usually no tenderness or respiratory distress in SMI. Radiographs may reveal dilated loops of proximal small bowel, but air-fluid levels are often absent (due to failure of the viscous meconium to layer out). A ground glass appearance also may be seen. The family history is positive for CF in 10% to 33% of infants.[85]

In contrast, CMI may have more varied presentations, ranging from completely asymptomatic patients who have incidental calcification on an abdominal film to patients with frank peritonitis or those in extremis. The incidence of CF is substantially lower in patients who present with CMI (15%–40%). CMI may result from an in utero perforation. The timing of the perforation dictates the clinical course. With an early in utero perforation, the hole is sealed and the baby is simply incidentally noted to have calcifications on a plain film but no obstruction or other symptoms. The findings are sometimes identified later, for example at herniorrhaphy. More often, perforations occurring later in fetal development result in peritonitis. Four types of meconium peritonitis are described: (1) adhesive, (2) meconium pseudocyst, (3) meconium ascites, and (4) infected meconium pseudocyst. Sterile bowel contents associated with the first 3 variants of meconium peritonitis do not produce an infection, rather, a chemical irritation that may be extreme. Radiographic findings of CMI are variable but include calcifications, free air, air-fluid levels, pseudocyst, ascites, and distended small bowel.

A water-soluble hyperosmolar contrast enema may be diagnostic (microcolon and ileal pellets) (**Fig. 8**) and therapeutic. Historically, more hyperosmolar solutions were used than are currently used at most institutions. Although the risk of dehydration and cardiovascular collapse is, therefore, much lower, adequate hydration is still essential.

All patients with MI should be tested for CF. Genetic tests are available, but because of the wide number of mutations, normal genetic screening does not rule out the diagnosis. The classic test is a sweat chloride, obtained by painless electrical stimulation of the skin to collect sweat (iontophoresis). The diagnosis is confirmed when sweat chloride levels are greater than 60 mmol/L in 100 mg of sweat; 60 mmol/L to 40 mmol/L is indeterminate and less than 40 mmol/L is normal. Sweat collection is difficult in newborns, and the test may not be able to be completed until a child is 1 or 2 months of age.

## Treatment

The treatment of SMI usually begins with hyperosmolar enemas as described previously. The number of attempts is limited: if there is no progress over a 48-hour period, or if more than 2 or 3 attempts do not result in significant improvement, operation is indicated. There has been a shift in the contrast materials used over time (less hyperosmolar agents) and in the number and duration of attempted reductions by radiologists—a recent multicenter review noted a decrease in successful reductions from approximately 40% to approximately 5% over the past 10 to 20 years.[48]

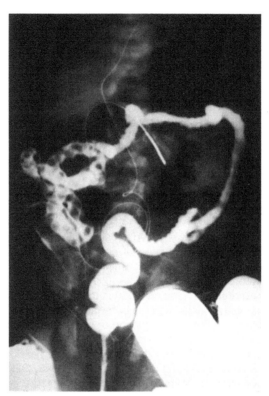

**Fig. 8.** A water-soluble hyperosmolar contrast enema may be diagnostic and therapeutic. The figure reveals a small microcolon with proximal ileal pellets. The radiograph also shows proximal small bowel dilation suggesting a distal obstruction.

A variety of operative techniques have been used for SMI. Generally, an enterotomy is made through a purse string suture in the dilated ileum above the area of the inspissated pellets. Irrigation is performed through a catheter inserted into the enterotomy with 2% to 4% N-acetylcysteine. The more soluble meconium is then manually milked out through the enterotomy. This process is repeated until the bowel is cleared.

Occasionally, the meconium is thick enough or requires enough trauma to the bowel that irrigation must be abandoned. An alternative is placement of a T-tube enterostomy, which allows for daily irrigation until clear (as well as radiographic access for contrast studies).[96] A variety of enterostomies and stomas were used historically, including the Santulli (distal bowel as the stoma with an end-to-side anastomosis from the proximal bowel), Bishop-Koop (essentially the reverse of the Santulli), or Mikulitz technique (where a double-barreled stoma is created, allowing access to the proximal and distal limbs).[97]

Surgery is almost always necessary for CMI; the procedure depends on the abnormality found. A pseudocyst is usually removed if possible, but the operation may be difficult with significant blood loss. One recent series found diffuse meconium peritonitis in 39%, fibroadhesive in 24%, and cystic type in 12% of CMI. Resection and primary anastomosis was possible in 22 of 31 patients.[98]

Elemental feeding and pancreatic enzyme supplementation are necessary. Careful attention to fluid and electrolyte status and pulmonary toilet is important. As discussed previously, diagnostic studies for CF should be obtained. The prognosis varies.

Survival has increased, ranging from 80% to 90% in CMI versus approximately 100% survival in SMI.

### Meconium Plug Syndrome

The incidence of meconium plug syndrome is estimated at approximately 1 in 500 live births. Symptoms are similar to those seen in SMI. Most patients have no underlying abnormality. Small left colon syndrome, CF, HD, and hypothyroidism (or other medical problems, such as maternal narcotic use), however, may all result in meconium plug syndrome. Usually the bowel is anatomically normal, and once the meconium plug is passed (often after water-soluble contrast enema), a patient has no further problems. It is usually recommended that babies are evaluated for CF and that a suction rectal biopsy is done. In the authors' experience, approximately 13% of such patients have HD and the incidence of CF is low.[99]

## HIRSCHSPRUNG DISEASE

The incidence of HD is estimated at approximately 1 in 5000 live births.[100,101] The male-to-female ratio is generally approximately 4 to 1, but in long-segment disease the ratio is equal.[102]

The familial incidence of HD is approximately 3.5% to 8% in most reports.[103] If total colonic disease is present in the family, however, there is a 13% to 20% incidence. If total intestinal aganglionosis (rare) is present, the familial incidence is approximately 50%. The disease is a gender-linked heterogeneous disorder of varying severity and incomplete penetrance. HD is thought a problem with molecular signaling, ultimately resulting in incomplete cephalocaudal migration of the intestinal neuroblasts. The migration begins at approximately 5 weeks' gestation and is usually complete by 12 weeks.[104]

Several genetic abnormalities have been identified, although most cases (80%) are sporadic. The expression and penetrance are variable. Mutations in the RET proto-oncogene (rearranged during transfection) on the long arm of chromosome 10 (10q11.2) account for most of the genetic abnormalities, but other gene mutations can cause the disease.[105–107] Because of the variability in the genetics (low penetrance, gender difference in penetrance and expression, and penetrance depending on the extent of aganglionosis), HD is more properly described as having susceptibility genes.

Approximately 12% of patients with HD have chromosomal abnormalities, most commonly trisomy 21. Overall, trisomy 21 is found in 4% to 16% of all patients with HD. Conversely, the incidence of HD in trisomy 21 is approximately 1 in 300, markedly higher than the general population incidence.[108] Associated abnormalities are present in 18% to 21%. These commonly include GI, central nervous system, genitourinary, musculoskeletal, craniofacial, skin, and other abnormalities. The incidence of these follows the order listed.[108]

Hereditary syndromes can be associated with HD; these are divided into neural cristopathies and non-neural cristopathies. The former consist of such entities as multiple endocrine neoplasia type 2A syndrome, congenital central hypoventilation, and Smith-Waardenberg syndrome. The latter consists of craniofacial dysmorphisms, limb anomalies, and other rare syndromes.

### Pathophysiology/Pathology

The basic pathophysiology is a functional obstruction with a patent intestine, due to a lack of peristalsis in abnormally innervated distal bowel. The adrenergic (excitatory) system exerts a stronger influence than the cholinergic (inhibitory) system, resulting in unopposed increased tone and contraction. Most cases (75%) of HD involve the colon distal to the rectosigmoid; total colonic aganglionosis occurs in 10% or less, and more proximal disease (including total intestinal aganglionosis) occurs rarely. The defect usually proceeds continuously from distal to proximal, with a transition zone of variable length at the junction with normal bowel.[109] Skip disease has been reported in fewer than 25 cases worldwide to date.[110]

### Clinical Presentation

The differential diagnosis in the newborn includes JIA, MI, meconium plug syndrome and hypoplastic left colon syndrome, and imperforate anus variants. The median age at diagnosis has been decreasing over the past several decades. Currently, approximately 90% of HD cases are identified in newborns[111] and 98% of term infants pass meconium in the first 24 hours of life.[112] Although traditional reports claimed that more than 90% of patients with HD failed to do so, more recent evidence suggests that up to 40% of HD newborns do pass meconium in the first 24 hours of life.[111] Prenatal diagnoses of HD are uncommon, except for total colonic disease.[113,114] Abdominal distention and bilious emesis are the other usual presenting features. A family history of HD is identified in approximately 10%. Perforation is a presenting symptom in less than 1% to 2% of newborns.

Diagnostic work-up usually includes a flat and lateral decubitus abdominal film, usually demonstrating dilated colon and or small bowel, occasionally with air-fluid levels. A contrast enema is the radiologic standard, demonstrating a transition zone between the smaller rectum and the proximally dilated ganglionated bowel (**Fig. 9**). It is important to avoid digital rectal examinations or washouts of the rectum before contrast studies, because this may decompress the bowel enough to mask identification of the transition zone. Although not commonly done in the United States, anorectal manometry in the newborn period is sometimes used as a screening test. A failure of the internal anal sphincter to relax with distention is characteristic of HD.

Definitive diagnosis requires tissue, usually obtained via a rectal suction biopsy in newborns. The sensitivity of this test in large series is approximately 90% to 95%, and the specificity is approximately 100% if done correctly.[115] Inadequate specimens are not infrequent, but complications are rare. Absent ganglion cells in the submucosal and myenteric plexus and increased acetylcholinesterase in parasympathetic nerve fibers in the lamina propria and muscularis mucosa are seen; abnormal nerve cells are identified. Hematoxylin-eosin stain confirmation of the diagnosis requires an experienced pathologist.[116]

### Treatment

Management of HD is surgical. The traditional approach for newborns is a leveling colostomy: an exploratory laparotomy is performed, with serial biopsies and frozen sections. When ganglion cells are definitively identified by frozen section histopathology, a colostomy is performed slightly proximal to this area (to avoid the transition zone). After a child has grown and gained adequate weight (usually at 6–12 months of age), a definitive pull-through procedure is performed.

One of 3 operations is usually selected for the definitive repair: (1) Duhamel procedure (retrorectal pull-through of ganglionated bowel with a stapled side-to-side anastomosis), (2) Soave endorectal pull-through (preservation of a short segment of muscular cuff), or (3) Swenson procedure (full-thickness endorectal pull-through).

Currently, many patients are managed by a single-stage pull-through procedure. Laparoscopic or transumbilical techniques are used to obtain frozen sections for

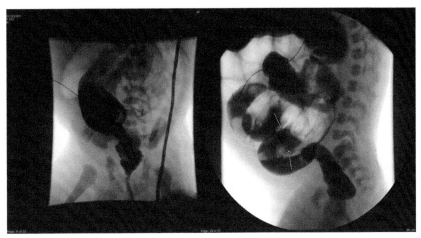

**Fig. 9.** Classic contrast enema of 2 patients demonstrating a transition zone (*arrows*) between the smaller rectum and the proximally dilated ganglionated bowel.

the level of ganglion cells. Either a laparoscopically assisted or a transrectal Soave pull-through is done with the ganglionated bowel.[117,118] This avoids the need for colostomy and its attendant costs and complications. Surgeons must completely rely on a frozen section diagnosis, however, and there is a potential for misdiagnosis or inappropriate leveling. Additionally, studies have demonstrated that the radiographic identification of the level of the transition zone is somewhat unreliable.[119] Contraindications to a single-stage procedure include suspected enterocolitis, significant concomitant disease, long-segment disease, trisomy 21, and lack of availability of experienced pathologic interpretation.[117] In the early postoperative period (after the pull-through procedure), avoidance of rectal temperature probes, examination, or medications is essential, and a sign at the bedside is helpful.

### Complications

Early complications include stricture anastomotic leak/abscess, early bowel obstruction, ischemia in the pull-through segment, and wound problems. Pull-through with the transition-zone bowel or aganglionic bowel is rare. Stomal complications with a staged procedure are common, and avoidance of these issues is an advantage of the single-stage procedure. Enterocolitis (the most life-threatening complication) can occur at any time and requires prompt recognition and vigorous resuscitation and treatment.

Late complications include soiling and incontinence (4%–10%), stricture (5%–10%, less common with the Duhamel procedure), and bowel obstruction (6%–10%).[120] Constipation is often ill defined, but milder forms are common after successful repair; preoperative and postoperative discussion with the family is helpful, because operation is often held out as the definitive cure for HD. The extent of knowledge of the disease is likely more limited than is believed, and the ganglionated normal bowel may eventually be found to harbor as-yet unrecognized abnormalities.

The long-term outcomes for traditional-staged versus single-staged operations are unclear. Some initial concerns regarding eventual continence have been raised, but the data are inconclusive.[121]

## IMPERFORATE ANUS

The incidence of ARMs is approximately 1 in 5000 live births, with a slight male predominance.

ARMs have a heterogeneous etiology, probably as a result of both genetic and environmental factors, although precise causation remains unknown. Several chromosomal abnormalities (trisomies 13, 18, and 21) and syndromic associations have been described, but most cases are sporadic.[122]

The incidence of associated anomalies is approximately 50% to 60%—the more proximal the anatomic ARM defect, the higher the risk of associated anomalies.[123] The most well-known association is VACTERL (vertebral, anal, cardiac, tracheal, esophageal, renal, and limb).

Cardiac anomalies should be ruled out by echocardiography and are seen in approximately one-third of patients.[124] The most common are atrial septal defect and patent ductus artery, followed by ventricular septal defect and tetralogy of Fallot.[123] GI anomalies are most commonly tracheoesophageal malformations (10%); duodenal atresia and HD are rare.[123,125] Genitourinary anomalies (vesicoureteric reflux, cryptorchidism, renal agenesis, and dysplasia) are the most common (30%–50%); their incidence depends primarily on the severity of the ARM and, to a lesser extent, the gender of the infant.[126] Bony lumbosacral vertebral anomalies are common (30%). Tethered cord and other spinal anomalies are less common. Gynecologic abnormalities in women with ARMs were historically often identified later in life, when menstrual or obstetric problems led to their identification. Increased awareness has led to earlier recognition and treatment.[127] Vaginal septations and agenesis and bicornate or malformed uterus are often seen.

ARMs are caused by faulty embryogenesis during the formation of the cloaca (sewer—a common cavity for the hindgut, tailgut, allantois, and mesonephric ducts) and the differentiation into normal adult structures between the third and ninth weeks of fetal development.[128]

ARMs constitute a diverse spectrum of anatomic variants. Although many classification systems exist, none is universally accepted. The Krickenbeck classification, widely used, is an international consensus system based on based on the fistula location (perineal, rectourethral, rectovesical, or vestibular), cloacal lesions, absent fistula (5% or less of patients), and anal stenosis.[129]

### Clinical Presentation

Typically, the deformity is recognized at birth. A fistula may be present to allow relief of the obstruction; sequential dilation may be necessary. Abdominal distention is usually present but may be mild. Evaluation of patients with an ARM should include an echocardiogram, renal and bladder US, spinal US, voiding cystourethrogram, and plain radiographs of the abdomen and lower spine. Invertograms to identify the distal extent of the rectum are often misleading and rarely indicated.

### Treatment

Operation is not usually urgent, and a delay of 24 to 48 hours when a perineal fistula is suspected but not confirmed (for example, a string of pearls—beading along the median raphe) is often beneficial.

The primary decision is whether or not a diverting colostomy is necessary. Infants with a perineal fistula can undergo primary repair: the timing in an otherwise healthy baby is often optional, with discharge and home dilations initially, followed by elective anoplasty. Alternatively, repair before discharge may be reasonable. Higher defects usually require a colostomy and mucus fistula. It is important to provide adequate separation between them to avoid a common bag for both and potential contamination of the urinary tract if a fistula is present.

ARMs are a widely variable constellation of anomalies, and extended discussion of the technical details of their surgical management is beyond the scope of this article. The standard procedure has been the posterior sagittal anorectoplasty, but laparoscopic repair (with or without a diverting colostomy) also has been used.[130,131]

Postoperative follow-up is important in these infants—early graded dilation as prophylaxis for stricture formation should continue for at least 4 to 6 months after definitive repair. Constipation is common, and the incidence is higher with lower defects. Continence is the major issue; barring surgical misadventure, this is dependent on the underlying anatomy of the defect. High defects with bowel to bladder fistulas, bony sacral ratios less than 0.3, and more severe ARMs have a poorer outcome. Longer-term urologic and sexual dysfunction is infrequent but related to defect severity.

## REFERENCES

1. Young JY, Kim DS, Muratore CS, et al. High incidence of postoperative bowel obstruction in newborns and infants. J Pediatr Surg 2007;42(6):962–5 [discussion: 962–5].
2. Okoye BO, Parikh DH, Buick RG, et al. Pyloric atresia: five new cases, a new association, and a review of the literature with guidelines. J Pediatr Surg 2000;35(8):1242–5.
3. Ilce Z, Erdogan E, Kara C, et al. Pyloric atresia: 15-year review from a single institution. J Pediatr Surg 2003;38(11):1581–4.
4. Bar-Maor JA, Nissan S, Nevo S. Pyloric atresia. A hereditary congenital anomaly with autosomal recessive transmission. J Med Genet 1972;9(1):70–2.
5. Nawaz A, Matta H, Jacobsz A, et al. Congenital pyloric atresia and junctional epidermolysis bullosa: a report of two cases. Pediatr Surg Int 2000;16(3):206–8.
6. Lestringant GG, Akel SR, Qayed KI. The pyloric atresia-junctional epidermolysis bullosa syndrome. Report of a case and review of the literature. Arch Dermatol 1992;128(8):1083–6.
7. Maman E, Maor E, Kachko L, et al. Epidermolysis bullosa, pyloric atresia, aplasia cutis congenita: histopathological delineation of an autosomal recessive disease. Am J Med Genet 1998;78(2):127–33.
8. Snyder CL, Mancini ML, Kennedy AP, et al. Multiple gastrointestinal atresias with cystic dilatation of the biliary duct. Pediatr Surg Int 2000;16(3):211–3.
9. Ducharme JC, Bensoussan AL. Pyloric atresia. J Pediatr Surg 1975;10(1):149–50.
10. Dalla Vecchia LK, Grosfeld JL, West KW, et al. Intestinal atresia and stenosis: a 25-year experience with 277 cases. Arch Surg 1998;133(5):490–7.
11. Kimura K, Mukohara N, Nishijima E, et al. Diamond-shaped anastomosis for duodenal atresia: an experience with 44 patients over 15 years. J Pediatr Surg 1990;25(9):977–9.
12. Tandler J. Zur Entwicklungsgeschichte des Menschlichen Duodenum in Fruhen Embryonalstadien. Morphol Jahrb 1900;29:187–216.
13. Kimble RM, Harding J, Kolbe A. Additional congenital anomalies in babies with gut atresia or stenosis: when to investigate, and which investigation. Pediatr Surg Int 1997;12(8):565–70.

14. Keckler SJ, Peter SD, Spilde TL, et al. The influence of trisomy 21 on the incidence and severity of congenital heart defects in patients with duodenal atresia. Pediatr Surg Int 2008;24(8):921–3.
15. Mustafawi AR, Hassan ME. Congenital duodenal obstruction in children: a decade's experience. Eur J Pediatr Surg 2008;18(2):93–7.
16. Escobar MA, Ladd AP, Grosfeld JL, et al. Duodenal atresia and stenosis: long-term follow-up over 30 years. J Pediatr Surg 2004;39(6):867–71.
17. Irving IM. Duodenal atresia and stenosis: annular pancreas. In: Irving IM, editor. Neonatal surgery. London: Butterworths; 1990. p. 424.
18. Grosfeld JL, Rescorla FJ. Duodenal atresia and stenosis: reassessment of treatment and outcome based on antenatal diagnosis, pathologic variance, and long-term follow-up. World J Surg 1993;17(3):301–9.
19. Jolleys A. An examination of the birthweights of babies with some abnormalities of the alimentary tract. J Pediatr Surg 1981;16(2):160–3.
20. Fonkalsrud EW, DeLorimier AA, Hays DM. Congenital atresia and stenosis of the duodenum. A review compiled from the members of the Surgical Section of the American Academy of Pediatrics. Pediatrics 1969;43(1):79–83.
21. Sajja SB, Middlesworth W, Niazi M, et al. Duodenal atresia associated with proximal jejunal perforations: a case report and review of the literature. J Pediatr Surg 2003;38(9):1396–8.
22. Bill AH Jr, Pope WM. Congenital duodenal diaphragm; report of two cases. Surgery 1954;35(3):482–6.
23. Bittencourt DG, Barini R, Marba S, et al. Congenital duodenal obstruction: does prenatal diagnosis improve the outcome? Pediatr Surg Int 2004;20(8):582–5.
24. Langer JC, Adzick NS, Filly RA, et al. Gastrointestinal tract obstruction in the fetus. Arch Surg 1989;124(10):1183–6 [discussion: 1187].
25. Bianchi DW, Crombleholme TM, D'Alton ME. Fetology. New York: McGraw-Hill Professional; 2000.
26. Britton JR, Britton HL. Gastric aspirate volume at birth as an indicator of congenital intestinal obstruction. Acta Paediatr 1995;84(8):945–6.
27. Rothenberg SS. Laparoscopic duodenoduodenostomy for duodenal obstruction in infants and children. J Pediatr Surg 2002;37(7):1088–9.
28. Spilde TL, St Peter SD, Keckler SJ, et al. Open vs laparoscopic repair of congenital duodenal obstructions: a concurrent series. J Pediatr Surg 2008;43(6):1002–5.
29. Weber TR, Lewis JE, Mooney D, et al. Duodenal atresia: a comparison of techniques of repair. J Pediatr Surg 1986;21(12):1133–6.
30. St Peter SD, Little DC, Barsness KA, et al. Should we be concerned about jejunoileal atresia during repair of duodenal atresia? J Laparoendosc Adv Surg Tech A 2010;20(9):773–5.
31. Paterson-Brown S, Stalewski H, Brereton RJ. Neonatal small bowel atresia, stenosis and segmental dilatation. Br J Surg 1991;78(1):83–6.
32. Feggetter S. A review of the long-term results of operations for duodenal atresia. Br J Surg 1969;56(1):68–72.
33. Kokkonen ML, Kalima T, Jääskeläinen J, et al. Duodenal atresia: late follow-up. J Pediatr Surg 1988;23(3):216–20.
34. Kumaran N, Shankar KR, Lloyd DA, et al. Trends in the management and outcome of jejuno-ileal atresia. Eur J Pediatr Surg 2002;12(3):163–7.
35. Moore KL, Persaud TV. The developing human. 8th edition. Philadelphia: Saunders; 2008.
36. Louw JH, Barnard CN. Congenital intestinal atresia; observations on its origin. Lancet 1955;269(6899):1065–7.

37. Nixon HH, Tawes R. Etiology and treatment of small intestinal atresia: analysis of a series of 127 jejunoileal atresias and comparison with 62 duodenal atresias. Surgery 1971;69(1):41–51.
38. Werler MM, Sheehan JE, Mitchell AA. Association of vasoconstrictive exposures with risks of gastroschisis and small intestinal atresia. Epidemiology 2003;14(3): 349–54.
39. Cywes S, Davies MR, Rode H. Congenital jejuno-ileal atresia and stenosis. S Afr Med J 1980;57(16):630–9.
40. Skandalakis J, Gray S, Ricketts R. The small intestines. 2nd edition. Baltimore (MD): Williams & Wilkins; 1994. p. 213–25.
41. Sweeney B, Surana R, Puri P. Jejunoileal atresia and associated malformations: correlation with the timing of in utero insult. J Pediatr Surg 2001;36(5):774–6.
42. Stollman TH, Wijnen RM, Draaisma JM. Investigation for cystic fibrosis in infants with jejunoileal atresia in the Netherlands: a 35-year experience with 114 cases. Eur J Pediatr 2007;166(9):989–90.
43. Grosfeld JL, Ballantine TV, Shoemaker R. Operative mangement of intestinal atresia and stenosis based on pathologic findings. J Pediatr Surg 1979;14(3): 368–75.
44. Baglaj M, Carachi R, Lawther S. Multiple atresia of the small intestine: a 20-year review. Eur J Pediatr Surg 2008;18(1):13–8.
45. Bilodeau A, Prasil P, Cloutier R, et al. Hereditary multiple intestinal atresia: thirty years later. J Pediatr Surg 2004;39(5):726–30.
46. Rescorla FJ, Grosfeld JL. Intestinal atresia and stenosis: analysis of survival in 120 cases. Surgery 1985;98(4):668–76.
47. Louw JH. Resection and end-to-end anastomosis in the management of atresia and stenosis of the small bowel. Surgery 1967;62(5):940–50.
48. Copeland DR, St Peter SD, Sharp SW, et al. Diminishing role of contrast enema in simple meconium ileus. J Pediatr Surg 2009;44:2130–2.
49. Benson CD, Lotfi MW, Brogh AJ. Congenital atresia and stenosis of the colon. J Pediatr Surg 1968;3(2):253–7.
50. Boles ET Jr, Vassy LE, Ralston M. Atresia of the colon. J Pediatr Surg 1976; 11(1):69–75.
51. Oldham KT, Arca MJ. Atresia, stenosis, and other obstructions of the colon. In: Grosfeld JL, O'Neil JA, Fonkalsrud EW, et al, editors. Pediatric surgery, vol. 2. Philadelphia: Mosby; 2006. p. 1493–500.
52. Powell RW, Raffensperger JG. Congenital colonic atresia. J Pediatr Surg 1982; 17(2):166–70.
53. Davenport M, Bianchi A, Doig CM, et al. Colonic atresia: current results of treatment. J R Coll Surg Edinb 1990;35(1):25–8.
54. Fairbanks TJ, Kanard RC, Del Moral PM, et al. Colonic atresia without mesenteric vascular occlusion. The role of the fibroblast growth factor 10 signaling pathway. J Pediatr Surg 2005;40:390–6.
55. Fairbanks TJ, Kanard RC, De Langhe SP, et al. A genetic mechanism for cecal atresia: the role of the Fgf10 signaling pathway. J Surg Res 2004;120(2):201–9.
56. Snyder CL, Miller KA, Sharp RJ, et al. Management of intestinal atresia in patients with gastroschisis. J Pediatr Surg 2001;36:1542–5.
57. Baglaj M, Carachi R, MacCormack B. Colonic atresia: a clinicopathological insight into its etiology. Eur J Pediatr Surg 2010;20(2):102–5.
58. Draus JM Jr, Maxfield CM, Bond SJ. Hirschsprung's disease in an infant with colonic atresia and normal fixation of the distal colon. J Pediatr Surg 2007; 42(2):e5–8.

59. Karnak I, Ciftci AO, Senocak ME, et al. Colonic atresia: surgical management and outcome. Pediatr Surg Int 2001;17(8):631–5.
60. Fishman SJ, Islam S, Buonomo C, et al. Nonfixation of an atretic colon predicts Hirschsprung's disease. J Pediatr Surg 2001;36(1):202–4.
61. Cox SG, Numanoglu A, Millar AJ, et al. Colonic atresia: spectrum of presentation and pitfalls in management. A review of 14 cases. Pediatr Surg Int 2005;21(10): 813–8.
62. Anderson N, Malpas T, Robertson R. Prenatal diagnosis of colon atresia. Pediatr Radiol 1993;23(1):63–4.
63. Pohlson EC, Hatch EI, Glick PL, et al. Individualized management of colonic atresia. Am J Surg 1988;155(5):690–2.
64. Watts AC, Sabharwal AJ, MacKinlay GA, et al. Congenital colonic atresia: should primary anastomosis always be the goal? Pediatr Surg Int 2003; 19(1–2):14–7.
65. Defore WW, Garcia-Rinaldi R, Mattox KL, et al. Surgical management of colon atresia. Surg Gynecol Obstet 1976;143(5):767–9.
66. Benawra R, Puppala BL, Mangurten HH, et al. Familial occurrence of congenital colonic atresia. J Pediatr 1981;99(3):435–6.
67. Kapfer SA, Rappold JF. Intestinal malrotation-not just the pediatric surgeon's problem. J Am Coll Surg 2004;199(4):628–35.
68. Kluth D, Jaeschke-Melli S, Fiegel H. The embryology of gut rotation. Semin Pediatr Surg 2003;12(4):275–9.
69. Kluth D, Kaestner M, Tibboel D, et al. Rotation of the gut: fact or fantasy? J Pediatr Surg 1995;30(3):448–53.
70. Smith SD. Disorders of intestinal rotation and fixation. In: Grosfeld JL, O'NeillL JA, Fonkalsrud EW, et al, editors. Pediatric surgery. 6th edition. Philadelphia: Mosby Elsevier; 2006. p. 1342–57.
71. Martin V, Shaw-Smith C. Review of genetic factors in intestinal malrotation. Pediatr Surg Int 2010;26(8):769–81.
72. Gross E, Chen MK, Lobe TE. Laparoscopic evaluation and treatment of intestinal malrotation in infants. Surg Endosc 1996;10(9):936–7.
73. Ford EG, Senac MO Jr, Srikanth MS, et al. Malrotation of the intestine in children. Ann Surg 1992;215(2):172–8.
74. Powell DM, Othersen HB, Smith CD. Malrotation of the intestines in children: the effect of age on presentation and therapy. J Pediatr Surg 1989;24(8):777–80.
75. Shimanuki Y, Aihara T, Takano H, et al. Clockwise whirlpool sign at color Doppler US: an objective and definite sign of midgut volvulus. Radiology 1996;199(1): 261–4.
76. Draus JM Jr, Foley DS, Bond SJ. Laparoscopic Ladd procedure: a minimally invasive approach to malrotation without midgut volvulus. Am Surg 2007; 73(7):693–6.
77. Mazziotti MV, Strasberg SM, Langer JC. Intestinal rotation abnormalities without volvulus: the role of laparoscopy. J Am Coll Surg 1997;185(2):172–6.
78. Bass KD, Rothenberg SS, Chang JH. Laparoscopic Ladd's procedure in infants with malrotation. J Pediatr Surg 1998;33(2):279–81.
79. Lessin MS, Luks FI. Laparoscopic appendectomy and duodenocolonic dissociation (LADD) procedure for malrotation. Pediatr Surg Int 1998;13(2-3):184–5.
80. Kidd J, Jackson R, Wagner CW, et al. Intussusception following the Ladd procedure. Arch Surg 2000;135(6):713–5.
81. Rescorla FJ, Shedd FJ, Grosfeld JL, et al. Anomalies of intestinal rotation in childhood: analysis of 447 cases. Surgery 1990;108(4):710–6.

82. Murphy FL, Sparnon AL. Long-term complications following intestinal malrotation and the Ladd's procedure: a 15 year review. Pediatr Surg Int 2006;22(4): 326–9.

83. Irish MS, Surgical Aspects of Cystic Fibrosis and Meconium Ileus. Medscape Reference 2011. Available at: http://emedicine.medscape.com/article/939603-overview. Accessed March 3, 2012.

84. Ziegler MM. Meconium ileus. In: Grosfeld JL, O'Neil JA, Fonkalsrud EW, et al, editors. Pediatric surgery, vol. 2. Philadelphia: Mosby Elsevier; 2006. p. 1289–303.

85. Dolan TF Jr, Touloukian RJ. Familial meconium ileus not associated with cystic fibrosis. J Pediatr Surg 1974;9(6):821–4.

86. Shigemoto H, Endo S, Isomoto T, et al. Neonatal meconium obstruction in the ileum without mucoviscidosis. J Pediatr Surg 1978;13(6):475–9.

87. Emil S. Meconium obstruction in extremely low-birth-weight neonates: guidelines for diagnosis and management*1. J Pediatr Surg 2004;39:731–7.

88. Kubota A, Shiraishi J, Kawahara H, et al. Meconium-related ileus in extremely-low-birth-weight neonates: etiological consideration from histological and radiological studies. Pediatr Int 2011;53(6):887–91.

89. Lai HJ, Cheng Y, Cho H, et al. Association between initial disease presentation, lung disease outcomes, and survival in patients with cystic fibrosis. Am J Epidemiol 2004;159(6):537–46.

90. Efrati O, Nir J, Fraser D, et al. Meconium ileus in patients with cystic fibrosis is not a risk factor for clinical deterioration and survival: the Israeli Multicenter Study. J Pediatr Gastroenterol Nutr 2010;50(2):173–8.

91. Johnson J-A, Bush A, Buchdahl R. Does presenting with meconium ileus affect the prognosis of children with cystic fibrosis? Pediatr Pulmonol 2010;45(10):951–8.

92. Munck A, Gérardin M, Alberti C, et al. Clinical outcome of cystic fibrosis presenting with or without meconium ileus: a matched cohort study. J Pediatr Surg 2006;41(9):1556–60.

93. Cystic Fibrosis Genetic Analysis Consortium. Cystic Fibrosis Mutation Database. 2011. Available at: http://www.genet.sickkids.on.ca/StatisticsPage.html. 2011. Accessed March 3, 2012.

94. Gallati S. Genetics of cystic fibrosis. Semin Respir Crit Care Med 2003;24(6): 629–38.

95. Harries JT. Meconium in health and disease. Br Med Bull 1978;34(1):75–8.

96. Mak GZ, Harberg FJ, Hiatt P, et al. T-tube ileostomy for meconium ileus: four decades of experience. J Pediatr Surg 2000;35(2):349–52.

97. Rescorla FJ, Grosfeld JL. Contemporary management of meconium ileus. World J Surg 1993;17(3):318–25.

98. Nam SH, Kim SC, Kim DY, et al. Experience with meconium peritonitis. J Pediatr Surg 2007;42:1822–5.

99. Keckler S, St Peter S, Spilde T, et al. Current significance of meconium plug syndrome. J Pediatr Surg 2008;43(5):896–8.

100. Amiel J, Sproat-Emison E, Garcia-Barcelo M, et al. Hirschsprung disease, associated syndromes and genetics: a review. J Med Genet 2008;45(1):1–14.

101. Suita S, Taguchi T, Ieiri S, et al. Hirschsprung's disease in Japan: analysis of 3852 patients based on a nationwide survey in 30 years. J Pediatr Surg 2005; 40(1):197–202.

102. Badner JA, Sieber WK, Garver KL, et al. A genetic study of Hirschsprung disease. Am J Hum Genet 1990;46(3):568–80.

103. Puri P. Hirschsprung's disease. In: Puri P, editor. Newborn Surgery. London: Arnold; 2003. p. 513–34.

104. Puri P, Shinkai T. Pathogenesis of Hirschsprung's disease and its variants: recent progress. Semin Pediatr Surg 2004;13(1):18–24.
105. Borrego S, Wright FA, Fernández RM, et al. A founding locus within the RET proto-oncogene may account for a large proportion of apparently sporadic Hirschsprung disease and a subset of cases of sporadic medullary thyroid carcinoma. Am J Hum Genet 2003;72(1):88–100.
106. Parisi MA, Kapur RP. Genetics of Hirschsprung disease. Curr Opin Pediatr 2000; 12(6):610–7.
107. Moore SW, Zaahl MG. Multiple endocrine neoplasia syndromes, children, Hirschsprung's disease and RET. Pediatr Surg Int 2008;24(5):521–30.
108. Moore SW. Congenital anomalies and genetic associations with hirschsprung's disease. In: Holschneider AM, Puri P, editors. Hirschsprung's disease and allied disorders. 3rd edition. Berlin: Springer-Verlag; 2008. p. 115–31.
109. White FV, Langer JC. Circumferential distribution of ganglion cells in the transition zone of children with Hirschsprung disease. Pediatr Dev Pathol 2000;3(3): 216–22.
110. O'Donnell AM, Puri P. Skip segment Hirschsprung's disease: a systematic review. Pediatr Surg Int 2010;26(11):1065–9.
111. Singh SJ, Croaker GD, Manglick P, et al. Hirschsprung's disease: the Australian Paediatric Surveillance Unit's experience. Pediatr Surg Int 2003;19(4): 247–50.
112. Clark DA. Times of first void and first stool in 500 newborns. Pediatrics 1977; 60(4):457–9.
113. Haeusler MC, Berghold A, Stoll C, et al. Prenatal ultrasonographic detection of gastrointestinal obstruction: results from 18 European congenital anomaly registries. Prenat Diagn 2002;22(7):616–23.
114. Belin B, Corteville J, Langer J. How accurate is prenatal sonography for the diagnosis of imperforate anus and Hirschsprung's disease? Pediatr Surg Int 1995;10: 30–2.
115. Lewis NA, Levitt MA, Zallen GS, et al. Diagnosing Hirschsprung's disease: increasing the odds of a positive rectal biopsy result. J Pediatr Surg 2003; 38(3):412–6.
116. Meier-Ruge W, Bruder E. Histopathological diagnosis and differential of Hirschsprung's disease in Hirschprung's diesease. In: Holschneider AM, Puri P, editors. Hirschsprung's disease. Berlin: Springer; 2008. p. 185–97.
117. Dasgupta R, Langer JC. Transanal pull-through for Hirschsprung disease. Semin Pediatr Surg 2005;14(1):64–71.
118. Georgeson KE, Cohen RD, Hebra A, et al. Primary laparoscopic-assisted endorectal colon pull-through for Hirschsprung's disease: a new gold standard. Ann Surg 1999;229(5):678–83.
119. Shayan K, Smith C, Langer JC. Reliability of intraoperative frozen sections in the management of Hirschsprung's disease. J Pediatr Surg 2004;39:1345–8.
120. Little D, Snyder C. Late complications of Hirschsprung's disease. In: Holschneide RA, editor. Hirschsprung's disease and allied disorders. 2nd edition. Berlin: Springer-Verlag; 2007. p. 377–89.
121. El-Sawaf MI, Drongowski RA, Chamberlain JN, et al. Are the long-term results of the transanal pull-through equal to those of the transabdominal pull-through? A comparison of the 2 approaches for Hirschsprung disease. J Pediatr Surg 2007; 42(1):41–7 [discussion: 47].
122. Marcelis C, de Blaauw I, Brunner H. Chromosomal anomalies in the etiology of anorectal malformations: a review. Am J Med Genet A 2011;155(11):2692–704.

123. Pena A, Levitt MA. Anorectal malformations. In: Grosfeld JL, O'Neil JA, Fonkalsrud EW, et al, editors. Pediatric surgery. Philadelphia: Mosby Elsevier; 2006. p. 1566–89.
124. Keckler SJ, St Peter SD, Valusek PA, et al. VACTERL anomalies in patients with esophageal atresia: an updated delineation of the spectrum and review of the literature. Pediatr Surg Int 2007;23(4):309–13.
125. Raboei EH. Patients with anorectal malformation and Hirschsprung's disease. Eur J Pediatr Surg 2009;19(5):325–7.
126. Ratan SK, Rattan KN, Pandey RM, et al. Associated congenital anomalies in patients with anorectal malformations—a need for developing a uniform practical approach. J Pediatr Surg 2004;39(11):1706–11.
127. Breech L. Gynecologic concerns in patients with anorectal malformations. Semin Pediatr Surg 2010;19(2):139–45.
128. Kluth D. Embryology of anorectal malformations. Semin Pediatr Surg 2010;19: 201–8.
129. Holschneider A, Hutson J, Peña A, et al. Preliminary report on the International Conference for the Development of Standards for the Treatment of Anorectal Malformations. J Pediatr Surg 2005;40(10):1521–6.
130. Georgeson KE, Inge TH, Albanese CT. Laparoscopically assisted anorectal pull-through for high imperforate anus–a new technique. J Pediatr Surg 2000;35(6): 927–31.
131. Sydorak RM, Albanese CT. Laparoscopic repair of high imperforate anus. Semin Pediatr Surg 2002;11(4):217–25.

# Congenital Abdominal Wall Defects and Reconstruction in Pediatric Surgery
## Gastroschisis and Omphalocele

Daniel J. Ledbetter, MD

### KEYWORDS

- Abdominal wall defect • Gastroschisis • Omphalocele • Prenatal • Congenital
- Newborn

### KEY POINTS

- Gastroschisis is a full thickness defect in the abdominal wall usually just to the right of a normal umbilicus.
- Omphalocele is a midline abdominal wall defect with herniated abdominal contents covered by a membrane that the umbilical cord inserts into.
- The treatment of patients with congenital abdominal wall defects is determined by the baby's size, the size of the defect and associated conditions.

This article on the evaluation and management of the two most common congenital abdominal wall defects, gastroschisis and omphalocele, may offer insights into the care of other patients with acquired abdominal wall defects after trauma, tumor resection, or major abdominal operations. The two scenarios in which congenital abdominal wall defects are most commonly presented to pediatric surgeons are the fetus with a prenatal diagnosis and the newborn. This article reviews the issues and options for management in each scenario. Most articles lump gastroschisis and omphalocele together. However, it is important to remember that they are separate and distinct conditions with many differences in anatomy, pathology, and associated conditions that explain their different treatment and markedly different outcomes. A brief summary of some important differences is shown in **Table 1**.

The author has nothing to disclose.
Division of Pediatric Surgery, Department of Surgery, Seattle Children's Hospital, University of Washington, 4800 Sand Point Way Northeast, PO Box 5371/W-7729, Seattle, WA 98105-0371, USA
*E-mail address:* dan.ledbetter@seattlechildrens.org

Surg Clin N Am 92 (2012) 713–727
doi:10.1016/j.suc.2012.03.010
0039-6109/12/$ – see front matter © 2012 Elsevier Inc. All rights reserved.

**Table 1**
Differences between gastroschisis and omphalocele

|  | Gastroschisis | Omphalocele |
|---|---|---|
| Covering membrane | No | Yes |
| Location of defect | Right of umbilicus | Midline including umbilicus |
| Umbilical cord insertion | Body wall at normal location | Omphalocele membrane |
| Herniated abdominal organs | Bowel | Bowel and sometimes liver |
| Associated anomalies | Uncommon | Very common |
| Prognostic factors | Condition of bowel | Associated anomalies |

## GASTROSCHISIS
### Definition

Gastroschisis is a full-thickness defect in the abdominal wall usually to the right of a normally inserted umbilical cord. Rarely, the defect is in a mirror-image position to the left of the umbilical cord.[1] A variable amount of intestine and occasionally parts of other abdominal organs are herniated outside the abdominal wall with no covering membrane or sac (**Fig. 1**).

### Embryology

The normal abdominal wall is formed by infolding of the cranial, caudal, and two lateral embryonic folds. As the abdominal wall is forming the rapid growth of the intestinal tract leads to its herniation through the umbilical ring into the umbilical cord from the 6th to the 10th week of gestation. By the 10th to 12th week of gestation, the intestine returns to the abdominal cavity in a stereotypical pattern that results in normal intestinal rotation and, later, fixation, and the abdominal wall is well formed.[2]

The cause of a gastroschisis is unknown. Several theories have been proposed to account for the unique body wall defect through which the bowel would eviscerate early in gestation, including a localized failure of mesoderm formation, rupture of the amnion at the umbilical ring, abnormal involution of the right umbilical vein, disruption of the right vitelline artery with localized body wall ischemia, and abnormal body wall folding.[3]

### Epidemiology

Although there are regional differences, the incidence of gastroschisis seems to be increasing worldwide and is approaching 3 to 4 per 10,000 births in endemic areas.[4,5]

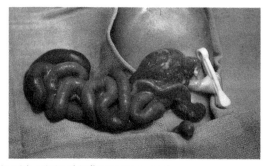

**Fig. 1.** Gastroschisis with minimal inflammatory peel.

The reason for the increasing incidence of gastroschisis is unknown and an increasing focus of investigation, in part because of the increasing burden to health care systems and the ultimate goal of prevention.[6,7] Most cases are sporadic with only unusual familial cases.[8] A major epidemiologic clue has been the strong association with young maternal age (most mothers are 20 years of age or younger)[4] but, as of yet, there is no clear cause of gastroschisis.[9]

### Associated Anomalies

Like any newborn with a congenital anomaly, newborns with gastroschisis are at increased risk for additional anomalies. Between 10% and 20% of newborns with gastroschisis have associated anomalies[9] and most the significant anomalies are in the gastrointestinal tract. About 10% of babies with gastroschisis will have intestinal stenosis or atresia[10] that results from vascular insufficiency to the bowel. This insufficiency could occur early at the time of gastroschisis development or, more likely, later from volvulus or compression of the mesenteric vascular pedicle against a narrowing abdominal wall ring. Serious associated anomalies, such as chromosomal abnormalities, are uncommon.[11] Thus, overall outcomes are related to the severity of bowel injury.

### Prenatal Diagnosis

Abdominal wall defects are often diagnosed before birth by ultrasound.[5] However the accuracy of routine prenatal ultrasound for diagnosing gastroschisis is less than perfect.[12] The specificity is high (more than 95%) but the sensitivity is lower because of differences in the experience and expertise of sonographers and the variable timing and different goals of prenatal ultrasound. Diagnostic errors may result from confusion with other rare abdominal wall disruptions (often away from the umbilicus, not covered by a membrane, and fatal) or the rare ruptured omphalocele that mimic a gastroschisis because of the lack of a covering membrane. However, probably the most common reason for diagnostic inaccuracy is that the abdominal wall is not seen well enough during studies done for screening for fetal number, position, and age. Directed ultrasound examination looking specifically for specific structural anomalies is much more accurate.[5] Such directed studies are often done if maternal serum screening shows an elevated alpha fetoprotein (AFP) or if there are abnormalities of fetal growth or amniotic fluid levels. AFP is the fetal analog of albumin and maternal serum AFP reflects the level of AFP in amniotic fluid. AFP testing was primarily developed to evaluate the fetus for chromosomal abnormalities and neural tube defects but when a fetus has gastroschisis, the maternal serum AFP is also almost always markedly elevated.[13]

### Prenatal Management

The prenatal diagnosis of gastroschisis often leads to the initial introduction of the pediatric surgeon to the patient and family. Although there currently is no fetal surgery for gastroschisis, a prenatal diagnosis allows the surgeon (and others) to counsel families about the condition, its treatment, and its prognosis. A fetus with gastroschisis is at risk for several adverse events in utero, including intrauterine growth retardation (IUGR), oligohydramnios, premature delivery, and even fetal death. In addition, the exposed bowel is vulnerable to a spectrum of injury. These adverse events are major determinants of prenatal and postnatal outcome so many prenatal investigations and interventions have been proposed to predict and prevent them. In addition, prenatal diagnosis of gastroschisis permits a transfer to high-risk obstetric care and a smooth transition to definitive postnatal care in a specialized center that will optimize the outcome.

The diagnosis of IUGR may include measurement of the fetal torso, which can be problematic in a fetus with gastroschisis because of the eviscerated intestine. Even with these difficulties of diagnosis, IUGR is diagnosed in 30% to 70% of these patients depending on the diagnostic criteria used.[14] The cause of fetal growth failure in gastroschisis is unknown. The cause is presumed to be due to increased losses of protein from the exposed viscera although inadequate supply of fetal nutrients is an alternative hypothesis. The recognition of IUGR will result in increased prenatal monitoring. Oligohydramnios may also complicate the gestation and, if moderately severe, it is associated with IUGR, fetal distress, and birth asphyxia. Severe cases of oligohydramnios associated with gastroschisis have been treated with amniotic fluid replacement with some success.[15]

In a fetus with gastroschisis, the exposed bowel is vulnerable to injury. The injury can range in severity from volvulus and loss of the entire midgut, to an intestinal atresia, to an inflammatory "peel" or serositis of the bowel that can make the bowel loops indistinguishable from one another (**Fig. 2**). The inflammatory peel is unique to gastroschisis, develops in some, but not all, cases after 30 weeks gestation, and is quite variable in severity. The cause is unknown but is proposed to be the result of bowel wall exposure to amniotic fluid, intestinal obstruction, or intestinal lymphatic obstruction. The degree of the inflammatory peel is difficult to quantify on both prenatal ultrasound and on postnatal physical examination; therefore, it has been difficult to correlate with any clinical outcome variables. Because bowel injury is the major predictor of postnatal morbidity, an improved understanding and prognostic testing would be valuable to identify high-risk patients but, as of yet, there are no prenatal ultrasound findings that reliably predict outcome.[16]

The most devastating complication in a fetus with gastroschisis is fetal death. It is typically late in gestation and may be caused by an in utero midgut volvulus or, possibly, by an acute compromise of umbilical blood flow by the eviscerated bowel. Unfortunately, there are no reliable prenatal predictors of this complication. These unpredictable, tragic cases have been a strong motivating force for those who argue for the early delivery of the fetus with gastroschisis.[17] Unfortunately, it is still unclear that a fetus with gastroschisis with a high risk of prenatal complications can be reliably identified[18] and it is unclear if the potential benefits of early delivery outweigh the risks of even moderate prematurity.[16,19,20]

Current recommendations for prenatal management of cases of gastroschisis include (1) follow-up ultrasounds every 3 to 4 weeks to assess fetal growth, amniotic fluid, and the condition of the bowel; (2) fetal nonstress once a week in fetuses less

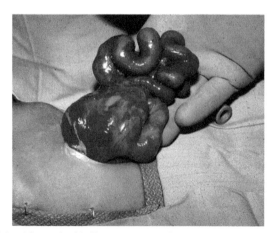

**Fig. 2.** Gastroschisis with marked inflammatory peel.

than 32-weeks gestation if there is an abnormality of fetal growth or amniotic fluid or progressive bowel dilation and, then, twice a week after 32-weeks gestation in all cases; (3) delivery at or near term, avoiding preterm (less than 37-weeks gestation) delivery; and (4) vaginal delivery unless there are other maternal or fetal indications for cesarean section.[16,21]

### Newborn Resuscitation and Medical Management

Similar to trauma patients with dramatic open wounds, the care of newborns with abdominal wall defects starts with an evaluation and management of airway, breathing, and circulation (ABCs) and, only then, attention is turned to the abdominal wall defect. Premature birth may lead to respiratory distress that requires endotracheal intubation, mechanical ventilation, and surfactant replacement. Vascular access is obtained for intravenous fluids and broad-spectrum prophylactic antibiotics. The umbilical artery and vein may be cannulated during resuscitation, even if they need to be removed before definitive surgical management. There may be marked heat loss because of evaporative losses and the increased exposed surface area of the viscera; therefore, it is important to dry the baby and maintain a warm environment.

After the ABCs of resuscitation, the exposed bowel must be protected from mechanical injury and fluid and heat losses from evaporation minimized. The easiest temporizing method is to place the exposed viscera and entire lower half the dried baby into a transparent plastic bag (bowel bag). This is fast, requires no special skills or experience, and allows for continuous evaluation of bowel perfusion. After the exposed bowel is covered, the baby is placed right-side down and the entire eviscerated mass of bowel is stabilized with support from the sides and from below, with care taken to avoid kinking the vascular pedicle. Part of a lower extremity can be brought out through a small hole in the plastic bag to provide a spot for intravenous access or heel-stick blood draw. Checking and maintaining serum glucose levels is part of any neonatal resuscitation but is especially important in babies with gastroschisis because associated prematurity and IUGR increase the risk of hypoglycemia. Gastric decompression is important to prevent distention of the gastrointestinal tract and minimize the risk of aspiration. Babies with gastroschisis may have high water losses from evaporation and third-space losses and may require twice maintenance volumes of fluids to maintain an adequate intravascular volume. A bladder catheter is useful to monitor urine output and guide the resuscitation.

### Surgical Management

Once the ABCs of resuscitation have been accomplished, the abdominal wall defect and the herniated viscera can be assessed and treated. The number one priority of surgical management is to prevent further bowel injury from ischemia and direct mechanical trauma during the initial procedure, the reduction of the intestine, and the eventual closure of fascia and skin. To achieve these goals, many different techniques have been described. Treatment and timing of treatment vary depending on the size of the defect, amount of eviscerated bowel, the size of the baby, and any associated problems.

First, the exposed viscera are inspected for intestinal atresia, intestinal necrosis, or vascular compromise, which is present in 10% to 15% of cases.[10] If there is vascular compromise because the abdominal wall opening is too small, the defect should be immediately surgically enlarged with care taken to avoid the adjacent umbilical vessels and mesentery. This can be done superiorly and slightly to the left, to avoid the umbilical vein, or directly to the right of the defect.

If an intestinal atresia is identified, the bowel is in good condition, and the abdomen can be closed without difficulty, combined primary repair of both defects can be done. However, such ideal circumstances are very uncommon. In the case of a distal atresia, another option is to form an end stoma and close the abdominal wall (see later discussion). This is only if the distal end can be identified but, often, the peel is thick enough to make this impossible. If an atresia is present or suspected and the condition of the bowel will not allow a safe anastomosis, which is often the case, the unrepaired bowel is simply reduced into the abdomen and the abdominal wall is closed. The baby is maintained with gastric decompression and parenteral nutrition for several weeks until repeat laparotomy and repair of the intestinal atresia.[22] This staging of the repair allows the inflammatory peel to resolve and the intra-abdominal pressure to stabilize before creating a vulnerable anastomosis.

A more difficult circumstance is that the bowel is necrotic or acutely injured. Similar to the case of intestinal atresia, when the bowel is in good condition, resection, anastomosis, repair, or stomas can be done and the abdominal wall closed. Another option is to close the bowel and treat the patient as if there was an atresia. Alternatively, a tube enterostomy can be placed into the dilated segment to provide decompression.

In most cases, the bowel is not acutely compromised and the first surgical decision is whether to immediately reduce the eviscerated bowel or to delay the reduction. Immediate reduction (and repair) has intuitive appeal and has some advantages compared with a delayed repair.[23] However, every comparison of primary versus delayed closure is subject to a large selection bias that makes it extremely difficult to interpret results. Overall outcomes are believed to be equivalent. If immediate reduction is performed, this can be accomplished at the bedside ("ward reduction") without anesthesia.[24] Others are concerned this method may increase the complication rate.[25]

Reduction can be delayed safely.[26] In the most popular method, at the initial resuscitation or soon thereafter, a prefabricated, a spring-loaded silo is placed in the defect to cover the exposed bowel (**Fig. 3**). These devices can be placed in the delivery room or at the bedside without anesthesia. However, as with primary reduction at the bedside without anesthesia, there is a concern that complications may be increased. The spring-loaded silo minimizes evaporative losses, prevents additional trauma, and

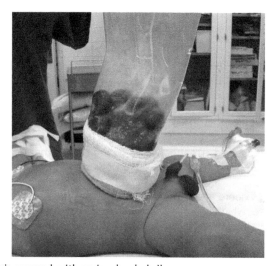

**Fig. 3.** Gastroschisis covered with spring-loaded silo.

allows for ongoing assessment of bowel perfusion. If the abdominal wall defect is too small to accommodate the device, the defect can be enlarged under local anesthesia and sedation. This procedure can be performed at the bedside or in the operating room.

The normal, spontaneous neonatal diuresis results in decreasing bowel wall edema and, with gravity alone, the bowel will begin to reduce into the abdomen. The amount of bowel in the bag will decrease in a few days. When the baby is otherwise stable and the spontaneous reduction of bowel into the abdomen has reached a plateau, the baby is taken to the operating room for an attempt at delayed primary reduction. Serial compressive reduction of the bowel with umbilical tape tied around the silo at the bedside has been advocated, but unplanned device displacement is relatively common with increasing manipulation.[27] One must balance risks and benefits of increased compression of the bowel or increased time in the silo, especially if this requires intubation, ventilation, and significant sedation.[28]

If primary reduction or delayed primary reduction is not successful, a formal silo may be sutured to the fascia and serial reduction done postoperatively. Many different methods of serial reduction have been described, but my preference is to use a specially designed wringer clamp with a guard that allows the sheets to be approximated while pushing the bowel down and away from the roller mechanism.[29] The incremental reduction steps are quick, easy, and easily reversible, and can be done multiple times during the day. The goal is to complete the reduction within a week to 10 days of placing the sutured silo. Otherwise, there is increased risk of infection and pressure creating a large "open abdomen." Once the viscera have been reduced to the level of the abdominal wall, the baby is returned to the operating room for removal of the silo and closure.[29]

After reduction of the bowel is complete the options for closing the abdominal wall are to close the skin, fascia, or both primarily, or to leave the skin, fascia, or both open and close a few days later (delayed primary closure). Other options include placement of a prosthetic patch (in the fascia, with or without skin closure) or to manage the open wound and allow secondary closure. One variation of the last strategy is to reduce the intestine primarily or in a delayed manner; then to cover the defect with the umbilical cord as a biologic dressing while the skin and umbilical ring fascia heals. This "sutureless" or "plastic" closure does result in a large number of umbilical hernias, many of which close spontaneously.[30] If the hernia does not close spontaneously, the eventual repair is more like a ventral incisional hernia repair than a typical umbilical hernia repair.

The decision of whether or not a baby can tolerate reduction and repair can be difficult and can be aided by measuring the intragastric pressure during attempted closure. A pressure of less than 20 mm Hg predicts successful closure without complications of excessive intra-abdominal pressure.[31] Other methods reported to help in the decision to reduce or close the abdomen are the splanchnic perfusion pressure (mean arterial pressure — intra-abdominal pressure)[32] and changes in central venous pressure, ventilatory pressures, and end-tidal $CO_2$.[31,33]

When there are so many proposed variations in treatment strategy (timing of reduction, timing and methods for fascial closure, and skin closure, using anesthesia or not) it is not clear that any single method or strategy is superior to any other method.[34] It is important to recognize factors that make it difficult to interpret the literature regarding gastroschisis, including (1) the small sample sizes of even multicenter studies; (2) the relatively low incidence of clearly defined end points, such as death; (3) the many factors besides operative techniques that influence end points, such as length of hospital stay, length of neonatal ICU stay, length of mechanical ventilation, and time to complete enteral feedings; (4) the lack of clinical detail in administrative data sets; (5) the inability to quantitate the degree of bowel injury prenatally or postnatally; and (6) the heterogeneous patient population that has been difficult to risk-stratify.

Even with these limitations, there are several observations that can help guide the management of individual patients. First, reduction and even some abdominal closures can be done without general anesthesia. However, the benefits of avoiding anesthesia must be balanced against the risk of damaging the bowel or compromising the procedure.[25] Second, bowel injury is possible with even with most "minimal" reductions and least invasive repairs so that, whatever technique is used, it is critical to avoid kinking the vascular pedicle and avoid traumatizing the bowel wall. Minimally invasive procedures do not necessarily equate to minimal patient risk.[28] Finally, whenever and wherever reduction is done and whatever repair is performed, it is still critical to assess intra-abdominal pressure and other markers of bowel perfusion.

The author's current recommendations are to place a spring-loaded silo during or immediately after neonatal resuscitation. Ideally, this can be done without intubation and general anesthesia. However, if the condition of the defect or the eviscerated bowel (bands or adhesions to the abdominal wall, abdominal wall defect too narrow, the mesenteric pedicle seems to kink, or the viability of the bowel is questionable), a more extensive operation with appropriate anesthesia should be done. If a formal operation is required, primary reduction may be attempted and, if successful with no significant elevation of intra-abdominal pressure, the abdominal fascia can be closed or left open using the umbilical cord as a biologic dressing.

If primary reduction is not possible then I allow for systemic stabilization, extubation, spontaneous diuresis, and auto reduction of the bowel in the silo. I avoid mechanical compression of the silo contents to prevent silo dislodgement. When the diuresis and spontaneous reduction is ceases the baby is taken to the operating room for an attempt at delayed primary reduction and closure with the same considerations noted above. If the bowel cannot be reduced, I replace the spring-loaded silo with sheeting sewn to the fascia and serially reduce the bowel as described.

### Outcomes

The outcome of patients with gastroschisis depends largely on the condition of the bowel. Survival is at least 90% to 95%, with most of the deaths in patients with massive bowel loss and intestinal necrosis.[35] The neonatal hospitalization is often prolonged, with only 40% being discharged within 1 month, 36% being in the hospital for 1 to 2 months, and 25% being hospitalized for more than 2 months.[36] Most of the neonatal hospitalization is spent waiting toleration of full enteral feedings. Even patients with relative short bowel syndrome early on often eventually achieve full enteral feedings after months to years of intestinal adaption.

A unique form of necrotizing enterocolitis, manifested by pneumatosis intestinalis on abdominal radiograph, may occur in the postoperative period after gastroschisis repair when feedings are being advanced.[37] Overall, long-term gastrointestinal function is usually good although occasional patients have inexplicable long-term intolerance of enteral feedings that seems due to severe dysmotility. In addition, there is a 5% to 10% long-term risk of adhesive obstruction in historical series.[38–40]

## OMPHALOCELE
### Definition

An omphalocele (also known as exomphalos) is a midline abdominal wall defect of variable size with the herniated viscera covered by a membrane consisting of peritoneum on the inner surface, amnion on the outer surface, and Wharton's jelly between the layers. The umbilical vessels insert into the membrane and not the intact body wall (**Fig. 4**). The defect may be centered in the upper, middle, or lower abdomen. The herniated viscera within the omphalocele include intestine, often part of the liver, and, occasionally, other organs depending on the size and location of the body wall defect.

### Embryology

In omphalocele, the intestine that is physiologically herniated into the umbilical cord in the 6th to 10th weeks does not return to the abdominal cavity. A variable amount of midgut and other intra-abdominal organs are herniated out of the defect depending on its relative size and location on the abdominal wall.[2] Predominately cranial fold deficits result in epigastric omphaloceles and, in their most severe form, may be associated with additional cranial fold abnormalities, such as anterior diaphragmatic hernia, sternal clefts, pericardial defects, and cardiac defects. When all occur together they are known as the Pentalogy of Cantrell.[41] The cause of this failure of intestinal return to the abdomen is unknown but is thought to be associated with defects in body wall folding. When the folding deficit involves the caudal fold, the omphalocele may be associated with bladder or cloacal exstrophy.[2]

### Epidemiology

Unlike gastroschisis, which seems to be increasing in incidence, the incidence of omphalocele has remained stable and ranges between 1.5 and 3 per 10,000 births. Most cases are sporadic but there are rare familial cases of omphalocele.[9]

### Associated Anomalies

In contrast to the relatively low risk of associated anomalies seen with gastroschisis, there is a very high (up to 50%–70%), incidence of associated anomalies with omphalocele. Chromosomal anomalies, notably trisomy 13, 14, 15, 18 and 21, are present in

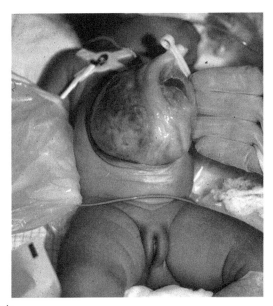

**Fig. 4.** Omphalocele.

up to 30% of cases. Cardiac defects are also common, being present in 30% to 50% of cases. Multiple anomalies are frequent and may be clustered into syndromic patterns.[42] One important pattern is the Beckwith-Wiedemann syndrome that may be present in up to 10% of cases of omphalocele. Beckwith-Wiedemann syndrome is marked by macroglossia, organomegaly, early hypoglycemia (from pancreatic hyperplasia and resulting excess insulin), and an increased risk of Wilms tumor, hepatoblastoma, and neuroblastoma later in childhood.[43] The size of the abdominal wall defect in omphalocele does not correlate with the presence of other anomalies.

### Prenatal Diagnosis

Similar to gastroschisis, the diagnosis of omphalocele is often made prenatally. Maternal serum AFP is often elevated but not to the same degree as gastroschisis.[13] This results in a lower sensitivity of maternal serum AFP elevations to detect omphalocele than for gastroschisis. As with gastroschisis, prenatal ultrasound done after the first trimester could potentially identify most cases of omphalocele and accurately distinguish omphalocele from gastroschisis. This would permit counseling of the family, appropriate obstetric follow-up, and a smooth introduction to postnatal care.

### Prenatal Management

Because of the high incidence of associated anomalies, the first step after diagnosis of fetal omphalocele is further diagnostic evaluation, including ultrasound evaluation for other structural defects, fetal echocardiography, and, possibly, chromosome determination. This information is critical in counseling families about the condition and prognosis.[44] A fetus with an omphalocele is at high risk for adverse outcomes including IUGR (5%–35%), premature delivery (5%–60%), and fetal death (usually due to severe associated anomalies).[45] There is usually no indication for early delivery although caesarian section is often done with large omphaloceles to prevent rupture or dystocia during labor.[46]

### Newborn Resuscitation and Medical Management

As in patients with gastroschisis, the initial management of newborns with omphalocele begins with the ABCs of neonatal resuscitation. Prematurity, associated pulmonary hypoplasia or the significant heart defects seen in omphalocele, may lead to early intubation and mechanical ventilation.[47] Monitoring serum glucose levels is part of any neonatal resuscitation but is especially important in babies with omphalocele because of associated prematurity, IUGR, and Beckwith-Wiedemann syndrome. Gastric decompression is initially used to prevent distention of the gastrointestinal tract within the omphalocele and prevent aspiration of gastric contents. Vascular access is obtained for intravenous fluids and broad spectrum prophylactic antibiotics. If needed, the umbilical artery and vein may be cannulated during resuscitation; however, with an omphalocele, these lines may be difficult to place because of the abnormal insertion and course of the umbilical vessels.

Once the ABCs have been accomplished, the abdominal wall defect can be assessed and treated. The omphalocele defect is inspected to ensure that the covering membrane is intact and nonadherent dressings are applied to prevent trauma to the sac. If the omphalocele sac is torn, repair can be attempted with absorbable sutures; however, this is often a short-term solution. If there is a large disruption that cannot be repaired, the patient will need to be treated as a patient with gastroschisis with temporary coverage and eventual reduction of the herniated contents and closure of the abdominal wall.

### Surgical Management

As with gastroschisis, the ultimate goal of the surgical care of a patient with an omphalocele is to reduce the herniated viscera back into the abdomen and close the fascia and skin to create a solid abdominal wall while minimizing risks to the baby. Treatment varies depending on the size and type of the defect, the size of the baby, and the associated problems. However, there is a fundamental difference compared with gastroschisis: if the covering sac is intact, there is no urgency to perform operative closure. As long as the viscera are covered with the omphalocele membrane, a complete evaluation for associated defects can be done and other problems treated before any operative intervention.

If, after diagnostic evaluation, the baby is in good condition and the defect is relatively small, an early, definitive repair can be done by excising the omphalocele membrane, reducing the herniated viscera, and closing the fascia and skin. Any omphalocele membrane adherent to the underlying liver can be left in place during the closure to avoid liver capsule injury.

Larger omphaloceles can be treated in the same manner as gastroschisis with excision of the membrane and sheeting sewn to the fascia to create a silo that can be serially reduced. However, I do not recommend removing an intact omphalocele membrane unless a primary reduction and primary fascial closure repair can be done easily. Several variations of reducing the contents of the omphalocele through an intact sac have been advocated. However, sometimes, the peritoneal attachments to the liver are in continuity with the omphalocele sac and traction on the sac can lead to disruption of the liver capsule and hemorrhage.

If primary closure is not likely to be easy, my preference is to treat the omphalocele sac with topical silver sulfadiazine (Silvadene) twice a day and allow the membrane to epithelialize and contract over the ensuing weeks to months.[48] Enteral feedings are usually tolerated during this process, even with the large hernia. Wound care can be done by the family at home and the baby followed in the outpatient clinic. When the sac is epithelialized and sturdy enough to withstand external pressure, compression is done with elastic bandages. The compression is slowly increased over time until the abdominal contents are reduced completely into the abdomen. After the omphalocele membrane has epithelialized, the omphalocele reduced completely, and the baby is well, the residual ventral hernia can be repaired electively. This can usually be accomplished within 6 to 12 months, but there is little risk in waiting even later because the remnants of the linea alba and rectus fascia become more readily identifiable and easier to bring together. The baby's rapid growth during the first year of life provides "tissue expansion" that makes primary repair possible. This strategy was initially advocated only for those patients with giant omphaloceles or serious associated problems; however, it is useful for any defect that cannot be easily closed or in any patient with significant operative risks. This strategy avoids problems of pulmonary compromise, wound breakdown, infection, and delayed enteral feedings that are encountered with a major operation in a vulnerable newborn. Many alternative strategies for omphalocele closure have been described, including skin flap mobilization and coverage, staged silo reduction and repair, reduction within the omphalocele membrane, amnion inversion, and fascial patches. Each technique may have utility in certain circumstances but topical treatment with silver sulfadiazine and delayed repair of the epithelialized ventral hernia has been safe and effective.[48,49] Systemic absorption of silver is a potential problem with silver sulfadiazine (and all silver containing wound care products).[41] However, no clinical toxicity has been reported, so this may be only a theoretical concern. Povidone-iodine has been used for topical treatment in the same way as silver sulfadiazine and, in a small series of patients, it was not associated with abnormal thyroid function tests.[50]

## Outcomes

The short-term and long-term outcomes of children with omphalocele are almost completely dependent on the type and severity of coexisting congenital anomalies and underlying medical conditions.

## SUMMARY

Gastroschisis and omphalocele are distinct congenital abdominal wall defects that require unique evaluation and management. The cause of gastroschisis is unknown, as well as why its incidence is increasing around the world. Most cases of gastroschisis are isolated problems although there is a 10% risk of associated intestinal atresia. Prenatal diagnosis is common and allows for follow-up of possible obstetric complications, counseling of the family, and planning for delivery and postnatal care. The surgical care of gastroschisis requires early coverage of the eviscerated bowel and either immediate or delayed reduction of the bowel back into the abdomen. Closure of the abdominal wall may be accomplished by immediate or delayed surgical closure, wound care and healing by secondary intention, or repair with a patch. The recovery of bowel function and initial hospital stay is usually 1 to 2 months but the long-term prognosis is excellent and mainly related to the severity of associated bowel injury.

The cause of omphalocele is also unknown but the incidence is stable. Unlike gastroschisis, most babies with omphalocele have other anomalies. The surgical correction of small defects is straightforward and, for larger defects, a strategy of topical treatment of the membrane with silver sulfadiazine and late repair after epithelialization and external reduction of the hernia contents has simplified management and optimized outcomes. The long-term prognosis of babies with omphalocele is related to the severity of coexisting congenital anomalies.

## REFERENCES

1. Suver D, Lee SL, Shekherdimian S, et al. Left-sided gastroschisis: higher incidence of extraintestinal congenital anomalies. Am J Surg 2008;195(5):663–6 [discussion: 666].
2. Sadler TW. The embryologic origin of ventral body wall defects. Semin Pediatr Surg 2010;19(3):209–14.
3. Feldkamp ML, Carey JC, Sadler TW. Development of gastroschisis: review of hypotheses, a novel hypothesis, and implications for research. Am J Med Genet A 2007;143(7):639–52.
4. Loane M, Dolk H, Bradbury I. Increasing prevalence of gastroschisis in Europe 1980–2002: a phenomenon restricted to younger mothers? Paediatr Perinat Epidemiol 2007;21(4):363–9.
5. Fillingham A, Rankin J. Prevalence, prenatal diagnosis and survival of gastroschisis. Prenat Diagn 2008;28(13):1232–7.
6. Castilla EE, Mastroiacovo P, Orioli IM. Gastroschisis: international epidemiology and public health perspectives. Am J Med Genet C Semin Med Genet 2008; 148C(3):162–79.
7. Keys C, Drewett M, Burge DM. Gastroschisis: the cost of an epidemic. J Pediatr Surg 2008;43(4):654–7.

8. Kohl M, Wiesel A, Schier F. Familial recurrence of gastroschisis: literature review and data from the population-based birth registry "Mainz Model". J Pediatr Surg 2010;45(9):1907–12.

9. Frolov P, Alali J, Klein MD. Clinical risk factors for gastroschisis and omphalocele in humans: a review of the literature. Pediatr Surg Int 2010;26(12):1135–48.

10. Owen A, Marven S, Johnson P, et al. Gastroschisis: a national cohort study to describe contemporary surgical strategies and outcomes. J Pediatr Surg 2010; 45(9):1808–16.

11. Ruano R, Picone O, Bernardes L, et al. The association of gastroschisis with other congenital anomalies: how important is it? Prenat Diagn 2011;31(4):347–50.

12. Barisic I, Clementi M, Hausler M, et al. Evaluation of prenatal ultrasound diagnosis of fetal abdominal wall defects by 19 European registries. Ultrasound Obstet Gynecol 2001;18(4):309–16.

13. Saller DN Jr, Canick JA, Palomaki GE, et al. Second-trimester maternal serum alpha-fetoprotein, unconjugated estriol, and hCG levels in pregnancies with ventral wall defects. Obstet Gynecol 1994;84(5):852–5.

14. Horton AL, Powell MS, Wolfe HM. Intrauterine growth patterns in fetal gastroschisis. Am J Perinatol 2010;27(3):211–7.

15. Sapin E, Mahieu D, Borgnon J, et al. Transabdominal amnioinfusion to avoid fetal demise and intestinal damage in fetuses with gastroschisis and severe oligohydramnios. J Pediatr Surg 2000;35(4):598–600.

16. Badillo AT, Hedrick HL, Wilson RD, et al. Prenatal ultrasonographic gastrointestinal abnormalities in fetuses with gastroschisis do not correlate with postnatal outcomes. J Pediatr Surg 2008;43(4):647–53.

17. Fitzsimmons J, Nyberg DA, Cyr DR, et al. Perinatal management of gastroschisis. Obstet Gynecol 1988;71(6 Pt 1):910–3.

18. Davis RP, Treadwell MC, Drongowski RA, et al. Risk stratification in gastroschisis: can prenatal evaluation or early postnatal factors predict outcome? Pediatr Surg Int 2009;25(4):319–25.

19. Engle WA. Morbidity and mortality in late preterm and early term newborns: a continuum. Clin Perinatol 2011;38(3):493–516.

20. Mozurkewich E, Chilimigras J, Koepke E, et al. Indications for induction of labour: a best-evidence review. BJOG 2009;116(5):626–36.

21. Brantberg A, Blaas HG, Salvesen KA, et al. Surveillance and outcome of fetuses with gastroschisis. Ultrasound Obstet Gynecol 2004;23(1):4–13.

22. Kronfli R, Bradnock TJ, Sabharwal A. Intestinal atresia in association with gastroschisis: a 26-year review. Pediatr Surg Int 2010;26(9):891–4.

23. Alali JS, Tander B, Malleis J, et al. Factors affecting the outcome in patients with gastroschisis: how important is immediate repair? Eur J Pediatr Surg 2011;21(2): 99–102.

24. Leadbeater K, Kumar R, Feltrin R. Ward reduction of gastroschisis: risk stratification helps optimise the outcome. Pediatr Surg Int 2010;26(10):1001–5.

25. Rao SC, Pirie S, Minutillo C, et al. Ward reduction of gastroschisis in a single stage without general anaesthesia may increase the risk of short-term morbidities: results of a retrospective audit. J Paediatr Child Health 2009;45(6):384–8.

26. Pastor AC, Phillips JD, Fenton SJ, et al. Routine use of a SILASTIC spring-loaded silo for infants with gastroschisis: a multicenter randomized controlled trial. J Pediatr Surg 2008;43(10):1807–12.

27. Aldrink JH, Caniano DA, Nwomeh BC. Variability in gastroschisis management: a survey of North American Pediatric Surgery Training Programs. J Surg Res 2011. [Epub ahead of print].

28. Lobo JD, Kim AC, Davis RP, et al. No free ride? The hidden costs of delayed operative management using a spring-loaded silo for gastroschisis. J Pediatr Surg 2010;45(7):1426–32.

29. Sawin R, Glick P, Schaller R, et al. Gastroschisis wringer clamp: a safe, simplified method for delayed primary closure. J Pediatr Surg 1992;27(10):1346–8.

30. Orion KC, Krein M, Liao J, et al. Outcomes of plastic closure in gastroschisis. Surgery 2011;150(2):177–85.

31. Yaster M, Scherer TL, Stone MM, et al. Prediction of successful primary closure of congenital abdominal wall defects using intraoperative measurements. J Pediatr Surg 1989;24(12):1217–20.

32. McGuigan RM, Mullenix PS, Vegunta R, et al. Splanchnic perfusion pressure: a better predictor of safe primary closure than intraabdominal pressure in neonatal gastroschisis. J Pediatr Surg 2006;41(5):901–4.

33. Puffinbarger NK, Taylor DV, Tuggle DW, et al. End-tidal carbon dioxide for monitoring primary closure of gastroschisis. J Pediatr Surg 1996;31(2):280–2.

34. Weinsheimer RL, Yanchar NL, Bouchard SB, et al. Gastroschisis closure—does method really matter? J Pediatr Surg 2008;43(5):874–8.

35. Molik KA, Gingalewski CA, West KW, et al. Gastroschisis: a plea for risk categorization. J Pediatr Surg 2001;36(1):51–5.

36. Lao OB, Larison C, Garrison MM, et al. Outcomes in neonates with gastroschisis in U.S. children's hospitals. Am J Perinatol 2010;27(1):97–101.

37. Oldham KT, Coran AG, Drongowski RA, et al. The development of necrotizing enterocolitis following repair of gastroschisis: a surprisingly high incidence. J Pediatr Surg 1988;23(10):945–9.

38. van Eijck FC, Wijnen RM, van Goor H. The incidence and morbidity of adhesions after treatment of neonates with gastroschisis and omphalocele: a 30-year review. J Pediatr Surg 2008;43(3):479–83.

39. South AP, Wessel JJ, Sberna A, et al. Hospital readmission among infants with gastroschisis. J Perinatol 2011;31(8):546–50.

40. Davies BW, Stringer MD. The survivors of gastroschisis. Arch Dis Child 1997; 77(2):158–60.

41. Cantrell JR, Haller JA, Ravitch MM. A syndrome of congenital defects involving the abdominal wall, sternum, diaphragm, pericardium, and heart. Surg Gynecol Obstet 1958;107(5):602–14.

42. Stoll C, Alembik Y, Dott B, et al. Omphalocele and gastroschisis and associated malformations. Am J Med Genet A 2008;146A(10):1280–5.

43. Cohen MM Jr. Beckwith-Wiedemann syndrome: historical, clinicopathological, and etiopathogenetic perspectives. Pediatr Dev Pathol 2005;8(3):287–304.

44. Porter A, Benson CB, Hawley P, et al. Outcome of fetuses with a prenatal ultrasound diagnosis of isolated omphalocele. Prenat Diagn 2009;29(7): 668–73.

45. Fratelli N, Papageorghiou AT, Bhide A, et al. Outcome of antenatally diagnosed abdominal wall defects. Ultrasound Obstet Gynecol 2007;30(3):266–70.

46. How HY, Harris BJ, Pietrantoni M, et al. Is vaginal delivery preferable to elective cesarean delivery in fetuses with a known ventral wall defect? Am J Obstet Gynecol 2000;182(6):1527–34.

47. Hershenson MB, Brouillette RT, Klemka L, et al. Respiratory insufficiency in newborns with abdominal wall defects. J Pediatr Surg 1985;20(4):348–53.

48. Lee SL, Beyer TD, Kim SS, et al. Initial nonoperative management and delayed closure for treatment of giant omphaloceles. J Pediatr Surg 2006;41(11): 1846–9.

49. Lewis N, Kolimarala V, Lander A. Conservative management of exomphalos major with silver dressings: are they safe? J Pediatr Surg 2010;45(12):2438–9.
50. Whitehouse JS, Gourlay DM, Masonbrink AR, et al. Conservative management of giant omphalocele with topical povidone-iodine and its effect on thyroid function. J Pediatr Surg 2010;45(6):1192–7.

# Pediatric Intestinal Failure and Vascular Access

Biren P. Modi, MD*, Tom Jaksic, MD, PhD

## KEYWORDS

- Intestinal failure • Short bowel syndrome • Intestinal rehabilitation • Pediatric
- Vascular access • Central venous catheter

## KEY POINTS

- Intestinal failure is a relatively new term that has superseded the traditional term, "short bowel syndrome."
- The multidisciplinary care of patients with intestinal failure includes focused medical care, with particular attention to nutritional, pharmacologic, gastrointestinal and surgical interventions.
- With advances in the multidisciplinary care of these complex patients, survival continues to improve.

Intestinal failure (IF) is a relatively new term that has superseded the traditional term, "short bowel syndrome" (SBS). A clinically measurable definition of IF is dependence on parenteral nutrition (PN) for longer than 90 days. Functionally, the umbrella of IF encompasses all states wherein the absorptive capacity of the intestine is inadequate to meet nutrition, hydration, electrolyte, and (in pediatrics) growth requirements of the patient.

These states are most commonly divided into three categories: traditional SBS, resulting from the loss of sufficient intestinal length to create IF; malabsorptive states such as microvillus inclusion disease; and motility disorders, such as intestinal pseudo-obstruction. In many cases, patients may fall into more than one category. For example, the child with gastroschisis and midgut volvulus loses a significant portion of their intestine and becomes "short." Intestinal rehabilitation in this patient, however, is often complicated by the dysmotility inherent in patients with gastroschisis.

Overwhelmingly, most patients with IF and the ones most often requiring surgical care are patients with true SBS who simply have insufficient intestinal mass to allow

The authors have no disclosures.
Department of Surgery and Center for Advanced Intestinal Failure (CAIR), Children's Hospital Boston and Harvard Medical School, Fegan 3, 300 Longwood Avenue, Boston, MA 02115, USA
* Corresponding author.
*E-mail address:* biren.modi@childrens.harvard.edu

for adequate nutrient absorption. Thus, in most instances and in the literature, the two terms are used relatively interchangeably.

## CAUSE

In the pediatric population, most IF is the result of intestinal resection secondary to acquired and congenital neonatal anomalies (**Table 1**).[1-6] The development of IF after resection is a multifactorial outcome and no single measurement is able to absolutely predict the ability to wean from PN and become enterally independent. The only consistent predictor in multiple pediatric outcomes analyses for the development of IF is the residual bowel length following resection.[7] As is evident in **Fig. 1**, the inaccuracy of bowel length measurement leads to a significant variance in the amount of bowel length required to wean from PN. Nonetheless, the residual bowel length is a useful predictor for the ability to achieve enteral independence, with 35 cm acting as an inflection point above which this overarching goal seems to be tenable in most neonates. Additional data have shown that the amount of residual bowel length not only predicts the ability to achieve enteral independence but also the duration of the requirement for PN.[7]

The presence of the ileocecal valve has been championed as an important variable, with potentially less bowel length necessary for achieving enteral independence if the ileocecal valve is present.[8] The overall body of data is conflicted concerning this point. As more is learned about the process of intestinal adaptation and the relative importance of the ileum in this process, it is likely that the ileocecal valve acts as a marker for presence of the terminal ileum, rather than having any functional importance in and of itself.[9]

### Epidemiology and Natural History

Population studies have demonstrated an incidence of SBS in Canada of approximately 24.5 per 100,000 live births. Premature neonates (born at <37 weeks gestation) made up most of these patients, with an incidence of 353.7 per 100,000 live births compared with only 3.5 per 100,000 live births in term infants. In this population study, mortality was significantly higher in patients with SBS (37.5%) compared with a matched control cohort (13.3%).[10]

The significantly higher incidence of SBS in premature neonates underscores both the prenatal physiology that can predispose to prematurity (eg, intrauterine volvulus, polyhydramnios) and the high percentage of SBS patients with necrotizing enterocolitis (NEC) as their underlying diagnosis (see **Table 1**). At Children's Hospital Boston, NEC comprises approximately 30% of our neonatal IF patients, with intestinal atresia (22%), gastroschisis (19%), and volvulus (17%) adding to those patients. The remaining patients have a variety of other diagnoses, including pseudo-obstruction and very-long-segment (ie, well into the small intestine) Hirschsprung disease.[4] As seen in **Table 1**, it is notable that single-institution series will differ in their relative preponderance of NEC based on the complexity of care offered by their neonatal unit. This is because the incidence of NEC is directly correlated with birth weight, with a 12% incidence in neonates born at 500–750 g, and a steady decrease in incidence with increasing birth weight.[11,12]

The intestine's reaction to the state of SBS is a process termed adaptation. Through adaptation, the intestine remodels in an attempt to increase its mucosal surface area and, therefore, its absorptive capacity to maximize intestinal function. Though the exact mechanisms for this process are not elucidated, the result is typically dilation of the shortened bowel. Longitudinal growth of the intestine is typically only achieved

**Table 1**
Distribution (by percentage) of underlying diagnoses in IF patients reported by multiple referral centers

| | Modi, 2008[4] | Diamond, 2007[2] | Cowles, 2010[1] | Javid, 2010[3] | Nucci, 2008[5] | Torres, 2007[6] |
|---|---|---|---|---|---|---|
| Total (N) | 54 | 54 | 93 | 49 | 389 | 51 |
| Necrotizing enterocolitis | 30% | 35% | 49% | 27% | 19% | 29% |
| Atresia | 22% | 19% | 13% | 18% | 12% | 12% |
| Gastroschisis | 19% | 22% | 16% | 31% | 20% | 35% |
| Volvulus | 17% | 6% | 4% | 10% | 15% | 12% |
| Pseudo-obstruction | 4% | NR | 12% | 6% | 9% | 4% |
| Other | 8% | 18% | 6% | 8% | 25% | 8% |

*Abbreviations:* N, number of patients in the study; NR, not reported.
*Data from* Refs. [1-6]

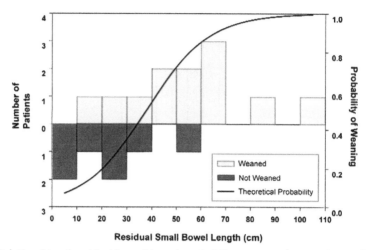

**Fig. 1.** Relationship of residual bowel length and ability to wean from PN in a cohort of IF patients. The solid line demonstrates the theoretical possibility of completely weaning from PN based on residual bowel length. (*Reproduced from* Andorsky DJ, Lund DP, Lillehei CW, et al. Nutritional and other postoperative management of neonates with SBS correlates with clinical outcomes. J Pediatr 2001;139(1):27–3; with permission.)

in proportion to somatic growth of the patient and is not enhanced by the short bowel state. Although over a period of months to years this process can result in an increase in mucosal surface area for nutrient absorption and can help a borderline patient, in patients with profound SBS it can also result in detrimental consequences, including dysmotility and small bowel bacterial overgrowth (see later discussion).

Outcomes in patients with SBS have improved dramatically in the last half-century owing to multiple major advances in care. The demonstration of complete intravenous nutritional supplementation in a canine model followed by the application of this novel therapy in adult and pediatric patients by Wilmore, Dudrick, and Rhoads in the 1960s turned a nearly uniformly fatal disease into a survivable one.[13] Unfortunately, with the advent of PN came the subsequent complications of PN: central venous catheter (CVC)-associated sepsis, and PN-associated liver disease, now referred to as IF-associated liver disease (IFALD). As a result, long-term survival in short bowel patients reached a plateau of approximately 75% for the next several decades.[2,7,14,15]

Recent concentration on this disease entity has led to the demonstration of significantly higher survival rates—close to 90% to 95%—due to the rise of centralized multidisciplinary centers for the care of IF patients, improvements in transplantation, and therapies directed at the major killers of these patients: sepsis and liver failure (see later discussion). Further improvements in these areas of clinical care will hopefully translate into further improvement in patient outcomes.

### Medical Management of IF

The multidisciplinary care of patients with IF includes focused medical care, with particular attention to nutritional, pharmacologic, gastrointestinal and surgical interventions. The goal of this care is enhancement of nutrition to allow for homeostasis as well as appropriate growth, optimization of pharmacologic therapy to assist in nutrition and to minimize symptoms and complications, and judicious surgical intervention. This intervention includes maintenance of central venous and enteral access when needed, definitive therapy for anatomic or postsurgical pathology, and, potentially, augmentation of native intestinal capacity via intestinal lengthening and tapering or, ultimately, transplantation.

## Parenteral Nutrition

As mentioned, adequate homeostasis and growth are the goal of nutrition therapy in IF. The mainstay of this therapy in the initial phases of management is PN. Since its advent in the late 1960s, PN has allowed for a previously fatal disease to become survivable.[13] The provision of calories, macronutrients, micronutrients, vitamins, and electrolytes via this route has become a specialized field that is best performed for IF patients by experienced dietitians, pharmacists, and physicians. Specific needs are met for each patient, as their PN is tailored around them.

Some considerations specific to IF patients include the propensity for low serum bicarbonate, due to losses in the stool or stoma output, and low serum sodium, due to losses and inadequate absorption. Close monitoring of these parameters allows for the use of acetate in solution to improve the acidosis secondary to bicarbonate loss and adequate provision of sodium to allow for normal levels necessary for adequate growth.[16] The measurement of urinary sodium and quantification of losses via measurement of stool electrolytes can assist in this management.

## Intestinal Failure Associated Liver Disease

Of particular interest in IF patients is the development of IFALD, which is a complicated pathology and seems to be linked to prematurity, sepsis, and PN—particularly the provision of lipids. IFALD is characterized by biochemical abnormalities, notably elevations in serum transaminases (especially alanine aminotransferase) and direct hyperbilirubinemia. Although cholestasis is the most commonly used surrogate for identification of IFALD, the presence and degree of liver damage is not completely reflected in this single test.[17]

Ongoing liver injury then results in elevations in the prothrombin time and international normalized ratio with eventual thrombocytopenia in the setting of portal hypertension and splenomegaly. Routine biochemical evaluation and constant vigilance for signs of hepatic dysfunction, jaundice, or portal hypertension are thus mandatory in the PN-dependent child. Appropriate therapy (see later discussion) may allow for reversal of IFALD, with resolution of cholestasis, and, later, normalization of alanine aminotransferase. If cirrhosis has not yet occurred, histopathological changes in the liver are typically reversible. A new, noninvasive method of determining liver function using the stable isotope $^{13}$C-methionine breath test has been reported and can be used to differentiate cirrhotic and noncirrhotic infants with IFALD.[18,19]

Although prematurity cannot be changed, the other causes of IFALD can be clinically addressed. The mainstay of lipid administration in the United States has been a soy-based lipid emulsion, which is rich in ω-6 fatty acids. Recent work has demonstrated that these ω-6 fatty acids are proinflammatory and may play a major role in the development of IFALD.[20] Current nutritional therapy is directed at limiting exposure to these proinflammatory fatty acids, via limitation of lipid administration to 1 g/kg/d or lower. This method has been demonstrated to be effective in at least delaying the onset of IFALD.[21] Though this tactic may limit hepatic toxicity, the loss of calories must be accounted for by increasing the portion of calories administered as glucose.

Another significant development in this field has been the demonstration that parenteral fish-oil supplements, which are rich in ω-3 fatty acids, have an antiinflammatory effect on the liver and may be useful in the treatment or prevention of IFALD.[22,23] The current and most widely used formulation (Omegaven, Fresenius Kabi, Bad Homberg,

Germany) is provided at 1 g/kg/d and is currently available only through compassionate-use protocols because it does not yet have US Food and Drug Administration (FDA) approval. Ongoing studies, including a randomized controlled trial currently being initiated, will determine the true utility of this formulation and potentially allow for FDA approval and standardization of its use.

### Catheter Associated Blood Stream Infections

Another common complication in IF patients with indwelling CVC access is catheter-associated blood stream infection (CABSI). Although the catheter is the pipeline for life-preserving therapy in the form of PN, it is also a nidus for significant infection, sepsis, and, potentially, death. No matter what the type and location of a CVC, appropriate care and preventative measures must be followed to minimize the risks of CABSI (see later discussion). Intensive care units have played particular attention to this issue, and data from adult and pediatric intensive care units, including neonatal intensive care units, have demonstrated continued improvements in rates of CABSI in these patient populations. In recent analyses, rates of CABSI average around 3 per 1000 catheter-days. Focused prevention protocols drop this rate to less than 1 per 1000 catheter-days. Specific populations at higher risk for CABSI include premature and low–birth weight infants in the neonatal ICU setting (approximately 4 per 1000 catheter-days) and IF patients (approximately 10 per 1000 catheter-days).[24,25] The special circumstances of IF patients that put them at higher risk include the use of high-dextrose PN, duration of need leading to a willingness to tolerate treatment of CABSI through the catheter rather than removal of the catheter, and abnormal intestinal mucosa leading to a higher incidence of bacterial translocation and seeding of the catheter. Specifically, the "shorter" a patient's intestine, the higher their apparent risk for CABSI. This is evident in the correlation between low serum citrulline levels and CABSI. Citrulline, which is a nonprotein amino acid component of the urea cycle, has circulating levels that directly correlate to the amount of functional intestinal mucosal mass because the intestinal mucosa is the source of nearly all serum citrulline.[26] Low serum citrulline levels have been demonstrated to correlate with an increased incidence of CABSI.[27]

Any child with IF and an indwelling CVC is at significant risk for CABSI and, accordingly, any fever, lethargy, or ileus in an IF patient must be presumed to be due to a CABSI until proven otherwise. The mainstay for this diagnosis is a blood culture drawn through the central line. Our practice has been to treat empirically with broad-spectrum intravenous antibiotics through the CVC until the blood culture is negative for 48 hours or an infection is demonstrated and the antibiotics can be tailored to the pathogen's sensitivities. If a child fails to clear their positive blood cultures over 3 serial days while on appropriate therapy or if they demonstrate any amount of systemic instability in the form of persistent fever, hypotension, or thrombocytopenia, we recommend CVC removal and a line holiday while the blood infection clears. Once peripheral blood cultures are clear for 72 hours, the patient can have a CVC replaced for ongoing administration of PN. In the special case of culture-proven fungemia, we recommend immediate line removal and evaluation for seeding of fungus using echocardiogram of the valves, ophthalmologic retinal examination, and abdominal ultrasound of the solid organs.

Multiple studies have looked at methods of reducing the risk of CABSI. These methods include protocols centered on checklists for the placement of CVCs and the changing of dressings.[28,29] Additional methods evaluated include the use of chlorhexidine-based cleansing solutions and chlorhexidine-impregnated dressings, the use of antimicrobial-impregnated CVCs, and the use of antibiotic locks.[30] Perhaps the most promising method, one that we have adopted in our IF population, is the use of 70% ethanol locks. This intervention is associated with a decrease in the rate of CABSI in IF patients from 9.9 per 1000 catheter-days to 2.1 per 1000 catheter-days with no demonstrated adverse effects. No known microbial pathogen has demonstrated resistance to ethanol, and ethanol has the ability to penetrate the biofilm that builds on CVCs, making it an excellent antimicrobial prophylactic agent.[25]

### Enteral Nutrition and Therapy

The therapy that is most efficacious at eradicating the risks and severity of IFALD and CABSI is the provision of enteral nutrition. Enteral nutrition improves the health of the intestinal mucosa, has been shown to diminish and eventually reverse IFALD, and can eventually obviate the indwelling CVC.[31] Postoperatively, once intestinal function has returned, attempts to feed the short bowel patient are mandatory, regardless of intestinal length. Any amount of enteral feeding can have dramatic effects on the patient's complication risk profile. We generally start with continuous feeding via either an indwelling nasogastric tube or a surgically-placed gastrostomy. Continuous feeding allows for a relatively uniform saturation of intestinal mucosal receptors and maximizes the function of the residual intestinal mucosal surface area. Although it is important to transition to enteral nutrition, high stool or stoma output can limit tolerance of enteral nutrition due to fluid and electrolyte disturbances or local skin irritation. Our general practice is to limit advancement of enteral nutrition once stool or stoma output reaches 2 mL/kg/h. Practices to limit stool output, such as continuous feedings, refeeding of stoma output into a mucus fistula, or pharmacologic therapy (see later discussion), can be used to maximize enteral tolerance in the face of high stool output.

If severe reflux is present, postpyloric feeds may be instituted. Although no consensus exists for the appropriate formulation of enteral feeding, both breast milk and elemental (amino-acid based) formulas have been shown to decrease duration of PN dependence in neonates with IF.[7]

An additional factor is the proper administration of micronutrients and vitamins that might be malabsorbed in patients without a terminal ileum. These include the fat-soluble vitamins (A, D, E, K) and vitamin $B_{12}$, as well as zinc. Because these are administered parenterally in patients on PN, patients may not become deficient in these factors for several months after the achievement of full enteral independence. The specifics of monitoring for these factors are detailed elsewhere, but it is paramount that any child with altered small bowel anatomy or function must have their vitamin and micronutrient levels watched carefully to avoid the dangerous and preventable side effects of their deficiency. In those patients with demonstrated deficiency, commercially-available enteral supplements are used to achieve normal levels. For vitamin $B_{12}$, only intramuscular or intranasal methods of supplementation are available.

### Small Bowel Bacterial Overgrowth

Small bowel bacterial overgrowth is an underappreciated entity in patients with IF and can occur in more than 50% of this patient population.[32] As the bowel dilates during adaptation and as this dilation leads to disordered motility, bacteria within the intestinal lumen have an ideal environment for overgrowth. Bacterial overgrowth leads to inflammation, which leads to mucosal injury, potentiates translocation, and produces gastrointestinal bleeding. In addition, the bacteria themselves can increase bile-acid deconjugation, leading to further malabsorption, and produce toxic by-products, such as D-lactic acid, leading to a specific syndrome of ataxia, mental status changes, and acidosis.[32,33]

Patients with new feeding difficulty, worsening of their disorganized motility, or development of more abdominal distention, pain, and possible gastrointestinal bleeding are potentially suffering from bacterial overgrowth. Typical treatment is empiric, with administration of an enteral antibiotic course for one week. Broad-spectrum antibiotics, effective against anaerobes and gram-negative bacteria, are used. Mainstays used in our patient population include metronidazole, ciprofloxacin, and the intravenous form of gentamicin administered enterally (typically has minimal systemic absorption). Use of probiotic medications to treat small bowel bacterial overgrowth has been reported. However, IF patients with indwelling CVCs have had devastating complications of CABSI traced back to the probiotic microbe being administered.[34] As a result, we advocate against the use of probiotics in this patient population.

Endoscopy can be used to help guide therapy, with quantitative duodenal aspirate cultures demonstrating the major bacteria species culpable for the patient's symptoms and allowing for tailored therapy. Endoscopy can also help in demonstrating other pathologic conditions, such as allergic enteritis or colitis, marginal ulceration or stricturing at surgical anastomoses, or more generalized intestinal inflammation that may benefit from antiinflammatory therapy.[35]

Surgical interventions in the form of tapering operations have been used for the treatment of small bowel bacterial overgrowth and its complications with some success. They serve, in general, as additional therapeutic options in patients who fail more conventional medical diagnostic and therapeutic maneuvers.[36]

### Pharmacotherapy

The use of specific pharmaceutical interventions to treat side effects of the short bowel state is an important adjunct to routine medical and surgical care. Patients with short bowel are known to have a hypergastrin state.[37] Although it is unclear if this translates into increased acid production, acid blockade in the form of proton-pump inhibitors is relatively innocuous and is strongly advocated, at least in the acute postoperative period.

Additionally, pharmaceutical agents that alter intestinal motility can be selectively used in appropriate clinical situations to modify intestinal motility and maximize intestinal function and absorption capacity. In the absence of mechanical or intestinal causes, patients with short bowel and high stool output that limits their enteral intake can benefit from the use of loperamide to decrease intestinal motility and maximize nutrient absorption.

Many patients with IF, outside of the true pseudo-obstruction patients, develop poor intestinal motility that limits their tolerance of enteral feeding due to vomiting, abdominal distention, or high gastric residuals. Promotility agents in this patient population, especially patients with gastroschisis who have a predilection to poor motility, can prove useful. In the past, agents such as cisapride and metoclopramide have been used with some success in this patient population. Unfortunately, metoclopramide now carries an FDA "black box" warning due to the risk of tardive dyskinesia secondary to prolonged use. Cisapride, due to cardiac arrhythmias, has been removed from the market, but can still be used on a per patient basis under a strictly monitored protocol through an application to the manufacturer. Cisapride's ability to promote both gastric and small intestinal motility makes it a particularly useful adjunct in the treatment of selected individuals despite its risk profile.[38,39] Additionally, erythromycin and azithromycin have been shown to invoke phase III of the migrating motor complex through their action on the motilin receptor, and have been used to improve antroduodenal motility in patients with gastroparesis despite a propensity toward tachyphylaxis.[40]

The use of hormonal modulation to maximize intestinal adaptation seems to be on the horizon as well. Specifically, glucagon-like peptide 2 (GLP-2) has been shown in animal models to increase bowel adaption. Its long-acting biodegradation-resistant analog, teduglutide, is currently being studied in prospective trials with the hope of demonstrating increased adaptation and improved intestinal function in IF patients.[41]

## SURGICAL THERAPY OF IF

Surgical therapy is an ongoing treatment option for patients with IF. From decision-making at the initial diagnosis, to maintenance of indwelling devices, to therapeutic interventions for the short bowel state, the role of surgery in the care of these patients remains paramount.

### Initial Management

The *sine qua non* of the initial surgical management of patients with potential IF is bowel conservation. The situational awareness of the surgeon to identify patients at risk for long-term intestinal dysfunction is required to have a defined surgical approach that ensures adequate life-saving therapy while conserving each centimeter of intestinal length possible. Although definitive surgical intervention with resection of frankly necrotic intestine is necessary, careful observation of marginal intestine can often mean the difference between eventual enteral independence and lifelong PN dependence. In the case of acute intestinal loss, such as midgut volvulus, this often centers on limited resection and multiple operative reevaluations ("second looks") to determine the true extent of intestinal injury. Temporary abdominal closures using silo devices can allow for ongoing observation of intestinal viability, aid in the decision-making to time re-exploration, and prevent the risk of abdominal compartment syndrome due to abdominal catastrophe.

The use of stomas and mucus fistulae can help in the eventual titration of enteral nutrition. Early stoma closure, however, has been shown to hasten the ability to wean from PN, and this known benefit must be balanced against other factors, such as lung disease in premature infants, other medical comorbidities, and the development of liver injury.[7]

### Vascular Access

Typically, at the time of diagnosis or shortly thereafter, patients with IF will require central venous access for both the administration of intravenous medications and the provision of PN. In considering the long-term care of IF patients, forethought in the management of vascular access in this population will allow for long-term access and prevent the development of access difficulties that can limit the ability to provide PN and lead to the need for intestinal or multi-organ transplant.

The placement of a CVC in these patients can occur in the operating room, the interventional radiology suite, or at the bedside. The type of catheter can include traditional cuffed CVCs, such as Broviac or Hickman lines, or noncuffed lines placed peripherally (peripherally-inserted central catheters [PICCs]) or used during cutdown procedures on central vessels.

Our practice, in the very small neonates, has been to use traditional surgical placement using cutdown approaches into branch vessels, such as the external jugular vein or the greater saphenous vein. This approach has the benefit of a traditional tunneled line without the risk of surgical injury to the major vessels. In no circumstance do we, or would we advocate, for the surgical ligation of a major vessel. In somewhat larger patients, we repeatedly use percutaneous approaches to minimize the risk of vessel injury. Finally, in patients that do develop significant thrombosis or occlusion of all of their central vessels, innovative methods of obtaining central venous access have been described, including transhepatic catheters, translumbar or percutaneous mammary catheters, and gonadal vein catheters.[42] Interventional radiology assistance is often quite helpful in these complex patients.

The loss of central venous access is a well-accepted indication for intestinal transplantation, and comprises up to 50% of referrals for intestinal transplantation.[42,43] A look at our own experience of 44 severe SBS patients demonstrates the use of 176 CVCs for a total of 13,781 catheter-days. At the very beginning of the study period (patients from 1999), two major vessels were ligated. None has been ligated since 1999. An additional two patients went on to have clinically significant thrombosis of a major vessel for an overall thrombosis rate of 1 per 6390 catheter-days. In addition, more than 25% of these catheters were PICCs while over 40% were placed percutaneously. Though 10 patients went on to transplantation evaluation, none required such evaluation due to loss of central venous access. This analysis demonstrates that the repeated use of percutaneously and peripherally placed CVCs is feasible in this patient population and minimizes the risk of vessel thrombosis or loss of central venous access.[44] Using these general guidelines, loss of central venous access should be an extremely rare indication for intestinal transplantation.

### Enteral Access

As outlined above, the use of gastric feedings to advance enteral nutrition in IF patients can allow for improved enteral tolerance and hasten weaning from PN. Most patients with IF require surgical gastrostomy tubes (percutaneous endoscopic gastrostomy, open gastrostomy, laparoscopic gastrostomy) for long-term enteral access. In addition, some patients may benefit from gastrojejunal tubes to allow for drainage of a poorly motile stomach while providing enteral nutrition via jejunal feeds. Appropriate care and appropriate surgical placement and/or revision of these tubes minimize the morbidities often associated with enteral feeding access while optimizing intestinal function.

### Lengthening and Tapering Operations

As noted above in the descriptions of intestinal adaptation, small bowel bacterial overgrowth, and CABSI, intestinal dilation in response to the short bowel state can be harmful. Surgical techniques for the tapering of dilated intestine, while concomitantly achieving intestinal lengthening, have been developed in response to this effect. Bianchi, in 1980, first described the longitudinal intestinal lengthening and tapering technique, which takes advantage of the two-leafed anatomy of the intestinal mesentery to longitudinally divide the intestine to essentially double its length and half its diameter.[45] Although a major breakthrough in the surgical treatment of short bowel, this technique was limited in its requirement for uniform bowel dilation and its technical difficulty. Additional techniques, including those espoused by Kimura and colleagues,[46–49] have been introduced but have suffered from similarly significant technical difficulty.

A novel technique introduced in 2003 overcame some of these obstacles in its simplicity. The serial transverse enteroplasty (STEP) procedure involves the sequential application of a linear stapling device from alternating sides of the dilated intestine, allowing for titration of the bowel diameter and both lengthening and tapering (**Fig. 2**). In this method, a uniform bowel diameter is created without the requirement of a uniform bowel diameter preoperatively, the bowel is placed at minimal ischemia risk (as opposed to the Bianchi and Kimura techniques), and the procedure can be

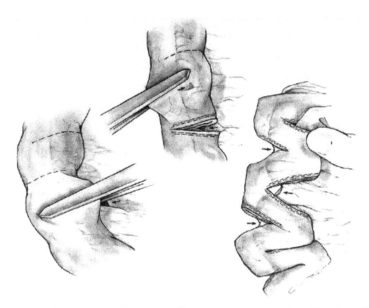

**Fig. 2.** STEP procedure. The small arrows indicate the alternating direction of application of the intestinal stapler. The intestine is oriented with the antimesenteric border facing the viewer and the mesentery going into the page, such that stapler applications are placed at 90° and 270° using the mesentery as the 0° reference point. (*Reproduced from* Kim HB, Fauza D, Garza J, et al. Serial transverse enteroplasty (STEP): a novel bowel lengthening procedure. J Pediatr Surg 2003;38(3):425–9; with permission.)

performed primarily, secondarily after a Bianchi, or repeated after a prior STEP (possibly multiple times).[50–52] It is fair to say that the STEP procedure has supplanted older techniques as the procedure of choice for autologous intestinal reconstruction in IF patients.

Large animal studies have demonstrated the efficacy of the STEP procedure in improving nutrient absorption, improving growth, and increasing plasma citrulline levels to demonstrate increased intestinal mucosal surface area.[53] Rodent models of the STEP procedure have also demonstrated an increase in GLP-2 post-STEP, suggesting that the procedure can further the effects of native intestinal adaptation.[54] Additionally, international registry data have proven this technique to be easily reproducible and demonstrated translation of the animal data into real patient populations.[55]

Furthermore, reports in the literature have demonstrated uses for the STEP procedure other than simple lengthening and tapering in patients with SBS. As hypothesized in the initial description of the procedure, the STEP procedure has been used with success as a primary option in neonates with marginal intestinal length and prenatal intestinal dilation secondary to atresia.[50,56,57] Other reports demonstrate the utility of the STEP procedure in the eradication of small bowel bacterial overgrowth, including overgrowth complicated by D-lactic acidosis.[36,53]

Our practice in the use of intestinal reconstruction surgery has been to maximize medical therapy and rehabilitation first. If the patient's ability to advance on enteral nutrition stagnates, then contrast studies are used to determine the presence of anatomic abnormalities that may be limiting enteral feeding and to assess the degree of bowel dilation. If there are no mechanical causes of the patient's plateau in enteral tolerance (eg, stricture), and the bowel is sufficiently dilated to suggest that adaptation has been maximized and dysmotility may be a factor, we consider the use of the STEP procedure for autologous intestinal reconstruction, to both lengthen and taper the dilated, short bowel. Using this algorithm, we have been able to demonstrate excellent short-term and long-term improvements in nutritional parameters and enteral tolerance in our IF patients.[58,59]

### Transplantation

The ultimate surgical intervention for the treatment of IF, and its complication IFALD, is transplantation. Although intestinal transplantation is certainly feasible and is performed routinely, it is not typically an option for neonates and young children. For patients in this young age group who develop IFALD, however, combined liver-intestine or complete multivisceral transplantation are options. These procedures are life-saving in the terminal cases of IFALD and have demonstrated improved overall survival in the last two decades, with 10 year patient and graft survival rates of 42% and 39%, respectively.[60] Nonetheless, as our ability to treat and potentially prevent IFALD has improved, these procedures continue to be an option of last resort. This is particularly true in light of the continued difficulty posttransplantation with complications such as life-threatening infections, chronic rejection, and posttransplant lymphoproliferative disorder. In older children without significant liver injury, isolated intestinal transplant remains an option, though it is still hampered by issues of rejection, limiting graft survival in the long-term, and actual decrease in long-term patient survival, though perhaps with an improved quality of life. In our program, the isolated intestinal transplant is reserved for older patients with the maturity to understand the complexity of their situation and the capacity to make an informed decision.

The decision for transplantation is a difficult one, and requires multidisciplinary discussions regarding likelihood of intestinal rehabilitation, determination of degree of liver injury and potential for reversal of IFALD, and individual patient risk factors in relation to transplantation. Early referral to centers specializing in intestinal rehabilitation has been shown to improve survival. This concept can be carried forward to early referral to centers with both intestinal rehabilitation expertise and transplantation capability, in order for informed decisions to be made for the management of these complex patients.

### SUMMARY

Emerging developments in the care of IF patients have drastically improved their overall prognosis in the last several decades, with recently reported survival rates over 90%. IF patients remain an extremely complex population who benefit from specialized, multidisciplinary care. Advances in the provision of parenteral and enteral nutrition, progress in the management of IFALD with parenteral fish oil and CABSI with ethanol lock therapy, and the availability of novel surgical interventions, such as the STEP procedure, have made this a dynamic health care field with the promise of ongoing improvements in outcomes for patients with IF.

### REFERENCES

1. Cowles RA, Ventura KA, Martinez M, et al. Reversal of intestinal failure-associated liver disease in infants and children on parenteral nutrition: experience with 93 patients at a referral center for intestinal rehabilitation. J Pediatr Surg 2010; 45(1):84–7 [discussion: 87–8].
2. Diamond IR, de Silva N, Pencharz PB, et al. Neonatal short bowel syndrome outcomes after the establishment of the first Canadian multidisciplinary intestinal

rehabilitation program: preliminary experience. J Pediatr Surg 2007;42(5): 806–11.

3. Javid PJ, Malone FR, Reyes J, et al. The experience of a regional pediatric intestinal failure program: Successful outcomes from intestinal rehabilitation. Am J Surg 2010;199(5):676–9.

4. Modi BP, Langer M, Ching YA, et al. Improved survival in a multidisciplinary short bowel syndrome program. J Pediatr Surg 2008;43(1):20–4.

5. Nucci A, Burns RC, Armah T, et al. Interdisciplinary management of pediatric intestinal failure: a 10-year review of rehabilitation and transplantation. J Gastrointest Surg 2008;12(3):429–35 [discussion: 435–6].

6. Torres C, Sudan D, Vanderhoof J, et al. Role of an intestinal rehabilitation program in the treatment of advanced intestinal failure. J Pediatr Gastroenterol Nutr 2007; 45(2):204–12.

7. Andorsky DJ, Lund DP, Lillehei CW, et al. Nutritional and other postoperative management of neonates with short bowel syndrome correlates with clinical outcomes. J Pediatr 2001;139(1):27–33.

8. Wilmore DW. Factors correlating with a successful outcome following extensive intestinal resection in newborn infants. J Pediatr 1972;80(1):88–95.

9. Gutierrez IM, Kang KH, Jaksic T. Neonatal short bowel syndrome. Semin Fetal Neonatal Med 2011;16(3):157–63.

10. Wales PW, de Silva N, Kim J, et al. Neonatal short bowel syndrome: population-based estimates of incidence and mortality rates. J Pediatr Surg 2004;39(5): 690–5.

11. Duro D, Kalish LA, Johnston P, et al. Risk factors for intestinal failure in infants with necrotizing enterocolitis: a Glaser Pediatric Research Network study. J Pediatr 2010;157(2):203–8, e201.

12. Fitzgibbons SC, Ching Y, Yu D, et al. Mortality of necrotizing enterocolitis expressed by birth weight categories. J Pediatr Surg 2009;44(6):1072–5 [discussion: 1075–6].

13. Wilmore DW, Dudrick SJ. Growth and development of an infant receiving all nutrients exclusively by vein. JAMA 1968;203(10):860–4.

14. Quiros-Tejeira RE, Ament ME, Reyen L, et al. Long-term parenteral nutritional support and intestinal adaptation in children with short bowel syndrome: a 25-year experience. J Pediatr 2004;145(2):157–63.

15. Spencer AU, Neaga A, West B, et al. Pediatric short bowel syndrome: redefining predictors of success. Ann Surg 2005;242(3):403–9 [discussion: 409–2].

16. Schwarz KB, Ternberg JL, Bell MJ, et al. Sodium needs of infants and children with ileostomy. J Pediatr 1983;102(4):509–13.

17. Fitzgibbons SC, Jones BA, Hull MA, et al. Relationship between biopsy-proven parenteralnutrition-associated liver fibrosis and biochemical cholestasis in children with short bowel syndrome. J Pediatr Surg 2010;45(1):95–9 [discussion: 99].

18. Duro D, Fitzgibbons S, Valim C, et al. [13C]Methionine breath test to assess intestinal failure-associated liver disease. Pediatr Res 2010;68(4):349–54.

19. Duro D, Duggan C, Valim C, et al. Novel intravenous (13)C-methionine breath test as a measure of liver function in children with short bowel syndrome. J Pediatr Surg 2009;44(1):236–40 [discussion: 240].

20. Lee S, Gura KM, Kim S, et al. Current clinical applications of omega-6 and omega-3 fatty acids. Nutr Clin Pract 2006;21(4):323–41.

21. Shin JI, Namgung R, Park MS, et al. Could lipid infusion be a risk for parenteral nutrition-associated cholestasis in low birth weight neonates? Eur J Pediatr 2008; 167(2):197–202.

22. Gura KM, Lee S, Valim C, et al. Safety and efficacy of a fish-oil-based fat emulsion in the treatment of parenteral nutrition-associated liver disease. Pediatrics 2008; 121(3):e678–86.

23. Puder M, Valim C, Meisel JA, et al. Parenteral fish oil improves outcomes in patients with parenteral nutrition-associated liver injury. Ann Surg 2009;250(3): 395–402.

24. Edwards JR, Peterson KD, Andrus ML, et al. National Healthcare Safety Network (NHSN) Report, data summary for 2006 through 2007, issued November 2008. Am J Infect Control 2008;36(9):609–26.

25. Jones BA, Hull MA, Richardson DS, et al. Efficacy of ethanol locks in reducing central venous catheter infections in pediatric patients with intestinal failure. J Pediatr Surg 2010;45(6):1287–93.

26. Windmueller HG, Spaeth AE. Source and fate of circulating citrulline. Am J Physiol 1981;241(6):E473–80.

27. Hull MA, Jones BA, Zurakowski D, et al. Low serum citrulline concentration correlates with catheter-related bloodstream infections in children with intestinal failure. JPEN J Parenter Enteral Nutr 2011;35(2):181–7.

28. Lee OK, Johnston L. A systematic review for effective management of central venous catheters and catheter sites in acute care paediatric patients. Worldviews Evid Based Nurs 2005;2(1):4–13 [discussion: 14–5].

29. Wheeler DS, Giaccone MJ, Hutchinson N, et al. A hospital-wide quality-improvement collaborative to reduce catheter-associated bloodstream infections. Pediatrics 2011;128(4):e995–1004 [quiz: e1004–7].

30. Huang EY, Chen C, Abdullah F, et al. Strategies for the prevention of central venous catheter infections: an American Pediatric Surgical Association Outcomes and Clinical Trials Committee systematic review. J Pediatr Surg 2011; 46(10):2000–11.

31. Javid PJ, Collier S, Richardson D, et al. The role of enteral nutrition in the reversal of parenteral nutrition-associated liver dysfunction in infants. J Pediatr Surg 2005; 40(6):1015–8.

32. Kaufman SS, Loseke CA, Lupo JV, et al. Influence of bacterial overgrowth and intestinal inflammation on duration of parenteral nutrition in children with short bowel syndrome. J Pediatr 1997;131(3):356–61.

33. Perlmutter DH, Boyle JT, Campos JM, et al. D-Lactic acidosis in children: an unusual metabolic complication of small bowel resection. J Pediatr 1983; 102(2):234–8.

34. Land MH, Rouster-Stevens K, Woods CR, et al. Lactobacillus sepsis associated with probiotic therapy. Pediatrics 2005;115(1):178–81.

35. Ching YA, Modi BP, Jaksic T, et al. High diagnostic yield of gastrointestinal endoscopy in children with intestinal failure. J Pediatr Surg 2008;43(5):906–10.

36. Modi BP, Langer M, Duggan C, et al. Serial transverse enteroplasty for management of refractory D-lactic acidosis in short-bowel syndrome. J Pediatr Gastroenterol Nutr 2006;43(3):395–7.

37. Williams NS, Evans P, King RF. Gastric acid secretion and gastrin production in the short bowel syndrome. Gut 1985;26(9):914–9.

38. Hyman PE, Di Lorenzo C, McAdams L, et al. Predicting the clinical response to cisapride in children with chronic intestinal pseudo-obstruction. Am J Gastroenterol 1993;88(6):832–6.

39. Raphael BP, Nurko S, Jiang H, et al. Cisapride improves enteral tolerance in pediatric short-bowel syndrome with dysmotility. J Pediatr Gastroenterol Nutr 2011; 52(5):590–4.

40. Di Lorenzo C, Lucanto C, Flores AF, et al. Effect of sequential erythromycin and octreotide on antroduodenal manometry. J Pediatr Gastroenterol Nutr 1999; 29(3):293–6.

41. Jeppesen PB, Gilroy R, Pertkiewicz M, et al. Randomised placebo-controlled trial of teduglutide in reducing parenteral nutrition and/or intravenous fluid requirements in patients with short bowel syndrome. Gut 2011;60(7):902–14.

42. Rodrigues AF, van Mourik ID, Sharif K, et al. Management of end-stage central venous access in children referred for possible small bowel transplantation. J Pediatr Gastroenterol Nutr 2006;42(4):427–33.

43. Kaufman SS, Atkinson JB, Bianchi A, et al. Indications for pediatric intestinal transplantation: a position paper of the American Society of Transplantation. Pediatr Transplant 2001;5(2):80–7.

44. Modi BP, Langer M, Ching YA, et al. Forty-four consecutive severe short bowel patients without loss of central venous access. Queenstown (New Zealand): Pacific Association of Pediatric Surgeons; 2007.

45. Bianchi A. Intestinal loop lengthening—a technique for increasing small intestinal length. J Pediatr Surg 1980;15(2):145–51.

46. Ienaga T, Kimura K, Hashimoto K, et al. Isolated bowel segment (Iowa model 1): technique and histological studies. J Pediatr Surg 1990;25(8):902–4.

47. Kimura K, Soper RT. Isolated bowel segment (model 1): creation by myoenteropexy. J Pediatr Surg 1990;25(5):512–3.

48. Yamazato M, Kimura K, Yoshino H, et al. The isolated bowel segment (Iowa model II) created in functioning bowel. J Pediatr Surg 1991;26(7):780–3.

49. Yoshino H, Kimura K, Yamazato M, et al. The isolated bowel segment (Iowa Model II): absorption studies for glucose and leucine. J Pediatr Surg 1991;26(12):1372–5.

50. Kim HB, Fauza D, Garza J, et al. Serial transverse enteroplasty (STEP): a novel bowel lengthening procedure. J Pediatr Surg 2003;38(3):425–9.

51. Kim HB, Lee PW, Garza J, et al. Serial transverse enteroplasty for short bowel syndrome: a case report. J Pediatr Surg 2003;38(6):881–5.

52. Piper H, Modi BP, Kim HB, et al. The second STEP: the feasibility of repeat serial transverse enteroplasty. J Pediatr Surg 2006;41(12):1951–6.

53. Chang RW, Javid PJ, Oh JT, et al. Serial transverse enteroplasty enhances intestinal function in a model of short bowel syndrome. Ann Surg 2006;243(2):223–8.

54. Kaji T, Tanaka H, Wallace LE, et al. Nutritional effects of the serial transverse enteroplasty procedure in experimental short bowel syndrome. J Pediatr Surg 2009; 44(8):1552–9.

55. Modi BP, Javid PJ, Jaksic T, et al. First report of the international serial transverse enteroplasty data registry: indications, efficacy, and complications. J Am Coll Surg 2007;204(3):365–71.

56. Cowles RA, Lobritto SJ, Stylianos S, et al. Serial transverse enteroplasty in a newborn patient. J Pediatr Gastroenterol Nutr 2007;45(2):257–60.

57. Wales PW, Dutta S. Serial transverse enteroplasty as primary therapy for neonates with proximal jejunal atresia. J Pediatr Surg 2005;40(3):E31–4.

58. Ching YA, Fitzgibbons S, Valim C, et al. Long-term nutritional and clinical outcomes after serial transverse enteroplasty at a single institution. J Pediatr Surg 2009;44(5):939–43.

59. Javid PJ, Kim HB, Duggan CP, et al. Serial transverse enteroplasty is associated with successful short-term outcomes in infants with short bowel syndrome. J Pediatr Surg 2005;40(6):1019–23 [discussion: 1023–4].

60. Mazariegos GV, Steffick DE, Horslen S, et al. Intestine transplantation in the United States, 1999-2008. Am J Transplant 2010;10(4 Pt 2):1020–34.

# Pediatric Malignancies
## Neuroblastoma, Wilm's Tumor, Hepatoblastoma, Rhabdomyosarcoma, and Sacroccygeal Teratoma

Katherine P. Davenport, MD[a], Felix C. Blanco, MD[a],
Anthony D. Sandler, MD[b],*

## KEYWORDS

- Pediatric malignancies • Wilm's tumor • Neuroblastoma • Hepatoblastoma
- Sacrococcygeal teratoma • Rhabdomyosarcoma

## KEY POINTS

- The aggressive behavior of high-risk neuroblastoma results in incomplete response to multimodality treatment.
- Multimodality therapies have led to improved prognosis and excellent cure rates for patients with Wilms tumor.
- Prognosis of hepatoblastoma is improved with combination of surgery and neoadjuvant therapy.
- The survival rate of children with rhabdomyosarcoma is improved with combination therapy.
- Sacrococcygeal teratoma is associated with significant perinatal concerns. Following complete en bloc excision, the overall prognosis is good.

## NEUROBLASTOMA

Neuroblastoma is the most common extracranial solid tumor in children. Despite the excellent prognosis of neuroblastoma when diagnosed early, the aggressive behavior of advanced-stage neuroblastoma results in a very poor prognosis, despite the use of multimodal therapy.

### Incidence

The incidence of neuroblastoma varies in different regions of the world, with a greater prevalence in developed countries of 1 in 7000 children.[1] The most common age at

The authors have nothing to disclose.
[a] Sheikh Zayed Institute for Pediatric Surgical Innovation, Children's National Medical Center, 111 Michigan Avenue NW, Washington, DC 20010, USA; [b] Department of Surgery, Sheikh Zayed Institute for Pediatric Surgical Innovation, Children's National Medical Center, 111 Michigan Avenue NW, Washington, DC 20010, USA
* Corresponding author.
*E-mail address:* ASandler@cnmc.org

presentation is 18 months and equally affects males and females. Neuroblastoma is more prevalent in children younger than 4 years (85%), declining to 8% at 9 years and 1.5% after 15 years of age.[2]

## Etiology

Through embryologic development, neuroblastic cells migrate from the neural crest to peripheral organs in the neck, chest, and abdomen. During this process, physiologic forces drive neuroblasts to differentiate into adult neuronal tissue that forms the sympathetic chain and adrenal medulla. Neuroblastoma is neuronal tissue derived from the neural crest that remains or becomes (de-)undifferentiated after reaching its peripheral location, adopting the appearance of small, round blue cells with neuritic processes.[3] Evidence of this embryologic development is seen in vestigial remnants of neuroblastoma tissue occasionally observed in the adrenal gland and sympathetic chains of otherwise normal newborns.[4]

No theory clearly explains the origin of neuroblastoma. Abnormalities in the rearrangement of chromosome 1p and 11q are reported.[5] Similarly, neuroblastoma was linked to neurofibromatosis and Hirschsprung disease that could explain its association with defects of neural crest development.[6]

## Distribution

Primary neuroblastoma tumors mainly originate in the following body compartments: craniofacial and neck in 1% to 3% of patients; mediastinum in 16% of patients; and retroperitoneum, with adrenal (48%) and extraadrenal (25%) locations.

## Classification and Staging of Neuroblastoma

The classification of neuroblastoma was for a long time based solely on the extension of the primary tumor, according to the International Neuroblastoma Staging System (INSS). Although useful and widely accepted, the INSS was unable to clearly assess the patient's risk status or to stage the patient in the preoperative setting, because the system was mainly based on operative findings. Furthermore, clinical trials using the INSS could not uniformly compare or assess the status of extraregional nodal disease.[7,8]

Briefly, the INSS includes[9]

- Stage 1: localized, unilateral tumor with negative lymph nodes, completely excised
- Stage 2A: localized, unilateral tumor with negative lymph nodes, incompletely excised
- Stage 2B: localized, unilateral tumor with ipsilateral positive lymph nodes, completely or incompletely excised
- Stage 3: unresectable, unilateral tumor infiltrating across the midline, with or without regional node involvement
- Stage 4: tumor with metastasis to distant lymph nodes, bone marrow, liver, skin, and other organs
- Stage 4S: localized tumor with metastasis to skin, liver, and bone marrow without involvement of cortical bone in infants younger than 1 year (<10% of cells are malignant).

To overcome some of the limitations of the INSS, the International Neuroblastoma Risk Group designed a staging system (INRGSS) to provide information about tumor resectability based on diagnostic imaging using CT scan or MRI.[7] The INRGSS includes image-defined risk factors (IDRFs) to characterize the extension of the tumor into adjacent structures, including major vascular structures and vital structures in the neck, chest, abdomen, and pelvis. Histologic confirmation of neuroblastoma through tissue biopsy and urinary or serum catecholamines or metabolites are an essential part of the system.[10] In addition, all children older than 6 months undergo bone marrow biopsy. When metastatic disease is found, it is evaluated using MIBG (metaiodoben-zylguanidine) scan, or [99]technetium scintigraphy if MIBG is equivocal.

The INRGSS not only allows the preoperative staging of neuroblastoma but also permits reassessment during its treatment.[10] The INRGSS includes localized tumor in one body compartment without involvement of vital structures according to IDFRs (L1); locoregional tumor with one or more IDFRs (L2); distant metastatic disease, including distant lymph nodes (M); and metastatic disease limited to skin, liver, and/or bone marrow in children younger than 18 months (MS).[7]

When encountered, malignant pleural effusion or ascites is only considered meta-static if distant from the primary tumor.

### Children's Oncology Group Risk Group Assignment

The Children's Oncology Group (COG) risk group assignment is widely accepted in the United States. It allows neuroblastoma to be classified into low-, intermediate-, and high-risk disease based on five characteristics: age, INSS stage, MYCN amplification, tumor cell ploidy (DNA index), and histopathology (Shimada classification: favorable and unfavorable based on presence of Schwannian components and mitosis). COG classification is discussed in this section.

#### Low-risk neuroblastoma

- INSS stage 1, any age, any pathologic stage or any DNA ploidy
- INSS stages 1 or 2, <365 days old, non amplified MYCN, any pathologic stage or any DNA ploidy
- INSS stage 1 or 2, >365 days old, non amplified MYCN, favorable pathology
- INSS stage 4S, <365 days, non amplified MYCN and favorable pathology and DNA ploidy.

#### Intermediate-risk neuroblastoma

- INSS stage 3, younger than 365 days, nonamplified MYCN and any pathology or DNA ploidy
- INSS stage 3, older than 365 days, nonamplified MYCN and favorable pathology
- INSS stage 4, older than 548 days, nonamplified MYCN, and any pathology or DNA ploidy
- INSS stage 4S, younger than 365 days, nonamplified MYCN, any pathology or DNA ploidy.

#### High-risk neuroblastoma

- INSS 2A/2B, older than 365 days, amplified MYCN unfavorable pathology
- INSS 3, younger than 365 days, amplified MYCN, any pathology or DNA ploidy
- INSS 3, older than 365 days, nonamplified MYCN, unfavorable pathology
- INSS 3, older than 365 days, amplified MYCN, any pathology
- INSS 4, younger than 365 days, amplified MYCN, any pathology or DNA ploidy
- INSS 4, older than 548 days, any MYCN, any pathology
- INSS 4S, younger than 365 days, amplified MYCN, any pathology or DNA ploidy.

MYCN genomic amplification and DNA ploidy are biologic markers that identify tumors with aggressive behavior and poor prognosis. MYCN promotes rapid tumor growth and is usually found in patients with advanced disease.

## Clinical Presentation

Most children diagnosed with neuroblastoma present with an incidentally discovered palpable abdominal mass. Often, the mass will compress the renal vessels, activate the renin-angiotensin axis, and cause hypertension. Rarely, hypertension is from the direct effect of catecholamine-secreting tumors.

When neuroblastoma tumors have paraspinal location with intraforaminal invasion, children may develop peripheral neurologic deficits, including paralysis and urinary or fecal incontinence.[11] Horner syndrome and superior vena cava syndrome are described in patients with high mediastinal lesions. These tumors, when extending into the neck, could cause airway compression.

Proptosis and periorbital ecchymosis (raccoon eyes) are manifestations of retroorbital or periorbital bone tumor infiltration.

Opsoclonus-myoclonus syndrome is manifested as ataxia and random eye movements, or "dancing eyes," and is considered an immune phenomenon with cross-reactivity of neuroblastoma antibodies with cerebellar or brain stem neuronal tissue.

Metastatic disease is manifested by hepatomegaly, subcutaneous nodules (blueberry muffin baby), and bone pain, which is caused by bone marrow infiltration.

Children younger than 365 days have a better prognosis with neuroblastoma; therefore age has prognostic and therapeutic implications. Most patients with advanced disease were diagnosed at an age older than 30 months.[12]

Neonatal neuroblastoma is found in a special subpopulation of children at birth. The incidence of neonatal neuroblastoma is as high as 10% in some series, and prenatal ultrasound can identify most cases at as early as 31 weeks' gestation.[13]

## Diagnosis

Elevation in serum lactate dehydrogenase and ferritin are markers of poor prognosis but have been replaced by biologic markers. Urine or serum catecholamines or metabolites are part of the initial diagnostic evaluation of patients with a retroperitoneal mass. Vanillylmandelic acid and homovanillic acid are two catecholamine metabolites frequently detected in the urine of children with neuroblastoma.

A CT scan is the preferred diagnostic test for neuroblastoma in children. Intratumoral hemorrhage and necrosis frequently give the heterogeneous radiologic appearance to neuroblastoma. Typically, coarse calcifications are present in 90% of cases (**Fig. 1**).[14] CT scan also provides information regarding local invasion and metastatic liver disease.

MRI provides excellent anatomic detail of the primary tumor, local invasion, and metastasis. It is helpful in assessing paraspinal tumors with intraspinal canal involvement. Unfortunately, MRI requires sedation in children.

[123]I-MIBG and [131]I-MIBG scans have a great affinity for neuroblastoma, with uptake in 90% of cases. It concentrates in primary and metastatic tumors in bone marrow and cortical bone, and is generally used to assess response to treatment.[15]

### Core needle biopsy

Core needle biopsy is performed in patients who have unresectable disease or those who are candidates for induction chemotherapy. Tumor biopsy could be omitted in patients with potentially resectable lesions based solely on clinical and typical radiologic features. Core needle biopsy provides enough tissue for histologic characterization and immunohistochemical and gene amplification studies, and has 88%

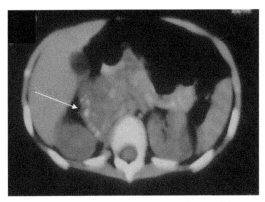

**Fig. 1.** Coarse calcifications are seen on CT evaluation of neuroblastoma (*arrow*).

accuracy, but often does not provide adequate tissue for research studies in which tissue processing is needed.[16]

### Bone marrow biopsy
Bone marrow biopsy is performed as part of the initial workup of a newly diagnosed neuroblastoma to exclude tumor invasion. The bone marrow specimen is usually obtained from iliac crest aspirates.

### Treatment
The guidelines provided by COG for risk stratification of neuroblastoma help outline treatment strategies for disease states.

### Low-risk neuroblastoma
In children with low-risk neuroblastoma, surgery alone is sufficient, with an expectation of excellent survival rates. The decision to operate without tissue diagnosis with the intent of upfront resection is based on the resectability of the tumor established by the risk factor analysis and radiologic features (ie, absent major vascular encasement). Grossly involved lymph nodes, usually adherent to the tumor, should be removed en block. Noninvolved regional nodes are usually sampled for staging purposes.

According to COG recommendations, chemotherapy is not needed when gross residual disease or positive regional lymph nodes are present after low-risk tumors with favorable histology are resected. Chemotherapy is reserved only for low-risk patients who are symptomatic from local invasion (cord compression) or with evidence of recurrent disease.

### Intermediate-risk neuroblastoma
Surgery and chemotherapy with cyclophosphamide, doxorubicin, cisplatin, and etoposide are the mainstay of treatment of patients with intermediate-risk neuroblastoma. Biopsy confirmation of the tumor is essential and is the first step to guide the management of locoregional disease. Induction chemotherapy is followed by local control of residual disease with surgery and radiation therapy. Surgery is performed even if the response to chemotherapy is not optimal, and should be aimed at obtaining clear margins without compromise to neurologic or organ function.

### High-risk neuroblastoma

High-risk neuroblastoma requires multimodal treatment starting with induction chemotherapy to control metastatic disease, and is followed by surgery and radiotherapy for local control. Irrespective of the response to chemotherapy, aggressive debulking of gross residual tumor and metastatic lesions is generally performed.

Topotecan, an inhibitor of topoisomerase I, is a new chemotherapeutic drug used alone or in combination with cyclophosphamide for induction chemotherapy in advanced or relapsed neuroblastoma.[17] The main side effect observed with topotecan is myelosuppression.

Myeloablative chemotherapy with etoposide, carboplatin, and melphalan followed by total body irradiation and autologous bone marrow transplantation has shown improved survival rates in high-risk neuroblastoma.[18]

Isotretinoin (13-*cis*-retinoic acid) is a maintenance biologic agent used mainly for minimal residual disease after surgical excision in patients with metastatic neuroblastoma. It has been shown to offer increased survival when added to usual maintenance regimens.[19]

### Neonatal Neuroblastoma

The routine use of ultrasound during pregnancy has allowed the identification of prenatal neoplasms, including neuroblastoma. After birth, adrenal masses detected by antenatal ultrasound should only be watched and monitored by ultrasound or MRI and urinary catecholamines. Their treatment should be individualized and therapy instituted when evidence of tumor growth is present on follow-up imaging or when these masses are large and symptomatic.

The survival of patients with neonatal neuroblastoma reaches almost 100%.

### 4S Neuroblastoma

4S is a special subset of neuroblastoma with limited metastatic disease in young children. Nonamplified MYCN 4S neuroblastoma tumors usually regress without treatment. Confirmation and risk assessment is performed through biopsy of the skin or liver lesions.

### Laparoscopic Resection of Neuroblastoma

Laparoscopic resection of adrenal neuroblastoma is an appropriate technique when feasible (large size and vascular invasion are relative contraindications).[20] The usual advantages of minimally invasive surgery, such as decreased need for analgesics, faster return of bowel function, and shorter hospital stay, apply to children with neuroblastoma. Laparoscopic biopsy of neuroblastoma is an attractive alternative for advanced tumors.

### Prognosis

The survival of patients with low and intermediate risk is excellent and approaches almost 90%. It drops off significantly to around 40% in patients with high-risk neuroblastoma. Survival decreases as the age of the child increases, with survival approaching 64% in children from 0 to 4 years of age and to only 30% in those aged 5 to 9 years.

## WILMS TUMOR

Wilms tumor is the most common pediatric renal tumor and constitutes 6% to 10% of all childhood cancer cases. Wilms tumor typically presents between the ages of 1 and

5 years and shows no gender predilection. Ninety-five percent of Wilms tumor cases are unilateral, and approximately 10% are associated with congenital syndromes, including WAGR (Wilms tumor, aniridia, genitourinary and mental retardation) syndrome, Beckwith-Wiedemann syndrome, Denys-Drash syndrome, and hemihypertrophy.[21] Routine radiographic screening of children with these predisposition syndromes for development of Wilms tumor is recommended until 5 years of age.[22]

## Presentation

Wilms tumor often presents as a palpable abdominal mass found incidentally or on routine physical examination. Although often asymptomatic, Wilms tumor may be associated with abdominal pain, hypertension, hematuria, loss of appetite, weight loss, or fever. Physical examination may reveal a nontender, large, firm abdominal mass, and a left-sided varicocele indicates compression of the renal vein by the tumor.[21,23]

## Diagnosis

The initial evaluation of a patient with an abdominal mass and suspected Wilms tumor includes radiographic examination. Abdominal ultrasound can confirm the site of origin, illustrate the nature of the mass (cystic vs solid), and show presence of intravascular tumor extension. CT and MRI allow for better characterization of the mass, evaluation of the contralateral kidney, and detection of vascular extension and metastases (most common locations are lymph nodes, lung, and liver) (**Fig. 2**). A chest radiograph is obtained for staging purposes and evaluates for pulmonary metastases.[21]

Pathologic variants of Wilms tumor impact prognosis through biologically different levels of aggressiveness, pattern of spread, recurrence, and response to therapy. Pathologic evaluation involves identification of anaplasia that distinguishes the classification of favorable or unfavorable histology. Most cases are of favorable type and respond to therapy with a favorable prognosis. The unfavorable type is present in approximately 10% of cases and includes the anaplastic, clear cell, and rhabdoid variants.

Surgical stage is determined by extent of surgical resection, preoperative or operative tumor rupture, and bilaterality (**Table 1**). Accurate staging of Wilms tumor is accomplished with preoperative imaging, histology, and surgical exploration. Staging correlates with prognosis and guides therapy.

**A**          **B**

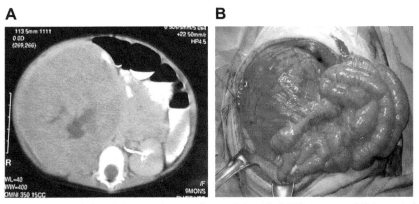

**Fig. 2.** A CT scan of the abdomen shows a large right-sided Wilms tumor (A) in an infant who subsequently underwent biopsy. (B) The tumor was not primarily resected secondary to size and adherence to surrounding structures.

| Table 1 Wilms tumor staging | |
|---|---|
| I | Unilateral tumor, without capsule extension or lymph node involvement<br>The tumor is completely removed without tumor spill |
| II | Unilateral tumor, with capsule extension or adherent to adjacent structures<br>No lymph node involvement<br>The tumor is completely removed without tumor spill |
| III | Unilateral tumor with lymph node involvement, preoperative tumor rupture,<br>  intraoperative tumor spill, incomplete resection, or tumor biopsy only |
| IV | Metastasis to lung, liver, bone, brain, or distant lymph node involvement |
| V | Bilateral tumors |

### Treatment

The treatment of patients in North America is based on surgical staging and radiographic evaluation for spread of disease. If Wilms tumor is unilateral and without extensive vascular involvement, resection of the tumor and involved kidney is the initial treatment recommendation. If the tumor is too large for resection the patient should undergo surgical biopsy, or if the tumor involves both kidneys then chemotherapy should be initiated to shrink the tumor, followed by nephron-sparing resection 6 to 9 weeks later.

### National Wilms tumor study group versus international society of pediatric oncology

The National Wilms Tumor Study Group (NWTS) and International Society of Paediatric Oncology (SIOP) groups use similar staging systems to guide treatment recommendations. The general treatment plan by NWTS is initial resection and biopsy if resection is not feasible, whereas the treatment scheme under SIOP recommends preoperative chemotherapy (optional biopsy) followed by resection. The driving force behind the SIOP preoperative chemotherapy recommendation was a high rate of operative rupture. Criticism for the SIOP method relates to uncertainty of diagnosis before chemotherapy initiation without a biopsy, whereas an argument against the NWTS method is that upfront surgery may be more difficult, leading to a higher rate of surgical complications and tumor recurrence. Outcomes are similar with either strategy, so the only relevant criticism of either may be against any protocol that overtreats the disease and could otherwise avoid unnecessary therapy.

### Operative treatment

The goals of operative therapy include confirmation of the diagnosis, assessment of other abdominal organs for evidence of metastatic spread, and complete resection of the tumor, kidney, ureter, and adjacent lymph nodes. Tumor nephrectomy is approached through a transverse or midline abdominal incision large enough to allow for removal of the specimen without rupture and dissection of associated lymph nodes. Intraoperative tumor rupture increases the risk of tumor recurrence and upstages the patient's status, necessitating postoperative radiation therapy.

At exploration, the tumor should only be biopsied if the tumor appears too large for complete resection, if tumor thrombus within the vena cava or right atrium is extensive, or if adjacent organs are involved that would prevent safe complete resection. The patient should then receive chemotherapy in an attempt to reduce the tumor volume in preparation for resection at a second operation.

### Adjuvant therapy

The goal of neoadjuvant therapy is to preserve renal parenchyma and thus function. Preoperative chemotherapy may provide tumor shrinkage to allow for a complete resection with less morbidity at eventual resection. Indications for preoperative chemotherapy include Wilms tumor in a solitary kidney, bilateral Wilms tumor, tumor in a horseshoe kidney, intravascular extension above the hepatic vena cava, and respiratory distress from extensive metastases.

Secondary to concern about the late effects of radiation therapy, the role of radiation therapy for Wilms tumor has evolved and is currently recommended only for stages III and IV Wilms tumor. Tumor spillage at surgery should be avoided to prevent upstaging of a tumor to stage III and mandating radiation therapy for the patient.

### Bilateral Wilms tumor

The goals of management in bilateral Wilms tumor are complete tumor excision and preservation of adequate kidney tissue to prevent renal failure. Patients should receive chemotherapy up front in attempt to shrink the tumors and preserve renal parenchyma at eventual resection. After chemotherapy, patients are reassessed with CT to evaluate response to treatment and determine operative feasibility. If amenable, the patient should undergo nephron-sparing resection. If tumor persists in both kidneys after chemotherapy, the patient may receive additional chemotherapy. If still not amenable to resection after additional treatment, bilateral nephrectomy with obligate dialysis and additional chemotherapy for 1 year, followed by renal transplant, is recommended.

### Intravascular involvement

Intravascular extension within the renal vein, inferior vena cava, or right atrium occurs in 4% of patients with Wilms tumor.[22] The goal of treatment is to remove both the kidney and the tumor within the vein if possible. Tumor thrombus often shrinks after a course of chemotherapy, allowing for safer, more complete resection; however, the thrombus is also prone to scarring and forming an adhesive communication to the vein. If the thrombus extends into the right atrium, cardiopulmonary bypass is needed.

### Recurrence

Patients with stage I or II Wilms tumor who experience recurrence may be treated with a more intense chemotherapeutic regimen. The treatment of recurrence in patients with later stage WT or adverse prognostic indicators with highdose chemotherapy and autologous stem cell transplant has been suggested; however the efficacy remains unknown.

### Long-Term Prognosis/Follow-up

Prognosis and long-term survival vary, but most children with Wilms tumor can be cured. Significant improvement in prognosis is secondary to improved multimodal therapies that offer less-aggressive strategies with lower morbidity and excellent cure rates. Current multimodal therapy yields a greater than 90% overall survival rate.[21] Early detection and aggressive therapy yields the best prognosis, and key elements for cure are accurate staging and complete resection.

Presence of intravascular extension does not affect the overall prognosis if it is resected. Additionally, the level of tumor within the vein does not affect survival. Key indicators of survival in these patients are tumor stage and type. The overall survival for patients with intravenous tumor involvement is 88%, 89%, and 62% for stages II, III, IV, respectively.

Recurrence of Wilms tumor is associated with significant mortality. Recurrence in favorable Wilms tumor subtypes has an overall survival of 50%, whereas recurrence of unfavorable types is associated with much lower survival rates.

Continuous follow-up care is necessary to monitor for recurrence, second malignancies, and side effects of adjuvant therapy. As treatment modalities improve, the overall incidence of chronic renal failure is declining. This improvement is credited to better therapies and delayed resection to preserve renal tissue. The risk of end-stage renal disease (ESRD) in unilateral Wilms tumor is low (0.2%–0.6%), whereas the risk of ESRD in bilateral Wilms is 5.4% to 12% at 20-year follow-up.[21]

The introduction of multimodal treatment has led to an exponential increase in the 5-year survival rate to greater than 90%. However, this successful treatment has also led to the development of late adverse effects, such as secondary malignancies and cardiac dysfunction. Awareness of the late consequences of cancer treatment is important, and early recognition may improve outcomes.[24] After treatment, patients are followed with imaging, examination, and laboratory evaluation for 5 years.

## HEPATOBLASTOMA

Primary liver tumors are rare, comprising less than 2% of all pediatric malignancies. Hepatoblastoma is the most common malignant liver tumor of early childhood, with an incidence of 1/1,000,000 cases per year in children younger than 15 years old (50–70 new cases per year in the United States).[25] It has a slight male predominance (1.7:1.0 male-to-female ratio) until 5 years of age, then gender differences disappear. Most cases of hepatoblastoma occur in children younger than 2 years, with a median age at diagnosis of 18 months.[26] Most arise in the right lobe of the liver and tend to be unifocal, and the most common site of metastases is the lung.[26]

Hepatoblastoma is associated with extreme prematurity, very-low-birth-weight (<1000 g), hemihypertrophy, and several genetic associations, including Beckwith-Wiedemann syndrome, Gardner syndrome, and familial adenomatous polyposis (FAP).[25,26] Childhood hepatoblastoma frequently involves associated mutations in the β-catenin gene, whose function is closely related to the development of FAP.

### Presentation

The presentation of hepatoblastoma can be varied and is related to size and location of the tumor. Patients are often asymptomatic, and a palpable abdominal mass is incidentally noted on examination by a parent or physician (**Fig. 3**). Patients may also present with weight loss, decreased appetite, failure to thrive, jaundice, anemia, pain, fever, or back pain. Tumor rupture is rare, but can present with hypovolemia secondary to hemorrhage.[26] The small cell variant of hepatoblastoma has a greater incidence of metastasis and is more likely to present with symptoms.[25]

### Diagnosis

Evaluation of hepatoblastoma includes a complete history and physical examination in addition to laboratory and imaging tests. Patients with hepatoblastoma may present with anemia and thrombocytosis (secondary to elevated cytokine release). An elevated serum alpha fetoprotein (AFP) level occurs in up to 90% of patients. This serum tumor marker parallels disease activity for hepatoblastoma, and can be used for both its diagnosis and surveillance. Normal AFP levels are elevated at birth, and do not reach a baseline until 6 months of age. A low AFP at the time of presentation is associated with poor survival outcome.[25]

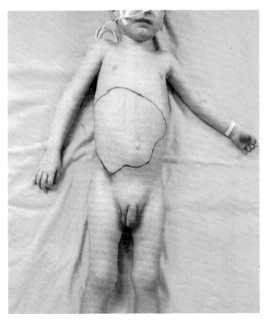

**Fig. 3.** Although often asymptomatic, hepatoblastoma may be large at presentation.

Multiple imaging modalities provide valuable information regarding location and relationship of the hepatoblastoma to its surrounding structures. Radiographic evaluation, including ultrasound, CT, and MRI, illustrates extent of tumor and feasibility of resection for preoperative planning. Abdominal ultrasound shows the character of the lesion, the extent of disease, and the patency of the hepatic vasculature. CT of the abdomen is helpful in confirming the diagnosis and staging the disease. It delineates the orientation of the mass regarding surrounding vasculature (inferior vena cava, hepatic veins, and the portal venous system) (**Fig. 4**). MRI of the abdomen provides greater detail of the tumor in relation to its surrounding hepatic anatomy. If malignancy is suspected, a chest CT and bone scan should be performed to evaluate for metastases and also aid in staging.

No current imaging technique allows for definitive diagnosis, and therefore a tissue biopsy is needed to confirm the diagnosis, either via a percutaneous, laparoscopic, or open approach. Hepatoblastoma has five histologic subtypes (fetal, embryonal, mixed mesenchymal, macrotubular, and small cell [anaplastic]),[27] and prognosis correlates with subtype. The pure fetal subtype has a better prognosis, whereas the small cell or anaplastic subtype is associated with a worse prognosis and greater incidence of metastases.[25]

### Staging

Two methods are used to determine hepatoblastoma staging. These systems determine treatment planning and predicted prognosis for patients with hepatoblastoma.

### COG

The COG staging method is a combined histologic and surgical staging system. COG staging is based on postoperative extent of disease and pre–chemotherapy treatment measures (**Table 2**).

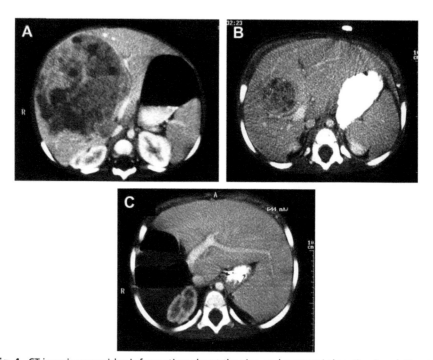

**Fig. 4.** CT imaging provides information about the size and anatomic location in relation to vascular structures. CT scans of a patient (*A*) with hepatoblastoma pretreatment, (*B*) after treatment with chemotherapy, and (*C*) after chemotherapy and surgical resection, with hypertrophy of the left lobe.

## SIOP/PRETEXT

The PRETEXT (pretreatment extent of disease) Grouping System was developed by the International Childhood Liver Tumour Strategy Group of the International Society of Paediatric Oncology Group (SIOPEL), and is based on pretreatment radiographic tumor findings. It is used to describe a patient's tumor extent before initiation of any therapy and is also used to assess tumor response and resectability before and after

**Table 2**
**Hepatoblastoma COG staging**

| Stage | Description | 5-Y Survival |
|-------|-------------|--------------|
| I | Complete resection<br>Clear margin<br>Pure fetal histology | 100% |
| IU | Complete resection<br>Clear margin<br>Unfavorable histology | 98% |
| II | Gross total resection with microscopic residual or perioperative rupture | 100% |
| III | Unresectable or resection with gross residual or lymph node involvement | 69% |
| IV | Metastatic disease | 37% |

neoadjuvant therapy.[28] PRETEXT is based on Cuinaud's system of liver segmentation. Segments are grouped into four sections, and PRETEXT level is derived from subtracting from four the highest number of continuous liver sections that are free of tumor. This number is roughly an estimate of difficulty anticipated with resection. In addition to describing the intrahepatic extent of tumors, this system also describes the presence of vascular involvement (obstruction, encasement, invasion of the inferior vena cava, hepatic veins, portal veins), extrahepatic abdominal disease, and metastases.

This system allows for a more effective comparison between studies conducted by different groups, has good interobserver reproducibility, and has been shown to hold good prognostic value in children with hepatoblastoma. Many studies use the PRETEXT system to describe imaging findings, although it is often not their main clinical staging system (**Table 3**).[29]

## Treatment

After evaluation and staging, definitive treatment plans are made through the collaboration of a multidisciplinary team of oncologists, surgeons, and radiologists.

### Treatment by Stage
**Stages I and II** For tumors of pure fetal histology (PFH), complete surgical resection followed by watchful waiting or combination chemotherapy is recommended. Children with completely resected PFH hepatoblastoma can achieve long-term survival without additional chemotherapy.[30] If undifferentiated small cell histology foci within an otherwise PFH tumor are identified, aggressive chemotherapy is used. Cisplatin-based therapies have resulted in a survival rate of approximately 90% for children with postoperative stages I and II disease.

### Stage III
Patients with stage III tumors should undergo chemotherapy followed by reassessment for surgical resectability. If amenable, the patient will undergo complete resection. For 75% of patients with initially unresectable disease, tumors can be made resectable after cisplatin-based preoperative chemotherapy.[31] If the primary tumor remains unresectable after chemotherapy, transplantation can be considered, in addition to alternative treatment options, such as transcatheter arterial chemoembolization (TACE).[32,33]

### Stage IV
The prognosis for patients who present with metastatic hepatoblastoma is poor; however, long-term survival and cure are possible. These patients undergo four courses of cisplatin-based chemotherapy, followed by reassessment for surgical resectability. If possible, the patient will undergo complete resection of the primary tumor and resection of extrahepatic metastases. Postoperatively, they will receive

| Table 3 SIOP PRETEXT staging | | |
|---|---|---|
| **Stage** | **Description** | **5-Y Survival** |
| PRETEXT 1 | Tumor only in 1 sector (3 adjoining sectors free) | 100% |
| PRETEXT 2 | 1 or 2 sectors involved (2 free) | 91% |
| PRETEXT 3 | Tumor involved 2 or 3 sectors (no adjoining sectors free) | 68% |
| PRETEXT 4 | Tumor in all 4 sectors (none free) | 57% |

two courses of the same chemotherapeutic regimen. If pulmonary metastases are present, resection of the metastasis is recommended.[34] However, if the tumor remains unresectable after the initial chemotherapeutic course but the extrahepatic disease is in complete remission, the patient may be evaluated for transplantation. If extrahepatic disease is not resectable after neoadjuvant chemotherapy, the patient may undergo radiation, TACE, or other nonstandard therapies (eg, irinotecan, high-dose combination chemotherapies). In a study of patients with metastases at presentation who tolerated neoadjuvant chemotherapy, the 5-year survival was 50%.[35]

### Operative Approach

The best chance for long-term cure is surgical resection of the primary tumor. Traditional hepatic resections or extended resections may be performed through either open or laparoscopic approach. Targeted margins of 2 to 3 mm of normal hepatic tissue are preferred. If this is unlikely to completely resect with clear margins, the patient should undergo preoperative chemotherapy with the goal of tumor volume reduction and subsequent complete resection.

### Chemotherapy

Most patients with hepatoblastoma require neoadjuvant chemotherapy in an attempt to reduce tumor size and allow for a safer conventional resection.[36] The potential downstaging effect of neoadjuvant chemotherapy may facilitate remission and convert unresectable tumors into resectable ones.[37] Adjuvant chemotherapy is also offered for patients with residual or microscopic disease after resection.[25]

### Transplant

Total hepatectomy with liver transplantation is a treatment option for unresectable hepatoblastoma confined to the liver. Two relative indications for transplantation in hepatoblastoma are localized disease to the liver and/or extrahepatic disease that is acutely chemosensitive and rendered inactive at the time of transplantation. After neoadjuvant chemotherapy for unresectable disease, patients are reassessed for surgical resection. If still unresectable, they may be offered transplantation, assuming the absence of extrahepatic disease at the time of transplantation. Predictive indicators of unresectability include age older than 3 years at presentation, bilobar or multifocal tumors, low AFP (<100 ng/mL), and tumor extension to the inferior vena cava, all three hepatic veins, or the bifurcation of the portal vein. Patients with these findings should be evaluated for transplantation early.[25]

Rescue transplantation also offers an alternative to patients with local recurrence, in which prognosis is poor. Rescue transplantation yields a 30% recurrence rate and a 30% survival rate.[25]

### Alternative Treatment Modalities

Alternative treatment modalities are available for otherwise unresectable disease. TACE provides greater concentration and targeted delivery of standard chemotherapeutic agents to the tumor. In addition to being a palliative resource, TACE has been shown to represent a curative therapeutic option when used to induce surgical resectability in pediatric patients.[38] Topotecan and irinotecan inhibit tumor growth and neovascularization and may be offered to patients with recurrent disease.[26]

### Metastases

The most common site of metastasis is the lung. Pulmonary metastases are chemosensitive and often disappear after the first few rounds of chemotherapy. If not resolved, however, metastasectomy is recommended before resection or transplantation.[26] Resection of lung metastases can be curative if the primary tumor is also controlled.[39]

### Long-Term Prognosis

The overall survival rate for children with hepatoblastoma is 70%. Patients with stage I or II tumors have cure rates greater than 90%, whereas those with stage III or IV disease have lower survival rates (60% and 20%, respectively).

Important prognostic factors for survival include tumor growth pattern, vascular invasion, serum AFP, and a fast decline in AFP posttreatment (>99% decline).[26] Contributors to improved prognosis include combination of surgery and (neo)adjuvant chemotherapy, early medical attention, aggressive therapy, complete resection of the primary tumor, and dedicated follow-up to evaluate for recurrence, therapy effects, and second malignancies.

Poor prognostic indicators include large tumor size, multifocality, extrahepatic disease, metastatic spread, small cell undifferentiated histology, AFP less than 100 ng/mL or greater than 1 million ng/mL, and a slow decline in AFP postresection.[40]

## RHABDOMYOSARCOMA

Rhabdomyosarcoma is a malignant soft tissue tumor of skeletal muscle origin and is the most common sarcoma in children. Rhabdomyosarcoma constitutes approximately 5% of all childhood cancers and more than 50% of the soft tissue sarcomas (STS) diagnosed in children.[41] Rhabdomyosarcoma typically presents before age 6, and has a slight increased prevalence in males.[42] The tumor can arise anywhere in the body, but is most commonly located in the head and neck, extremities, trunk, and genitourinary tract. Most cases occur sporadically, but rhabdomyosarcoma can occur in families with cancer-related syndromes, such as Li-Fraumeni, neurofibromatosis type 1, and Beckwith-Wiedemann syndromes. Rhabdomyosarcoma is a curable disease, with a greater than 60% 5-year survival rate.

### Presentation

Presenting symptoms are frequently the consequence of the tumor interfering with the function of surrounding tissues or structures. Symptoms are dependent on tumor location. Head and neck rhabdomyosarcomas represent 40% of cases, and patients may present with diplopia, exophthalmos, headache, congestion, nasal discharge, cranial nerve palsy, bleeding, obstruction, dysphagia, and/or loss of hearing or vision. Genitourinary rhabdomyosarcomas constitutes 20% of cases and presents with urinary tract obstruction or constipation. Extremity rhabdomyosarcomas contributes to the remainder of cases and may present with a painful mass that is often mistaken for injury.[43] Approximately 15% of rhabdomyosarcomas present with distant metastatic disease.[41]

### Diagnosis

Lack of clear-cut symptoms often leads to a delay in diagnosis. Early diagnosis is important because rhabdomyosarcoma spreads quickly. A complete family history is important because of the association between rhabdomyosarcoma and familial cancer-related syndromes.[43] Radiographic evaluation through ultrasound, CT, and MRI helps determine the extent of disease and its relationship to surrounding structures and vasculature, and aids in surgical planning.

Accurate diagnosis depends on incisional biopsy of the tumor. For extremity masses, the direction of the incision must be longitudinal to allow for incorporation by a subsequent wide local excision.[41] Open biopsy allows for ample tissue sample, which is necessary for accurate diagnosis and appropriate staging. Rhabdomyosarcoma has several histologic subtypes, including embryonal, alveolar, undifferentiated small cell, and botryoid. The embryonal subtypes are associated with more favorable outcomes, whereas the alveolar or undifferentiated subtypes are associated with a worse prognosis.

### Treatment

Risk categorization and treatment strategies depend on rhabdomyosarcoma staging that incorporates distant disease, TNM classification, and postsurgical clinical grouping.[44] Stage I tumors include any size tumor at a favorable site (orbit, vagina, uterus, superficial head and neck, paratesticular regions), without distant metastases. Stage II tumors include those smaller than 5 cm at unfavorable sites (extremities, bladder, retroperitoneal, or parameningeal head and neck), without evidence of metastases. Tumors at unfavorable locations greater than 5 cm are stage III. Tumors at unfavorable locations with evidence of nodal disease are stage IV.[43]

All children with rhabdomyosarcoma require multimodality therapy. If possible, initial surgical resection is recommended, followed by chemotherapy. The goal of surgical resection is removal of the tumor with negative (uninvolved) margins and lymph node sampling, with a focus on organ preservation.[44] The margin of resection varies and is dependent on the proximity to adjacent organs and neurovascular structures.[43] Most pediatric rhabdomyosarcomas are chemosensitive at presentation, with initial response rates of 85%. Radiation plays a role in local control for residual microscopic postoperative disease, and in the neoadjuvant setting for tumors that abut vital organs (eg, the orbit or bladder).[41]

### Long-Term Prognosis

The survival rate of children with rhabdomyosarcoma is improved with combination therapy (surgery, chemotherapy, radiation).[44] Overall, more than 60% of pediatric patients with rhabdomyosarcoma have long-term survival with combined modality therapy. Additionally, if diagnosed with early-stage tumors, the survival rate increases to 80%.

Prognosis is related to risk of disease that is dependent on patient age, site of origin, histology, and the extent of tumor at diagnosis. Age younger than 10 years is favorable. Rhabdomyosarcoma tumors originating from the orbit, nonparameningeal head and neck, and the genitourinary system (excluding bladder or prostate) have better prognosis. The most favorable histology subtypes include botryoid and spindle cell, whereas intermediate prognosis is anticipated with embryonal and pleomorphic subtypes; and the worst prognosis is associated with alveolar and undifferentiated types. Tumors smaller than 5 cm and those that are completely excised have a better prognosis.

Regional lymph node involvement and metastases at diagnosis are associated with a poor prognosis.[42] Metastatic disease has the worst prognosis, and the prognostic significance of metastases is augmented by tumor histology, patient age, and primary site. Younger age (<10 years) and embryonal histology are associated with a better 5-year survival rate, whereas age older than 10 years or with alveolar histology yields a much poorer outcome. In general terms, the survival rate is greater than 90% for patients with low-risk disease, 55% to 70% for those with intermediate-risk disease, and less than 50% for those with high-risk disease.

## SACROCOCCYGEAL TERATOMA

Sacrococcygeal teratoma (SCT) is the most common pediatric teratoma and is one of the most common tumors in newborns, with a prevalence of 1/21,000 births.[45] Most

SCTs are benign, but malignant or immature characteristics may be present, and the incidence of malignancy is often associated with the patient's age at diagnosis. Although more commonly found in females, the likelihood of malignancy is slightly increased in males.[46] Tumors that are benign at birth may become malignant after several months, and the incidence of malignancy increases if resection is delayed.[47]

### Presentation

SCT arises from the coccygeal region and typically presents with an obvious external presacral mass; however, a spectrum of intrapelvic and external tumor components exists. SCT with a large intrapelvic component may lead to urinary obstruction and, if present in utero, may lead to significant morbidity in the neonatal period. Patients may require intensive care due to prematurity, high-output cardiac failure, disseminated intravascular coagulation, or tumor rupture and bleeding.[48]

### Diagnosis

SCTs are occasionally identified during routine fetal screening. Doppler ultrasound evaluation and MRI allow for evaluation of the tumor extent and identification of patients at risk for serious fetal complications.[45] Prenatal diagnosis is accompanied with important implications for both the fetus and the mother and requires close ultrasound surveillance in the perinatal period. Despite an overall good prognosis for infants with SCT, these patients are at high risk for perinatal complications, including death that could occur secondary to tumor rupture, preterm labor caused by polyhydramnios, and high-output cardiac failure.[49]

The most common presentation for neonatal SCT is an obvious midline or paramedian mass at birth. The overlying skin is often normal, but may contain evidence of hemangioma, necrosis, or ulceration. Intrapelvic tumors may present later in life with obstructive symptoms that are related to the mass effect of the tumor.

Evaluation of a patient with SCT must include a thorough physical examination, including digital rectal examination to palpate the normal presacral space.[46] Imaging studies assist in the assessment of tumor size, location, and vascularity. Plain pelvic radiographs may show calcifications or bony erosions. Abdominal ultrasound is helpful in evaluating the size and consistency of the intrapelvic component. CT/MRI better illustrates anatomy and assessment of the vasculature but requires sedation (**Fig. 5**).

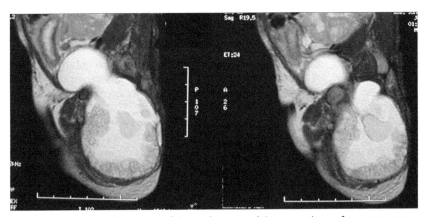

**Fig. 5.** MRI illustrates the intrapelvic and extrapelvic extension of a sacrococcygeal teratoma.

Serum AFP levels are elevated in patients with malignant SCT but are critical for follow-up and detection of postoperative malignant recurrence.[49]

## Treatment

### Prenatal diagnosis treatment concerns

Antenatal diagnosis of SCT is accompanied by concerns for the fetus both in utero and perinatally. Development of hydrops or placentomegaly has poor prognosis and is an indication for urgent intervention,[1] with potential delivery via Caesarean section. Polyhydramnios can be seen with large tumors and may lead to premature labor. A fetus should not be delivered vaginally if the mass is larger than the fetal biparietal diameter.[48]

### Preoperative management

Neonates with SCT require stabilization before early surgical resection. Secure vascular access with arterial monitoring is necessary, and blood type and cross should be performed on all patients. Resection of massive SCT can pose a significant risk if baseline hemodynamic instability is present and uncontrolled bleeding occurs.[50]

### Operative details

At surgery, the patient undergoes general endotracheal anesthesia, bladder catheterization, and skin preparation from the lower chest to toes. The patient is placed in the prone position with towel rolls under the shoulders and anterior superior iliac crests. Vaseline packing or intermittent placement of a Hegar dilator may be placed in the rectum to facilitate identification intraoperatively (**Fig. 6**).[48]

A chevron incision is made with the apex over the low sacrum and carried down to the fascia. The tumor is approached along its tissue planes after elevating skin and muscle flaps. The vasculature should be meticulously controlled as the mass is defined. En bloc excision of the mass, including the coccyx, is performed with careful identification of tumor extent, as it may infiltrate into the spine. Failure to remove the coccyx leads to a higher recurrence rate.[48] After resection, the levator muscle complex is secured to the presacral fascia and the wound is closed. A drain may be placed and excess skin is removed before a layered closure.[46]

Most tumors are completely resectable via a sacral approach. Abdominal exploration is indicated for tumors with wide intrapelvic extension identified by preoperative imaging or if bleeding occurs from tumor rupture or vascular injury during the sacral approach.[46] The abdomen is approached through a transverse, infraumbilical incision, to allow for mobilization of the intrapelvic component and ligation of the middle sacral vessels.

Rapidly growing sacrococcygeal teratomas are highly vascularized tumors and more likely to exhibit hemodynamic consequences.[45] High-output cardiac failure in the setting of SCT not only requires intensive perinatal care, but also contributes additional risk to the operation. Hemodynamic control and "damage control" operations have been described for these patients in which bleeding is controlled initially and resection can be delayed.[50]

The laparoscopic approach for vascular control in neonatal SCT may be an evolving technique. This less-invasive and rarely needed approach allows ligation of the arterial supply to preempt potential operative bleeding. Laparoscopic vascular control is potentially useful, but mistaken arterial division secondary to anatomic distortion and endosurgical limitations could be catastrophic.[51]

### Postoperative management

Postoperatively, the patient should initially remain in the prone position. The bladder catheter may be removed after 24 hours, and drains should be removed as soon as

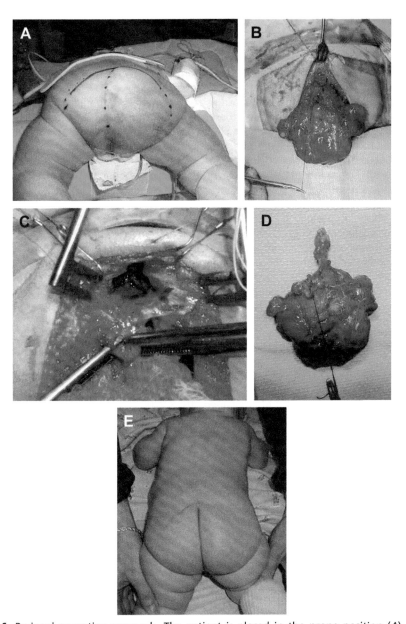

**Fig. 6.** Perineal operative approach. The patient is placed in the prone position (*A*) and a chevron incision is made with the apex over the sacrum (*B*). Skin and muscle flaps are raised (*C*) and the tumor is removed en bloc with the coccyx (*D*). Postoperative well-healed appearance of the incision (*E*).

reasonable. Serum AFP levels should be checked prior to discharge and then every 3 months for the first year, every 6 months for the following 2 years, and yearly until the fifth year to monitor for recurrence.[49] Physical examination is also performed at each visit.

### Long-Term Prognosis

Dedicated postoperative follow-up is necessary for timely identification and treatment of complications and recurrence. SCT may result in significant morbidity, either directly related to the tumor or as a consequence of surgical intervention.[45] Long-term bladder and bowel dysfunction occurs after SCT resection and should be evaluated as needed. Neuropathic bladder may be treated with clean intermittent catheterization, and bowel dysfunction is managed with bowel management programs for fecal incontinence.[49] Although common among all SCT's, higher-grade SCT should raise suspicion for possible urologic sequelae, and careful evaluation and management of the genitourinary tract should be included in prenatal and preoperative counseling.[52] Variable degrees of urinary incontinence and constipation can occur in patients who have undergone a combined abdominosacral approach for resection.[47]

Thorough follow-up care is also necessary to monitor for recurrence, even in the setting of benign tumors. If clinical suspicion is raised or the AFP trend is elevated, the patient should undergo CT/MRI to evaluate for recurrence.[46]

In the absence of prematurity and peripartum complications, the overall prognosis is good and is dependent on the presence of malignancy and completeness of resection, including the coccyx.[48] Even patients with malignant SCT have survival rates greater than 80% due to advances in platinum-based multimodal therapy.

### REFERENCES

1. Woods WG, Gao RN, Shuster JJ, et al. Screening of infants and mortality due to neuroblastoma. N Engl J Med 2002;346(14):1041–6.
2. Navalkele P, O'Dorisio MS, O'Dorisio TM, et al. Incidence, survival, and prevalence of neuroendocrine tumors versus neuroblastoma in children and young adults: nine standard SEER registries, 1975-2006. Pediatr Blood Cancer 2011; 56(1):50–7.
3. Thiele CJ. Neuroblastoma. In: Masters J, editor. Human cell culture. Lancaster (United Kingdom): Kluwer Academic Publishers; 1998. p. 21–53.
4. Shuangshoti S, Shuangshoti S, Nuchprayoon I, et al. Natural course of low risk neuroblastoma. Pediatr Blood Cancer 2012;58:690–4.
5. Gilbert F, Balaban G, Moorhead P, et al. Abnormalities of chromosome 1p in human neuroblastoma tumors and cell lines. Cancer Genet Cytogenet 1982;7(1):33–42.
6. Nemecek ER, Sawin RW, Park J. Treatment of neuroblastoma in patients with neurocristopathy syndromes. J Pediatr Hematol Oncol 2003;25(2):159–62.
7. Monclair T, Brodeur GM, Ambros PF, et al. The International Neuroblastoma Risk Group (INRG) staging system: an INRG Task Force report. J Clin Oncol 2009; 27(2):298–303.
8. Kushner BH, LaQuaglia MP, Kramer K, et al. Radically different treatment recommendations for newly diagnosed neuroblastoma: pitfalls in assessment of risk. J Pediatr Hematol Oncol 2004;26:35–9.
9. Brodeur GM, Pritchard J, Berthold F, et al. Revisions of the international criteria for neuroblastoma diagnosis, staging, and response to treatment. J Clin Oncol 1993; 11(8):1466–77.
10. Cohn SL, Pearson AD, London WB, et al. The International Neuroblastoma Risk Group (INRG) classification system: an INRG Task Force report. J Clin Oncol 2009;27(2):289–97.
11. Brodeur GM, Maris JM. Neuroblastoma. In: Pizzo PA, Poplack DG, editors. Principles and practice of pediatric oncology. 5th edition. Philadelphia: Lippincott Williams & Wilkins; 2006. p. 933–70.

12. London WB, Castleberry RP, Matthay KK, et al. Evidence for an age cutoff greater than 365 days for neuroblastoma risk group stratification in the Children's Oncology Group. J Clin Oncol 2005;23(27):6459–65.
13. Kostyrka B, Li J, Soundappan SV, et al. Features and outcomes of neonatal neuroblastoma. Pediatr Surg Int 2011;27(9):937–41.
14. Xu Y, Wang J, Peng Y, et al. CT characteristics of primary retroperitoneal neoplasms in children. Eur J Radiol 2010;75(3):321–8.
15. Naranjo A, Parisi MT, Shulkin BL, et al. Comparison of [123]I-metaiodobenzylguanidine (MIBG) and [131]I-MIBG semi-quantitative scores in predicting survival in patients with stage 4 neuroblastoma: a report from the Children's Oncology Group. Pediatr Blood Cancer 2011;56(7):1041–5.
16. Hussain HK, Kingston JE, Domizio P, et al. Imaging-guided core biopsy for the diagnosis of malignant tumors in pediatric patients. Am J Roentgenol 2001; 176(1):43–7.
17. Park JR, Scott JR, Stewart CF, et al. Pilot induction regimen incorporating pharmacokinetically guided topotecan for treatment of newly diagnosed high-risk neuroblastoma: a Children's Oncology Group Study. J Clin Oncol 2011;29(33): 4351–7.
18. Berthold F, Hero B, Kremens B, et al. Long-term results and risk profiles of patients in five consecutive trials (1979–1997) with stage 4 neuroblastoma over 1 year of age. Cancer Lett 2003;197(1-2):11–7.
19. Matthay KK, Villablanca JG, Seeger RC, et al. Treatment of high-risk neuroblastoma with intensive chemotherapy, radiotherapy, autologous bone marrow transplantation, and 13-cis-retinoic acid. Children's Cancer Group. N Engl J Med 1999;341(16):1165–73.
20. International Pediatric Endosurgery Group. IPEG guidelines for the surgical treatment of adrenal masses in children. J Laparoendosc Adv Surg Tech A 2010; 20(2):vii–vix.
21. Hollwarth ME. Wilms' tumor. In: Puri P, Hollworth M, editors. Pediatric surgery: diagnosis and management. Heidelberg (Germany): Springer; 2009. p. 709–15.
22. Shamberger RC. Renal tumors. In: Holcomb GW, Murphy JP, Ostlie DJ, editors. Ashcraft's pediatric surgery. 5th edition. Philadelphia: WB Saunders; 2010. p. 853–71.
23. Vieira C, Leite MT, Ribeiro RC, et al. Renal tumor and trauma: a pitfall for conservative management. Int Braz J Urol 2011;37(4):514–8.
24. Levitt G. Renal tumours: long-term outcome. Pediatr Nephrol, in press.
25. Paran TS, La Quaglia MP. Hepatic tumors in childhood. In: Puri P, Hollworth M, editors. Pediatric surgery: diagnosis and management. Heidelberg (Germany): Springer; 2009. p. 727–32.
26. Andrews WS. Lesions of the liver. In: Holcomb GW, Murphy JP, Ostlie DJ, editors. Ashcraft's pediatric surgery. 5th edition. Philadelphia: WB Saunders; 2010. p. 903–9.
27. Zimmerman A. The emerging family of hepatoblastoma tumours: from ontogenesis to oncogenesis. Eur J Cancer 2005;11:1503–14.
28. Roebuck DJ, Aronson D, Clapuyt P, et al. 2005 PRETEXT: a revised staging system for primary malignant liver tumours of childhood developed by the SIOPEL group. Pediatr Radiol 2007;17:123–32.
29. Aronson DC, Schnater JM, Staalman CR, et al. Predictive value of the pretreatment extent of disease system in hepatoblastoma: results from the International Society of Pediatric Oncology Liver Tumor Study Group SIOPEL-1 study. J Clin Oncol 2005;23(6):1245–52.

30. Malogolowkin MH, Katzenstein HM, Meyers RL, et al. Complete surgical resection is curative for children with hepatoblastoma with pure fetal histology: a report from the Children's Oncology Group. J Clin Oncol 2011;29(24):3301–6.

31. Reynolds M, Douglass EC, Finegold M, et al. Chemotherapy can convert unresectable hepatoblastoma. J Pediatr Surg 1992;27(8):1080–3.

32. Xianliang H, Jianhong L, Xuewu J, et al. Cure of hepatoblastoma with transcatheter arterial chemoembolization. J Pediatr Hematol Oncol 2004;26(1):60–3.

33. Malogolowkin MH, Stanley P, Steele DA, et al. Feasibility and toxicity of chemoembolization for children with liver tumors. J Clin Oncol 2000;18(6):1279–84.

34. Perilongo G, Brown J, Shafford E, et al. Hepatoblastoma presenting with lung metastases: treatment results of the first cooperative, prospective study of the International Society of Paediatric Oncology on childhood liver tumors. Cancer 2000;89(8):1845–53.

35. Pritchard J, Brown J, Shafford E, et al. Cisplatin, doxorubicin, and delayed surgery for childhood hepatoblastoma: a successful approach–results of the first prospective study of the International Society of Pediatric Oncology. J Clin Oncol 2000;18(22):3819–28.

36. Tiao GM, Bobey N, Allen S, et al. The current management of hepatoblastoma: A combination of chemotherapy, conventional resection, and liver transplantation. J Pediatr 2005;146:204–11.

37. Tsay PK, Lai JY, Yang CP, et al. Treatment outcomes for hepatoblastoma: experience of 35 cases at a single institution. J Formos Med Assoc 2011; 110(5):322–5.

38. Li JP, Chu JP, Yang JY, et al. Preoperative transcatheter selective arterial chemoembolization in treatment of unresectable hepatoblastoma in infants and children. Cardiovasc Intervent Radiol 2008;6:1117–23.

39. Schnater JM, Aronson DC, Plaschkes J, et al. Surgical view of the treatment of patients with hepatoblastoma: results from the first prospective trial of the International Society of Pediatric Oncology Liver Tumor Study Group. Cancer 2002;94: 1111–20.

40. Schnater JM, Kohler SE, Lamers WH, et al. Where do we stand with hepatoblastoma? a review. Cancer 2003;98(4):668–78.

41. Merchant MS, Mackall CL. Current approach to pediatric soft tissue sarcomas. Oncologist 2009;14(11):1139–53.

42. Kapoor G, Das K. Soft tissue sarcomas in children. Indian J Pediatr, in press.

43. Carachi R. [Soft tissue sarcoma]. In: Puri P, Hollworth M, editors. Pediatric surgery: diagnosis and management. Heidelberg (Germany): Springer; 2009. p. 717–24.

44. Zhao M, Feng C, Wang JW, et al. [Childhood rhabdomyosarcoma: a retrospective review of 23 cases]. Zhongguo Dang Dai Er Ke Za Zhi 2011;13(8):657–60 [in Chinese].

45. Gucciardo L, Uyttebroek A, De Weyer I, et al. Prenatal assessment and management of sacrococcygeal teratoma. Prenat Diagn 2011;31(7):678–88.

46. Warner B. Pediatric surgery. In: Townsend C, Beauchamp R, Evers M, et al, editors. Sabiston textbook of surgery, the biologic basis of modern surgical practice. 18th edition. Philadelphia: Saunders; 2008. p. 2080–9.

47. Barakat MI, Abdelaal SM, Saleh AM. Sacrococcygeal teratoma in infants and children. Acta Neurochir (Wien) 2011;153(9):1781–6.

48. Laberge J, Puligandla P, Shaw K. Teratomas, dermoids, and other soft tissue tumors. In: Holcomb GW, Murphy JP, Ostlie DJ, editors. Ashcraft's pediatric surgery. 5th edition. Philadelphia: WB Saunders; 2010. p. 915–35.

49. Paran TS, Puri P. Sacrococcygeal teratoma. In: Puri P, Hollworth M, editors. Pediatric surgery: diagnosis and management. Heidelberg (Germany): Springer; 2009. p. 697–701.
50. Smithers CJ, Javid PJ, Turner CG, et al. Damage control operation for massive sacrococcygeal teratoma. J Pediatr Surg 2011;46(3):566–9.
51. Solari V, Jawaid W, Jesudason EC. Enhancing safety of laparoscopic vascular control for neonatal sacrococcygeal teratoma. J Pediatr Surg 2011;46(5):e5–7.
52. Le LD, Alam S, Lim FY, et al. Prenatal and postnatal urologic complications of sacrococcygeal teratomas. J Pediatr Surg 2011;46(6):1186–90.

# Vascular Anomalies in Pediatrics

R. Dawn Fevurly, MD, Steven J. Fishman, MD*

## KEYWORDS

- Arteriovenous malformation • Hemangioma • Lymphatic malformation
- Kaposiform hemangioendothelioma • Vascular anomaly • Vascular malformation
- Venous malformation

## KEY POINTS

- Vascular anomalies are divided into lesions secondary to endothelial hyperplasia (vascular tumors) and vascular dysmorphogenesis (vascular malformations).
- Infantile hemangiomas are vascular tumors with a unique life cycle consisting of a proliferative growth phase followed by slow involution, resulting in replacement of the tumor with fibrofatty tissue.
- Kasabach-Merritt phenomenon describes profound thrombocytopenia associated with the vascular tumors kaposiform hemangioendothelioma and tufted angioma.
- Malformed lymphatic channels, or lymphatic malformations, may be associated with disfigurement, bleeding, or infections, and treatment may involve sclerotherapy or surgical excision.
- Venous malformations range from varicosities to networks of channels, expand over time, and may be associated with a variety of syndromes.
- Disorganized, directly communicating arteries and veins harbor arteriovenous malformations that may be inherited or sporadic, and often require intervention over time.

## INTRODUCTION

Most vascular anomalies involve the skin and are noted at birth. For centuries, vascular birthmarks were referred to by vernacular names derived from folk beliefs that a mother's emotions or patterns of ingestion could indelibly imprint her unborn fetus. Old medical texts are dotted with references to brightly colored foods appropriated to describe the appearance of an unusual cutaneous lesion. Depending on culture and sensitivity, the mother was blamed for eating too much or too little red fruit during her pregnancy. The present-day use of such terms as "cherry," "port-wine stain," and "strawberry" can be referenced to this false doctrine of maternal impressions.[1]

Virchow may be credited with the first effort to categorize vascular anomalies on the basis of histologic features.[2] Unfortunately, a lack of specificity or identifying features

Department of Surgery, Vascular Anomalies Center, Children's Hospital Boston, Harvard Medical School, 300 Longwood Avenue, Boston, MA 02115, USA
* Corresponding author.
E-mail address: steven.fishman@childrens.harvard.edu

Surg Clin N Am 92 (2012) 769–800
doi:10.1016/j.suc.2012.03.016
0039-6109/12/$ – see front matter © 2012 Elsevier Inc. All rights reserved.

continued to plague the field. Overlapping clinical, vernacular, and histopathologic terms contributed to persistent confusion, often resulting in misdiagnosis, incorrect treatment, and misdirected research.[3] A reliable system of classification for vascular anomalies was ultimately developed by Mulliken and Glowacki, who divided vascular anomalies into 2 major categories: hemangiomas and malformations.[4] In 1996, this division was modified to tumors and malformations and was formally accepted by the International Society for the Study of Vascular Anomalies.[5] Vascular tumors consist of lesions secondary to endothelial hyperplasia, incorporating both hemangiomas and less common pediatric vascular tumors. Vascular malformations arise by dysmorphogenesis and exhibit normal endothelial cell turnover.[3] Use of this division provided a clinically useful method of diagnosis and prognosis, as well as a guide to therapy. Despite this system, some anomalies seem to span both categories. It is hoped that with continued investigation into the biology and pathogenesis of these lesions, a more comprehensive molecular classification will soon be developed.

## HEMANGIOMAS AND OTHER VASCULAR TUMORS
### Incidence

Hemangiomas represent the most common infantile tumor with a documented perinatal incidence of 1.0% to 2.6%. Over the first year of life the incidence increases, with approximately 4% of all Caucasian infants affected.[6] Dark-skinned babies are less frequently affected. A female to male ratio of 3:1 to 5:1 has been observed.[3] Preterm infants with low birth weight (<1000 g) have an increased incidence of hemangioma, possibly as high a 30%, and with every 500-g decrease in birth weight, the risk of developing an infantile hemangioma increases by 40%.[7,8] No clear genetic tendency toward hemangioma formation exists, and studies have demonstrated no difference in the frequency of coexpression in monozygotic and dizygotic twins.[9–11] A positive family history in a first-degree relative, however, increases the risk of hemangioma formation 2-fold.[8] Additional risk factors include older maternal age, placental abnormalities, and multiple gestations.[12]

### History and physical examination

Hemangiomas typically appear in the neonatal period, generally around the first or second week of life. Approximately 30% to 50% of hemangiomas are nascent at birth, presenting as a premonitory pink macular stain, pale spot, telangiectasia, or purplish ecchymotic patch.[3] The typical cutaneous or superficial hemangioma permeates the dermis so that the skin becomes raised, bosselated, and vivid crimson in color, inspiring its common name of strawberry hemangioma (**Fig. 1**). Deeper hemangiomas located in the lower dermis, subcutis, or muscle may present as raised bluish lesions with indistinct borders manifesting at 2 to 3 months of life or later. These tumors were sometimes referred to historically as cavernous hemangiomas.[1,4] This term is a misnomer, and should be avoided to prevent confusion with venous malformations (VMs) or lymphatic malformations (LMs) sharing the same historical appellation.

Hemangiomas are most commonly located in the head and neck region (60%), followed in frequency by the trunk (25%) and extremities (15%).[13] Approximately 80% of hemangiomas are focal lesions.[3,14] An increased risk of complications and need for treatment correlates with size, with larger lesions 11 times more likely to experience complications and 8 times more likely to require treatment.[15] Nearly one-fifth of hemangiomas proliferate in multiple sites. These infants are more likely to also have hemangiomas of the gastrointestinal (GI) tract and those exhibiting more than 5 lesions

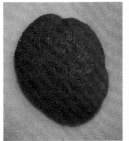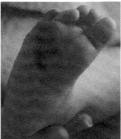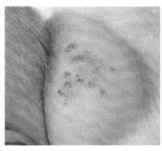

**Fig. 1.** Infantile hemangioma (IH). (*Left*) Proliferating-phase cutaneous IH on the trunk. (*Middle*) Foot IH. (*Right*) Deep IH over the back of the neck.

display a significantly increased risk of hepatic hemangiomas.[16] Infants with hepatic hemangioma(s) typically present at 1 to 16 weeks postnatally with hepatomegaly, congestive heart failure, anemia, or 1 or more asymptomatic masses. Multiple GI hemangiomas can manifest as infantile anemia and bleeding.

In contrast to the typical postnatal (infantile) hemangioma, congenital hemangiomas evolve in utero and present fully grown at birth. Such hemangiomas may be detected via prenatal screening as early as the 12th week of gestation and are often solitary.[17] Further characterization divides these hemangiomas into rapidly involuting congenital hemangiomas (RICH) or noninvoluting congenital hemangiomas (NICH).[17,18] Appearance varies, but the lesions most commonly present as raised gray to violaceous telangiectasias or ectatic veins, often surrounded by a pale halo. Occasionally a congenital hemangioma exhibits a depression or area of central necrosis.[19] Large focal hepatic masses, detected antenatally or in early infancy, are now recognized to be RICH rather than infantile hemangioma.[20] Under ultrasonographic evaluation, RICH and NICH are fast-flow lesions, and frequently exhibit large tubular vessels not seen in infantile hemangiomas. In addition, the presence of calcification suggests a congenital origin.[21]

### Clinical course

The infantile hemangioma exhibits unique biological behavior: it grows rapidly during the first 6 to 12 months of life (the proliferative phase), enters a second stage of growth proportionate with that of the child, and then enters a phase of slow regression (involuting phase) lasting 1 to 7 years during which the endothelial matrix of hemangiomas is replaced by loose fibrous or fibrofatty tissue (**Fig. 2**). Cellular studies have demonstrated that maximum apoptosis occurs at 2 years.[22] Regression is complete in half of the children by age 5, in 70% of children by age 7, and in the remainder by age 10 to 12 years. In the involuted phase, nearly normal skin is restored in approximately 50% of children.[23] Otherwise, the involved skin is damaged with telangiectasias, crepe-like laxity (secondary to destruction of elastic fibers), and yellowish discoloration or scarred patches (present if ulceration occurred during the proliferative phase).[3] If the tumor was formerly large and protuberant, fibrofatty residuum and redundant skin may remain.

Congenital hemangioma, defined as a tumor fully grown at birth, differs from the common postnatal infantile hemangioma in its clinical course. In RICH, regression begins early, with full involution by 9 to 14 months (**Fig. 3**).[17] Alternatively, NICH grow proportionally with the child but undergo no involution.[18]

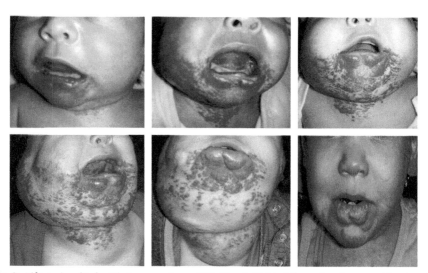

**Fig. 2.** Life cycle of infantile hemangioma (IH). (*Top left*) IH at 2 weeks of age, corticosteroid therapy initiated. (*Top middle*) Following 2 weeks of therapy. (*Top right*) Age 2 months, after 6 weeks of corticosteroid therapy. (*Bottom left*) Continued proliferation of IH. (*Bottom middle*) Age 11 months, rebound growth following weaning of corticosteroid. Propranolol therapy initiated. (*Bottom right*) Age 18 months, following propranolol therapy. (*From* Kulungowski AM, Fishman SJ. Vascular anomalies. In: Coran A, Adzick NS, Krummel T, et al, editors. Pediatric surgery (7th edition). Mosby; 2012. p. 1615; with permission.)

### Etiology and pathogenesis

Despite its overwhelming incidence, little is known about the pathogenesis of infantile hemangioma. Evidence supports the development of hemangiomas from clonal expansion of endothelial stem/progenitor cells subject to either abnormal local cellular signals or an initial somatic mutation favoring rapid expansion.[11,24,25] However, the source of these endothelial progenitors remains elusive. Some studies suggest that a population of resident angioblasts, arrested in an early stage of vascular development, gives rise to these endothelial cells.[26] A second theory suggests that these

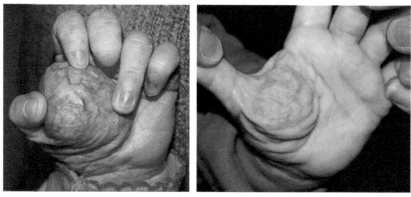

**Fig. 3.** Rapidly involuting congenital hemangioma (RICH). (*Left*) Hand RICH at 12 days of age. (*Right*) Follow-up at 5 months of age, demonstrating significant involution of lesion.

endothelial cells are of placental origin because they coexpress several markers: GLUT1, merosin, Lewis Y antigen, Fcγ-RIIb, indoleamine 2,3-deoxygenase, insulin-like growth factor 2, and type III iodothyronine deiodinase.[10,27–31] A small embolic nidus of placental endothelial cells may reach fetal tissues through the permissive right to left shunt of fetal circulation. This process could, in part, explain the 3-fold increased risk of hemangiomas observed in infants subjected in utero to chorionic villus sampling, as local placental injury might predispose the shedding of cells into the fetal circulation.[32]

Another theory emerges from more recent findings. Endothelial cells derived from hemangioma express vascular endothelial growth factor A (VEGF-A), VEGF receptors (VEGFRs), TIE2, and angiopoietin-2.[30,33,34] VEGF-A is the predominant growth factor in endothelial proliferation and migration, and binds to 2 major receptors: VEGFR1 and VEGFR2. VEGFR1 primarily acts as a decoy receptor, binding with high affinity to VEGF-A, whereas VEGFR2 activation promotes migration, proliferation, adhesion, and survival.[35] In infantile hemangioma endothelial cells, VEGFR2 signaling is consti-tutively expressed and VEGFR1 levels are decreased.[33] Mice lacking VEGFR1 die as embryos because of overgrowth of endothelial cells and disorganized blood vessels, characteristics seen in hemangiomas.[36] Genetic analysis of DNA from patients with hemangioma reveals sequence changes in VEGFR2, possibly representing risk-factor mutations in infantile hemangiomas.[37] These results point to evidence for infan-tile hemangioma resulting from deregulation of angiogenesis.[38]

The clinical characteristics of growth and involution of the infantile hemangioma are mirrored in its cellular course. During the proliferative phase, hemangiomas overex-press such proangiogenic molecules as fibroblast growth factor 2 (FGF-2), VEGF-A, and matrix metalloproteinases. With the exception of FGF-2, these molecules are downregulated during involution.[38,39] At the same time, angiogenesis decreases as endothelial cells undergo apoptosis. Involution is also marked by the appearance of mast cells and the induction of the angiogenesis inhibitors interferon-β and tissue inhibitor of metalloproteinases.[22] Proapoptotic markers mitochondrial cytochrome b and homer-2a are also expressed.[22,40] However, other key elements to under-standing the behavior of hemangiomas, including the trigger toward involution, its female predominance, and its trophism, remain a mystery.

### Associated malformative anomalies

Historical association of hemangiomas with a wide variety of syndromes is most likely secondary to misappellation of another vascular lesion. However, certain true heman-giomas do occasionally occur in association with other malformations. A disorder known as PHACES syndrome consists of a cervicofacial hemangioma with associated structural anomalies of the brain (eg, posterior fossa abnormality), cerebral vascula-ture (eg, aneurysms, hypoplasia, or absence of carotid or vertebral vessels), eye (eg, cataracts, optic nerve hypoplasia), aorta (eg, coarctation), and chest wall defects (eg, sternal clefts).[41–44] Lumbosacral tumors may signal underlying occult spinal dys-raphism (eg, lipomeningocele, tethered spinal cord).[41,42] In patients with sacral hemangioma, ultrasonography can be used to screen infants younger than 4 months, whereas magnetic resonance imaging (MRI) is usually necessary in older children. In addition, there are rare reported incidences whereby pelvic and perineal hemangioma is associated with urogenital and anorectal anomalies.[43]

### Differential Diagnosis

#### Kasabach-Merritt phenomenon

In 1940, radiologist Kasabach and pediatrician Merritt reported a child with profound thrombocytopenia, petechiae, and bleeding in the presence of a "giant hemangioma."[43] Only recently has it become known that persistent, profound thrombocytopenia is never associated with common hemangioma of infancy. Instead, the so-called Kasabach-Merritt phenomenon (KMP) occurs with a more invasive type of infantile vascular tumor called kaposiform hemangioendothelioma (KHE) or tufted angioma (TA).[45–47] Both tumors are typically present at birth. Unlike infantile hemangioma, KHE and TA are unifocal and involve the trunk, shoulder, thigh, or retroperitoneum. KHE presents equally in both sexes, whereas TA may demonstrate a male predominance.[48] The overlying skin is deep red-purple in color with surrounding ecchymosis and occasionally generalized petechiae (**Fig. 4**). Thrombocytopenia unresponsive to platelet transfusion can be profound (fewer than 10,000 cells/μL). Platelets are likely trapped intralesionally, supported by absence of hemolysis on peripheral blood smears, and platelet transfusions can result in rapid expansion of the tumor.[49–51] The child with Kasabach-Merritt thrombocytopenia is at risk for intracranial, pleural-pulmonic, intraperitoneal, or GI hemorrhage with an associated mortality of 20% to 30%.[52] MRI demonstrates enhanced signal on T2-weighted images and dilated feeding/drain vessels as in other vascular tumors. KHE specifically demonstrates a poorly defined tumor margin with extension across tissues and small vessels relative to tumor size.

Histopathologic examination differs according to underlying cause. KHE demonstrates an aggressive cellular pattern of infiltrating sheets or nodules of slender epithelial cells, and slit-like vascular spaces filled with hemosiderin and fragments of red blood cells. TA, while macroscopically similar to KHE, is histologically composed of small tufts of capillaries (cannonballs) in the middle to lower dermis.[47,53]

Treatment of KMP consists of corticosteroids (2–3 mg/kg/d), platelet transfusions only in episodes of active bleeding or in preparation for a surgical procedure, and, occasionally, cryoprecipitate for correction of hypofibrinogenemia.[54] Heparin should be avoided as it can stimulate tumor growth and aggravate platelet trapping. Vincristine has emerged as a safe and effective method of treatment, resulting in increased platelet counts and fibrinogen levels.[55,56] Vincristine blocks formation of microtubules

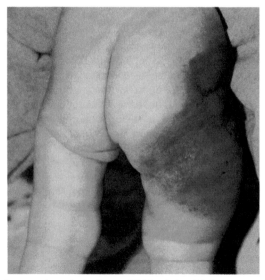

**Fig. 4.** Kaposiform hemangioendothelioma (KHE) of the thigh.

in cells, induces apoptosis in tumor endothelial cells, and inhibits blood flow, resulting in tumor necrosis.[57] Interferon-α is an effective antiangiogenic agent in KMP, but neurologic side effects such as spastic diplegia have been noted.[58,59] Sirolimus has recently shown promising results in KHE with KMP, prompting an ongoing clinical trial.[60,61] For KHE without KMP, treatment must be based on size of tumor, medication side effects, and possible sequelae of persistent tumor (eg, muscle fibrosis joint contracture).[62,63]

### Pyogenic granuloma

Hemangiomas can be confused with a very common, cutaneous vascular growth known as a pyogenic granuloma (**Fig. 5**). Pyogenic granulomas are small lesions rarely appearing before 6 months of age (average age 6.7 years) and are sometimes associated with port-wine stains.[64] The lesions grow rapidly, erupting through the skin on a stalk or pedicle. Epidermal breakdown with crusting is the norm associated with recurrent, often copious, bleeding. The treatment includes curettage or full-thickness excision, shave excision with cautery, cautery alone, or laser phototherapy.[65,66] Failure of complete excision leads to a high recurrence rate.[64]

### PTEN hamartoma tumor syndrome

PTEN hamartoma tumor syndrome results from mutation of *PTEN*, a gene encoding a tumor-suppressor protein involved in cell-cycle regulation. Mutations are responsible for 2 disorders that predispose to cancer: Bannayan-Riley-Ruvalcaba syndrome (BRRS) and Cowden syndrome (CS).[67] BRRS is a congenital disorder with common clinical findings of macrocephaly, penile freckling, macrosomia at birth, lipomas, hamartomatous intestinal polyposis, proximal myopathy, and variable degrees of developmental delay. CS is generally identified in adulthood with a range of mucocutaneous manifestations and leads to an increased risk for tumor development in the breast, thyroid, and endometrium. Associated vascular anomalies tend to be fast-flow lesions radiographically, but disordered growths of blood vessels, adipose tissue, and fibrous tissue histopathologically.[68] Given the increased risk of cancer, patients

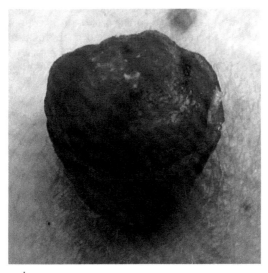

**Fig. 5.** Pyogenic granuloma.

with fast-flow lesions should undergo clinical and genetic evaluation for *PTEN* mutations.

### Other

Multifocal hemangiopericytoma is another uncommon congenital vascular tumor that can present with low-grade thrombocytopenia.[69] Other rare lesions that can masquerade as congenital hemangiomas include nasal glioma and infantile fibrosarcoma.[65]

### Treatment

Most hemangiomas are small, regressing without need for cosmetic or therapeutic intervention. These lesions should be allowed to undergo proliferation and involution under careful observation by a pediatrician with gentle and sympathetic parental education and reassurance, recognizing the anguish caused by the appearance of a tumor on their previously unblemished infant. Referral to a specialty center should occur in the event of equivocal diagnosis, dangerous location, large size, rapidity of growth, or potential for other complications.

### Ulceration

Spontaneous epithelial breakdown, crusting, ulceration, and necrosis occur in 5% of cutaneous hemangiomas, most commonly around the lips, parotid glands, or anogenital region.[70,71] Ulceration most frequently takes place during the proliferative phase, possibly due to rapid expansion, exceeding the elastic capability of the skin (**Fig. 6**).[72,73] Initial treatment should involve the application of a petroleum-based antibiotic salve along with viscous lidocaine to assist with pain control. If eschar is present, sharp debridement and wet-to-dry dressing changes are used to stimulate granulation tissue. Ulceration of larger than several millimeters is an indication for referral. Superficial ulcerations usually heal within days to weeks, whereas a deep ulceration can take several weeks. Pharmacologic treatment with corticosteroid or flashlamp pulsed-dye laser can accelerate healing.[74] Total resection should be considered if the resultant scar would be equivalent to removal of an involuted area later in childhood.

### Endangering complications

Fatal or significantly morbid complications caused by hemangioma are usually associated with cervicofacial or visceral lesions.[45] A periorbital hemangioma can block the visual axis and cause deprivation amblyopia, or extend into the retrobulbar space causing ocular proptosis. Similarly, a hemangioma of the upper eyelid can distort the growing cornea, producing astigmatic amblyopia. Such cases should be referred for immediate evaluation by a pediatric ophthalmologist. Even a small hemangioma

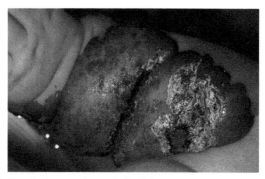

**Fig. 6.** Ulcerating infantile hemangioma (IH) of the arm.

can obstruct the subglottis, with symptoms of hoarseness initially and, later, biphasic stridor around 6 to 8 weeks of age. Approximately one-half of these infants have cutaneous cervical hemangioma, often in the "beard distribution."[75] GI hemangiomas may cause GI bleeding, symptomatically controlled with pharmacologic treatment, endoscopy, or surgery. Hepatic hemangiomas may cause high-output cardiac failure, hypothyroidism (due to expression of a deiodinase that inactivates thyroid hormone), hepatomegaly, and abdominal compartment syndrome (**Fig. 7**).[29] Complicated hemangiomas may require management by transfusion, parenteral nutrition, and antiangiogenic drug therapy to hasten involution.

### Pharmacologic therapy

Until recently, the mainstay of pharmacologic treatment of infantile hemangiomas was corticosteroids. In 2008, following a serendipitous finding of a dramatic decrease of proliferation of a nasal hemangioma in a patient with obstructive hypertrophic cardiomyopathy treated with propranolol, a small case series of systemic propranolol treatment in infantile hemangiomas demonstrated halting of hemangioma growth and a decreased time to involution.[76,77] Following this study, a multitude of publications have emerged supporting these findings.[78,79] Within the first 1 to 3 days of propranolol therapy, a palpable softening and change in color is noted, likely secondary to the inhibition of vasodilation.[76,80] Tumor growth arrest occurs as a result of reduced expression of VEGF, basic fibroblast growth factor, and matrix metalloproteinase 2/9, effectively blocking proangiogenic signals.[80] Propranolol induces apoptosis in proliferating endothelial cells, providing a possible explanation for regression.[81,82] This finding is supported by the accelerated rate of reduction of hemangiomas with the use of propranolol past the proliferation phase.[83] Following a cardiology consultation, dosing of 0.5 to 0.7 mg/kg 3 times a day (total daily dose of 2–3 mg/kg/d, divided 3 times a day) is recommended, with treatment durations averaging 20 weeks.[79,84] As chronic use may lead to withdrawal symptoms of tachycardia, hypertension, angina, and myocardial infarction, cessation should involve tapering over a 2-week period.[84,85] Side effects of use included bradycardia, hypotension, hypoglycemia, GI complaints, and bronchospasm but, given the low dose used, were infrequent.[78,84,86,87] A role for topical β-blockers, such as timolol maleate, has shown modest results.[88]

Small, well-localized cutaneous hemangiomas may be considered for intralesional injection of corticosteroid. Triamcinolone (25 mg/mL) is injected slowly at low pressure, with the periphery of the lesion compressed to minimize the chances of embolization through a draining vein. Three to 5 mg/kg is injected 3 to 5 times at a 6- to 8-week interval. Topical treatment has produced more modest results, with only 35% of patients displaying a good result to clobetasol propionate 0.05% or

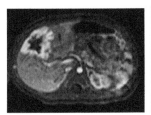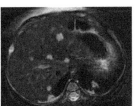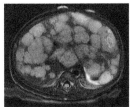

**Fig. 7.** Axial T2 magnetic resonance (MR) images of hepatic hemangioma. (*Left*) Focal hepatic hemangioma displaying a heterogeneous appearance and central involution. (*Middle*) Multifocal hepatic hemangioma. (*Right*) Diffuse hepatic hemangioma with near total replacement of liver parenchyma.

betamethasone dipropionate 0.05% (Diprolene AF 0.05%; Schering-Plough, Kenilworth, NJ).[89]

Systemic therapy using oral prednisolone, 2 to 3 mg/kg/d each morning for 2 to 3 weeks, is still useful as an alternative to propranolol for treatment of large, problematic, or life-threatening hemangiomas. It can be administered without fear of bradycardia, hypotension, or hypoglycemia. For an acute situation such as an upper airway constriction, an equivalent dose of intravenous corticosteroid is recommended. Approximately 30% of hemangiomas demonstrate accelerated regression in response to corticosteroids, approximately 40% have stabilized growth, and the remaining 30% demonstrate no response at all.[90] Corticosteroids have recently been shown to suppress VEGF-A expression in hemangioma-derived skin cells, effectively limiting their vasculogenic potential and providing a possible mechanism of action.[91] Signs of responsiveness occur within several days to 1 week after initiation of the treatment and include a diminished rate of growth, fading color, and softening of the tumor. Treatment typically is terminated around 10 months of age, and may be tapered toward the end of the treatment course over weeks or months to minimize steroid-associated complications. Side effects of treatment include Cushingoid facies (71%), growth delay (35%), personality changes (29%), gastric irritation (21%), hirsutism (13%), and hypertension.[92–94]

Recombinant interferon-α (interferon-α2a or-α2b) had been a second-line therapy for hemangioma, but has fallen out of favor because of the risk of spastic diplegia.[95–98] Vincristine has been effective in some children unresponsive to interferon and is now chosen by some practitioners as an alternative agent for both hemangioma and KHE.[55,99]

### Embolic therapy
Embolization may be indicated for hemangiomas that cause severe congestive heart failure and do not respond sufficiently to drug therapy. Hepatic hemangiomas are the most common lesions that necessitate embolization, only when macrovascular shunts are present. Antiangiogenic therapy is continued even after successful embolization.

### Laser therapy
Despite widespread interest, true indications for laser therapy for hemangiomas are relatively few. Previous investigators advocated treatment to prevent tumor growth and subsequent complications.[100] However, flashlamp pulsed-dye laser only penetrates 0.75 to 1.2 mm into the dermis, typically affecting only a superficial portion of a hemangioma. While lightening surface color, proliferation is not affected. Small, flat lesions can be successfully treated, but these same lesions would regress naturally with little to no scar. Moreover, overzealous use of the laser can result in ulceration, partial-thickness skin loss, and consequent scarring. Two well-accepted indications for laser use are the obliteration of persistent telangiectasias in involuting/involuted hemangiomas and excision of a unilateral subglottic hemangioma with a continuous-wave carbon dioxide laser.[101]

### Surgical therapy
Surgical excision of a hemangioma may be indicated at any stage of its life cycle. A well-localized, pedunculated hemangioma, particularly one demonstrating ulceration or recurrent episodes of bleeding, may be removed during the tumor's proliferative phase (during infancy). Similarly, problematic hemangiomas of the upper eyelid unresponsive to medical therapy should be considered for surgical excision to prevent the attendant changes in vision. Persistently bleeding focal or multifocal GI hemangiomas may be considered for removal, although such lesions are often patchy in distribution and difficult to manage surgically or endoscopically.[102]

As children progress through their preschool years and develop a sense of physical awareness, consideration should be given to staged or total excision of a large or protuberant involuting-phase hemangioma. Excision in early childhood may be considered if: (1) it is obvious that resection is inevitable, (2) the scar would be the same if the excision were postponed until the involuted phase, and (3) the scar is easily hidden. Most commonly, it is preferred to wait until late childhood to remove the hemangiomatous residuum of the involuted phase. Protrusive hemangiomas frequently leave unsightly expanded skin and fibrofatty tissue. Staged resection is often indicated to minimize distortion and recreate a cosmetically acceptable outcome.

There is almost no role for surgical intervention in the treatment of hepatic hemangiomas. Asymptomatic lesions without shunt can be observed. Lesions with shunts can be treated with propranolol or steroids and, if necessary, shunt embolization. Hepatic artery ligation should be chosen only if a skilled interventional radiologist is unavailable in such situations. Diffuse lesions always manifest acquired hypothyroidism and should be treated with aggressive thyroid replacement.[29,103] In rare instances, massive hepatomegaly causing compartment syndrome refractory to pharmacotherapy should stimulate evaluation for liver transplantation.

## VASCULAR MALFORMATIONS

Vascular malformations are localized or diffuse errors of embryonic development affecting any segment of the vascular tree including arterial, venous, capillary, and lymphatic vessels. It is useful to subcategorize vascular malformations by the predominant type of channel abnormality and flow characteristics. According to this distinction, 2 major categories exist: (1) slow-flow anomalies (capillary malformations [CMs], LMs, and VMs) and (2) fast-flow anomalies (arteriovenous malformations [AVMs] and arteriovenous fistulae). Complex, combined vascular malformations also exist. Congenital vascular malformations are present in approximately 1.2% to 1.5% of the population.[104] Most vascular malformations are sporadic (ie, nonfamilial), but some exhibit classic Mendelian inheritance.[105,106] Although much of the pathogenesis of vascular malformations remains unelucidated, recent strides have been made in understanding the development of the blood vascular and lymphatic systems, opening the door for greater insight into observed aberrancies.

### Embryology and Development of the Vascular and Lymphatic Systems

During embryogenesis, the development of the vascular system occurs by 2 separate, but related, processes: vasculogenesis and angiogenesis.[53] Vasculogenesis describes the formation of the vessels from blood islands, whereas angiogenesis entails the formation of new blood vessels from preexisting vessels via sprouting. Mesodermally derived hemangioblasts congregate to form primary blood islands around the third week of development. The inner cells of the blood islands become hematopoietic stem cells while those at the periphery differentiate into endothelial cell precursors called angioblasts. Proliferating angioblasts form a capillary-like network of tubes that constitute the primary vascular plexus. Angiogenesis then allows for reorganization of this plexus into a functional vascular system with sprouting of new vessels and capillaries.[107]

Early in embryogenesis, the fate of endothelial precursors to differentiate into distinct cell types can be detected via unique markers.[108] Arterial endothelial cells express ephrin-B2, whereas venous endothelial cells express its receptor, Eph-B4[109] The recruitment of periendothelial cells to the vessel wall results in stabilization through the inhibition of endothelial proliferation and migration, and by the stimulation of the production of extracellular matrix and the deposition of a basement membrane. The angiopoietin/TIE, platelet-derived growth factor B, and transforming growth factor (TGF) receptor systems regulate this periendothelial cell–endothelial cell interaction.[110]

Development of the lymphatic system begins in the sixth to seventh week of embryogenesis, only after the establishment of functional blood vessels.[111] Existing veins give rise to lymph sacs, which then bud to form lymphatic vessels.[112,113] Endothelial cells along the anterior cardinal vein initiate this process via the expression of lymphatic vessel endothelial hyaluronan receptor (LYVE-1).[114] A subpopulation of these cells then expresses the transcription factor prospero-related homeobox 1 (PROX-1) in a polarized fashion, which serves as a master regulator of lymphatic endothelial differentiation.[115] As lymphatic endothelial cells express the VEGFR3 they are drawn to its ligand, VEGF-C, which directs budding and migration.[116] Further remodeling allows for formation of the peripheral lymphatic network.[111]

### Capillary Malformation

Still commonly referred to as port-wine stains, CMs are dermal vascular anomalies that occur in 0.3% of newborns, with an even gender distribution (**Fig. 8**).[117] CM must be differentiated from the fading macular stain nevus flammeus neonatorum ("angel kiss" on the forehead or "stork bite" on the nuchal area), a transient dilation of dermal vessels that is the most common vascular birthmark. CMs are present at birth, occur anywhere on the body, and can be localized or extensive; they are composed of dilated, ectatic capillary-to-venule sized vessels in the superficial dermis. Histopathology demonstrates a paucity of surrounding normal nerve fibers.[118] With age the vessels gradually dilate, probably accounting for the darkening color and tendency to nodular ectasias. Cutaneous CM is often associated with hypertrophy of the subcutaneous tissue, muscle, and bone; CMs located on the extremity may be associated with leg-length discrepancy. Although CMs are usually sporadic, a familial pattern of autosomal dominant inheritance with incomplete penetration has been

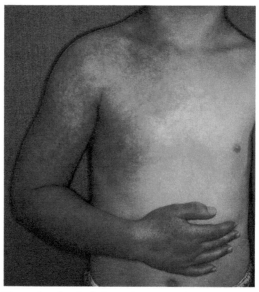

**Fig. 8.** Capillary malformation (CM) of the right arm and chest.

reported. Linkage analysis identified a locus on chromosome 5q13-15 termed CMC1, with the causative gene a negative regulator of ras termed RASA1.[119,120]

A CM can be a signal of underlying structural abnormality. A midline occipital CM can overlie an encephalocele or ectopic meninges. A CM over the cervical or lumbo-sacral spine can be a clue to occult spinal dysraphism or tethered cord. CM of the ophthalmic and maxillary branches of the trigeminal nerve distribution should alert to Sturge-Weber syndrome, an associated vascular anomaly of the ipsilateral choroid and leptomeninges. Clinical manifestations include seizures, contralateral hemiplegia, and variable developmental motor and cognitive delay. CM may also be observed in complex-combined vascular malformations.

Treatment of CM is primarily for cosmetic reasons. Flashlamp pulsed-dye laser is currently the treatment of choice, with significant lightening of skin observed in approximately 70% of patients. Better outcomes are observed in early, thin CMs located on the face. The optimal timing is controversial.[121,122] Beginning treatment before 6 months of age has shown promising early results.[123] Soft-tissue and skeletal hypertrophy often require surgical strategies.

### Telangiectasias

Tiny acquired capillary vascular marks, commonly known as spider nevus or spider telangiectasias, typically appear on preschool and school-aged children. Epidemiologic studies suggest they may be present in nearly half of all children, with an equal gender distribution. Spontaneous disappearance is possible, but pulsed-dye laser successfully removes the lesion.

Cutaneous marbling of the skin of Caucasian infants placed at a low temperature, so-called cutis marmorata or livido reticularis, is an accentuated pattern of normal cutaneous vascularity that improves with age as the skin thickens. In one rare congenital pathologic disorder, the newborn has a distinctive deep purple, serpiginous, reticulated vascular staining pattern called cutis marmorata telangiectatica congenital (CMTC). CMTC occurs in a localized, segmental distribution, usually involving the trunk and extremities.[124] Histopathologic findings include dilated capillaries in the papillary dermis and proliferation of blood vessels in the reticular dermis.[125] Neonatal ulceration of the depressed purple areas can occur, in addition to hypoplasia of the affected limb and subcutaneous tissues. Stenosis of the common iliac and femoral arteries has also been observed.[126] Almost all infants with CMTC demonstrate steady improvement during the first year of life. In time, venous dilation becomes more prominent and persists in to adulthood, together with residual cutaneous atrophy and staining.[1]

Hereditary hemorrhagic telangiectasia (HHT; Osler-Weber-Rendu syndrome) is an autosomal dominant disorder estimated to occur at a frequency of 1 to 2 per 100,000 of the Caucasian population. HHT results from mutations in endoglin, activin receptor–like kinase 1 or, rarely, Smad4, which modulate TGF-$\beta$ signaling in vascular endothelial cells.[127–129] Diagnosis is based on family history and the presence of 3 separate manifestations: mucocutaneous telangiectasia (such as on the fingertip, lips, oral mucosa, or tongue), spontaneous recurrent nosebleeds, and visceral involvement (GI tract, pulmonary, hepatic, cerebral, or spinal AVM).[130] Affected individuals often suffer from recurrent nasal and GI bleeding, with one-third presenting with chronic anemia.[130,131]

### Lymphatic Malformations

Historically termed lymphangioma or cystic hygroma, slow-flow vascular anomalies of the lymphatic system consist of localized or diffuse malformations of lymphatic channels best characterized as microcystic (diameter <1 cm), macrocystic (diameter >1 cm), or combined. Such size classification is advantageous, as it often determines whether the cavity can be successfully aspirated and compressed. LMs most commonly appear as ballotable masses with normal overlying skin, although a blue hue may result if large underlying cysts are present. Less common dermal involvement is manifest as puckering or deep cutaneous dimpling. LMs in the subcutis or submucosa manifest as tiny vesicles. Intravesicular bleeding is evidenced by tiny, dark-red, dome-shaped nodules. Histologically, LMs are thin-walled vessels lined by lymphatic endothelial cells, which are immunopositive for podoplanin (D2-40) and LYVE-1.[132] Lumens may be empty or filled with a proteinaceous fluid containing macrophages and lymphocytes.[133]

Prenatal ultrasonography can detect macrocystic LM in the late first trimester. Fetal cystic hygroma is noted around the same time, with septated forms of the nuchal region associated with an increased risk of aneuploidy, chromosomal abnormalities, cardiac malformation, and perinatal death.[134,135] However, most prenatally diagnosed LMs are not detected until the second or third trimesters.[136] Typical LMs of the anterior cervicofacial region are not associated with chromosomal abnormalities. Those LMs not diagnosed prenatally are generally evident at birth or before age 2 years, but occasionally can manifest suddenly in older children and adults. Radiologic documentation is best performed by MRI, although ultrasonography is a useful auxiliary method for confirming the presence of macrocystic LM. LMs, such as hemangiomas and VMs, demonstrate hyperintense signal intensity in T2-weighted and turbo-STIR (short-tau inversion recovery) images.[137] Rim enhancement following contrast application is noted. Microcystic lesions have an intermediate signal in T1 sequences and an intermediate to high signal on T2 sequences. Macrocystic lesions show low intensity on T1 images and high intensity on T2 images (**Fig. 9**). Although conventional contrast lymphangiography is rarely performed, it may be useful for determining the precise location of lymphatic or chylous leaks in a patient with a diffuse thoracic lymphatic anomaly.[138]

LMs are most commonly located in the axilla/chest, cervicofacial region (70%–80%), mediastinum, retroperitoneum, buttocks, and anogenital areas.[137] LMs in the forehead and orbit cause proptosis and localized overgrowth. Facial LM is the most common basis for macrocheilia, macroglossia, macrotia, and macromala. Cervicofacial LM is associated with the overgrowth of the mandibular body, causing an open bite and underbite (**Fig. 10**).[139] LMs in the floor of the mouth and tongue are characterized by vesicles, intermittent swelling, bleeding, and the possibility of oropharyngeal obstruction. Cervical LMs involve the supraglottic airway, and tracheostomy may be necessary early in infancy. Mediastinal LMs often accompany cervical LMs and/or axillary LMs. Diffuse thoracic lymphatic anomalies or rare abnormalities of the thoracic duct or cisterna chili can manifest as recurrent pleural and pericardial chylous effusion or chylous ascites. Anomalous lymphatics in the GI tract can cause hypoalbuminemia as the result of chronic protein-losing enteropathy. LMs in an extremity cause diffuse or localized swelling or gigantism with both soft-tissue and skeletal overgrowth. Pelvic LMs are accompanied by bladder outlet obstruction, constipation, or recurrent infection.

Progressive osteolysis, caused by diffuse soft-tissue and skeletal LM, is called Gorham-Stout syndrome, known also as disappearing bone disease or phantom bone disease.[140] Radiologic features demonstrate radiolucent foci in the intramedullary or subcortical regions resembling osteoporosis.[141] Affected areas may be throughout the skeleton, but most commonly involve the shoulder, facial, spinal, and pelvic bones.[142] Histopathologic features reveal replacement of bone with

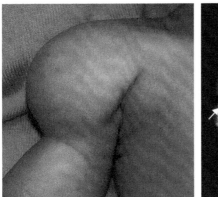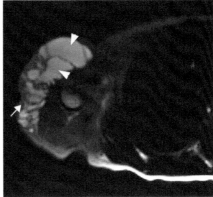

**Fig. 9.** Lymphatic malformation (LM). (*Left*) LM of right shoulder. (*Right*) Axial T2 MR image of same LM demonstrating mixture of macrocysts (*arrowheads*) and microcysts (*arrow*).

multiple thin-walled blood vessels or vascular spaces.[143] Gradual and often complete resorption of the bone develops, leading to pathologic fractures.[133] Course and prognosis is highly variable, with multiple varieties of treatment attempted.

Lymphedema should also be included as a type of LM. Congenital lymphedema (Milroy disease) is an autosomal dominant disorder presenting early in life with localized areas of edema, primarily below the knees. The initial superficial lymphatics of these areas are thought to be hypoplastic or absent, although superficial lymphatics are observed in nonedematous areas. A mutant, inactive VEGFR3 receptor is to blame, with both hereditary and sporadic mutations noted.[144–146] A rare form of edema, known as generalized lymphatic dysplasia, commonly includes systemic involvement, such as intestinal lymphangiectasia, ascites, pleural or pericardial

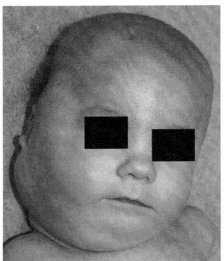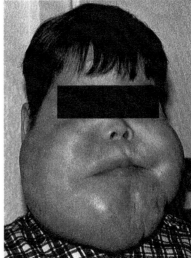

**Fig. 10.** Cervicofacial lymphatic malformation (LM). (*Left*) Cervicofacial LM in an infant. (*Right*) Extensive cervicofacial LM requiring tracheostomy.

effusions, and pulmonary lymphangiectasia.[144] Late-onset lymphedema is divided into lymphedema distichiasis syndrome (LDS) and Meige disease. LDS is a late-onset (post puberty to mid-50s) autosomal dominant disorder with variable penetrance and phenotype. Affected patients demonstrate distichiasis, meaning a double row of eyelashes. Patients with this disorder suffer not only from defective lymphatic valves leading to impairment in drainage and subsequent edema, but defective venous valves leading to distal reflux and varicose veins.[147,148] The putative gene is FOXC2, a member of the forkhead/winged helix family of transcription factors, which is thought to play a role in somite development.[149] Meige disease presents as bilateral lower-extremity edema often developing at or after puberty. It is more common in females (3:1 female/male ratio), and an associated gene or locus has yet to be identified.[150]

### Treatment

The 2 main complications of LMs are intralesional bleeding and infection. Bleeding, spontaneous or the result of local trauma, causes rapid, painful enlargement of an LM. The LM becomes firm and ecchymotic. Analgesia, rest, and time are generally sufficient. Prophylactic antibiotics should be prescribed if there is a large collection of intraluminal blood. Hemorrhage and infection can transform a macrocystic lesion into a microcystic and scarred lesion.

LMs often swell in the event of a viral or bacterial infection. Most often this is a harmless event, likely related to change in flow or alterations in lymphocytic component in the walls of the anomalous channels. Bacterial cellulitis, however, is a more dangerous condition. An infection in a cervicofacial LM can cause obstruction of the upper airway and dysphagia. Prolonged intravenous antibiotic therapy is frequently indicated, with choice of antibiotic agents based on the presumption of oral pathogens in the head and neck or enteric organisms in the trunk or perineum.

The 2 strategies for treating lymphatic anomalies are sclerotherapy and surgical resection. Sclerotherapy works through obliteration of the lymphatic lumen by endothelial destruction with subsequent sclerosis/fibrosis (**Fig. 11**). Success depends on the damage inflicted on the endothelial and deeper muscular and connective tissue layers. Macrocystic LM is more likely than microcystic tissue to shrink after an injection of sclerosant. Common sclerosants include ethanol, sodium tetradecylsulfate, bleomycin, and doxycycline.[151–153] Technically, sclerotherapy involves entering the cystic cavity by direct puncture, aspiration of fluid, and injection of sclerosant. Typically several sessions are required with any sclerosant, with most effective results in macrocystic lesions. Superficial lymphatic vesicles may be treated via intravesicular injection. Complications of sclerotherapy include necrosis of overlying skin, local neuropathy, and cardiopulmonary toxicity related to overdose.

Resection is the only way to potentially "cure" LM. Staged excision is often necessary and total excision is often possible. In each resection a surgeon should focus on a defined anatomic region, attempt to limit blood loss, perform as thorough a dissection as possible, and be prepared to operate as long as necessary. Even with such an intensive approach to resection, the recurrence rate is reported to be 40% after an incomplete excision and 17% after a macroscopically complete excision.[154] Cutaneous wart-like lymphatic vesicles may develop within the scar, but are easily treated by intravesicular sclerotherapy, cauterization, laser coagulation, or excision.

### Venous Malformations

VMs are the most common of all vascular anomalies, and are frequently misdiagnosed as hemangiomas or mislabeled as cavernous hemangiomas. These slow-flow lesions

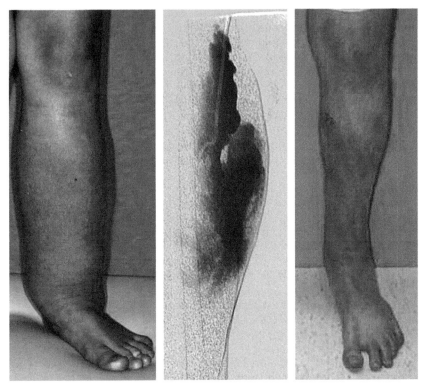

**Fig. 11.** Sclerotherapy for lymphatic malformation (LM). (*Left*) Left leg LM before sclero-therapy. (*Middle*) Contrast introduction into LM demonstrating cavity during sclerotherapy procedure. (*Right*) Left leg LM following sclerotherapy.

are present at birth but are not always immediately evident. The typical description of a VM is of a blue, soft, and compressible lesion, but can vary from simple varicosities to networks of channels within an organ (**Fig. 12**). Most are solitary, but multiple lesions may exist. VMs enlarge proportionally with the child and slow expansion occurs over time. Histologically VMs are composed of thin-walled, dilated, sponge-like abnormal channels with surrounding smooth muscle distorted into clumps. This mural muscular

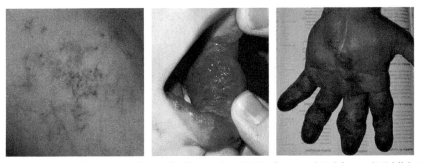

**Fig. 12.** Venous malformation (VM). (*Left*) Localized VM of antecubital fossa. (*Middle*) VM of the lip. (*Right*) Extensive VM of the hand.

abnormality is likely responsible for the tendency of VMs toward gradual expansion. Microscopy often reveals evidence of clot formation, fibrovascular ingrowth and phleboliths. Phlebothrombosis is common and can be painful.

Complications of VMs depend on their location. VMs of the head and neck may distort facial features and cause exophthalmia, dental malalignment, and obstructive sleep apnea. Limb-length discrepancies, painful hemarthrosis, and degenerative arthritis may be seen in extremity VMs. Intraosseous VMs may cause structural weakening and subsequent pathologic fractures. GI tract lesions may cause chronic bleeding and anemia.[155] Bowel VMs may be present throughout but are more commonly found encompassing the entire left colon, rectum, and surrounding pelvic and retroperitoneal structures.[3,102,156] A rectal VM associated with ectasia of mesenteric veins is a risk factor for portomesenteric venous thrombosis.[157]

Most VMs are sporadic. Half of these may be traced to a loss-of-function mutation in TIE2, a receptor tyrosine kinase involved in vascular remodeling.[158,159] An autosomal dominant inheritance pattern of VMs is seen in familial cutaneous mucosal VM, which occurs in 1% to 2% of VMs. This condition exhibits millimeter- to centimeter-sized dome-shaped lesions in the skin and GI mucosa that progress over time.[105] Dysregulation of TIE2 is likely to blame.[160,161] As histopathologic examination reveals a lack of an inner elastic membrane in lesional vessels, it is postulated that local uncoupling of endothelial smooth muscle cell signaling may occur.[162,163] Glomuvenous malformations (GVMs) are also inherited in an autosomal dominant manner, and account for 5% of all lesions. Clinically GVMs are multiple blue nodular dermal lesions with a cobblestone-like appearance. GVMs tend to localize on the extremities, are poorly compressible, and often involve pain with compression.[164] Histologically, GVMs consist of ectatic, dilated blood vessels surrounded by cuboidal epithelioid glomus cells expressing smooth muscle actin and vimentin.[53] The lesions are caused by loss-of-function mutations in glomulin, which derails the differentiation of vascular smooth muscle cells.[165]

Blue-rubber bleb nevus syndrome is a rare, sporadic disorder composed of cutaneous and GI VMs. Cutaneous lesions can occur anywhere on the body, but there is a predilection for the trunk, palms, and soles of the feet (**Fig. 13**).[166] There is often a large, dominant VM present. Lesions increase in size and become more apparent with age. GI lesions are most frequently located in the small bowel and, in addition to bleeding, may provide a lead point for intussusception or volvulus. Capsule endoscopy has been effectively used to visualize these bowel lesions.[167] Complications include consumptive coagulopathy and iron-deficiency anemia secondary to bleeding episodes.[168]

Like other vascular malformations, VMs are best imaged by MRI. Lesions demonstrate bright T2 signal and more uniform enhancement with contrast in comparison with LMs, another slow-flow lesion. Phleboliths can manifest as signal voids. Flow-sensitive sequences should show no evidence of arterial flow. Magnetic resonance venography (MRV) is useful for the evaluation of an extensive VM of the extremities, and direct phlebography is sometimes helpful as a presurgical planning tool.

### Treatment

Indications for treatment of VMs include pain, functional deficits, bleeding, and cosmetic appearance. Elastic support stockings are indispensable in the treatment of extremity VM. Low-dose aspirin (81 mg/d or every other day) helps to minimize phlebothromboses. However, as with LMs, the mainstay of therapy for VMs is sclerotherapy and surgical resection. Sclerosing agents induce direct endothelial damage, thrombosis, and scarring. Multiple pharmacologic agents have been used, including

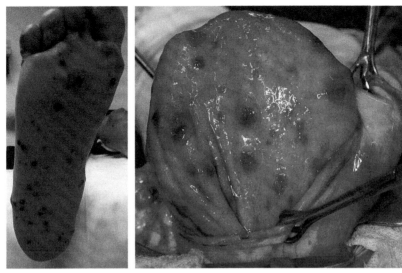

**Fig. 13.** Blue-rubber bleb nevus syndrome (BRBNS). (*Left*) Characteristic dome-shaped lesions on the plantar aspect of the foot. (*Right*) Serosal view of intestinal VMs.

bleomycin, doxycycline, 1% sodium tetradecylsulfate, and OK-432.[137] Unfortunately, VMs often recanalize and recur, requiring multiple treatments.[169] Complications include blistering, full-thickness necrosis, nerve injury, hemolysis, pulmonary hypertension, and cardiac and renal toxicities.[170]

Excision of a VM is usually successful for small, well-localized lesions. For GVMs in particular, excision may be beneficial because of their poor response to compression and often localized presentation.[164] Sclerotherapy is frequently used to shrink large VMs before surgical resection. Staged subtotal resections may be required. Surgical resection of GI VMs are indicated in cases of chronic bleeding, anemia, and transfusion dependence. Multifocal GI lesions are best treated via wedge excision (sometimes numbering in the hundreds) and polypectomy.[171,172] Bowel resections should be minimized and used only in segments in which there is a high density of VMs. Diffuse, chronically bleeding, colorectal VMs may be treated with colectomy, anorectal mucosectomy, and coloanal pull-through.[173] Patients with rectal and/or vaginal VM associated with an ectatic inferior mesenteric vein (IMV) should be anticoagulated and considered for ligation of the proximal IMV to prevent portomesenteric thrombosis.[157]

### Arteriovenous Malformations

AVMs are fast-flow malformations consisting of disorganized arteries and veins that directly communicate (shunts), thus bypassing the high-resistance capillary bed. The shunt is the epicenter, or nidus, of the AVM. Most often AVMs are latent during infancy and childhood and expand during adolescence, manifesting as a warm, pink patch in the skin with an underlying thrill or bruit. Later, cutaneous consequences may include ischemic changes, ulceration, pain, and intermittent bleeding. The hormonal changes of puberty or local trauma seem to trigger expansion.[174] The natural history of AVMs can be documented by a clinical staging system introduced by Schobinger (**Table 1**).[175]

Although most AVMs are sporadic, heritable forms have been identified. The autosomal dominant disorder capillary malformation–arteriovenous malformation

| Table 1 | |
|---|---|
| Schobinger clinical staging system for AVMs | |
| **Stage** | **Description** |
| I (Quiescence) | Pink-bluish stain, warmth, and arteriovascular shunting by continuous Doppler scanning or 20 MHz color Doppler scanning |
| II (Expansion) | Same as stage I plus enlargement, pulsations, thrill, and bruit and tortuous/tense veins |
| III (Destruction) | Same as stage II plus either dystrophic skin changes, ulceration, bleeding, persistent pain, or tissue necrosis |
| IV (Decompensation) | Same as stage III plus cardiac failure |

(CM-AVM) involves a randomly distributed CM along with a fast-flow lesion. CM-AVM is caused by mutations in *RASA1*. Such conditions include Parkes Weber syndrome, intracranial or extracranial AVM, and aneurysmal malformation of the vein of Galen.[176]

Ultrasonography and Doppler imaging detect the fast flow of the AVM. Dilated feeding arteries and draining veins appear as areas of contrast enhancement on computed tomography, signal flow voids (black tubular structures) on MRI, and signal enhancement (white tubular structures) on MR angiography (MRA). Muscle hypertrophy, bony changes, and increased fat may also be present. The nidus is often difficult to discern, but superselective angiography may aid in its delineation.[3]

### Treatment

Angiographic embolization alone or in combination with surgical excision is the mainstay of treatment for AVM. Conventional dogma dictates that intervention should be delayed until there are symptoms or endangering signs (eg, recurrent ulceration refractory to treatment, pain, bleeding, increased cardiac output [Branham's sign] or Schobinger stage III–IV). Children with stage I or II AVMs should undergo a diagnostic evaluation followed by annual examination for signs of expansion. Intervention is rarely indicated in infancy, except in instances of AVM related postnatal congestive heart failure. Treatment often begins when AVMs of stage III and greater develop. Efforts to treat the AVM should be directed toward the nidus. Ligation or proximal embolization of feeding vessels should never be attempted, as this causes the rapid recruitment of flow from nearby arteries to supply the malformation, and may preclude future embolization.[169] Rather, the usual strategy is arterial embolization for the temporary occlusion of the nidus 24 to 72 hours before surgical resection. If the arteries are tortuous or if the feeding arteries have been ligated, sclerotherapy may play a role in conjunction with local arterial and venous occlusion. Whenever possible, the lesion should be resected completely. Intraoperative frozen sectioning of the resection margins can be helpful, but the most accurate way to determine whether resection is complete is by observation of the pattern of bleeding from the wound edges. Unfortunately, many AVMs are not localized and may permeate throughout the deep craniofacial structures or the soft and skeletal tissues of an extremity. In these instances, embolization is usually palliative and surgical resection is rarely indicated (**Fig. 14**).

### Combined (Eponymous) Vascular Malformations

Combined (or complex) vascular malformations are often associated with the overgrowth of soft tissue and the skeleton. Many are named after the physicians who are credited with the most memorable description of the condition.

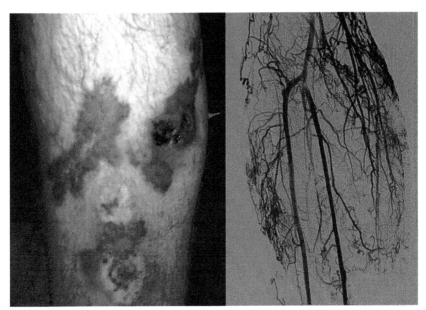

**Fig. 14.** Arteriovenous malformation (AVM) of the calf. (*Left*) Late-stage AVM revealing discoloration and ulceration of the overlying skin. (*Right*) Angiography of calf demonstrating multiple areas of AVM.

### Slow-flow anomalies

Klippel-Trenaunay syndrome is a well-described combined capillary-lymphaticovenous malformation (CLVM) associated with soft-tissue and skeletal hypertrophy of the lower extremity (88%), upper extremity (29%), and/or trunk (23%) (**Fig. 15**).[177] CLVM is typically evident at birth by the presence of an enlarged extremity, multiple CMs geographically arranged in a lateral distribution, lymphatic vesicles, and visible varicosities.[3] Often the CM component is macular in the newborn, becoming studded with lymphatic vesicles as the child ages. Persistent embryologic veins become prominent because of incompetent valves, while a deep venous component may be absent. Lymphatic hypoplasia is present in more than 50% of patients with associated lymphedema or isolated lymphatic microcysts, although lymphatic hyperplasia has been described.[1,178] Pelvic involvement is frequently asymptomatic but can be associated with constipation, bladder outlet obstruction, and recurrent infection. Venous anomalies of the lower extremities often extend into the pelvis, and may connect with femoral and iliac veins or the inferior vena cava. This connection can result in pulmonary embolism in 4% to 25% of cases.[157]

MRI and MRV are the primary imaging modalities. The venous system is reliably observed with MRV, particularly the anomalous venous channels present in the extremity. A large lateral vein of Servelle is often present. Microcystic LM, macrocystic LM, or a combination of LM may be seen. Plain radiographs are useful in evaluating and following limb-length discrepancies. Venography may be used to map venous drainage for planned interventions.

Management is fundamentally conservative. Compression therapy forms the basis of treatment and is typically initiated after the child is walking. Limb length is followed by serial radiographs. For discrepancies between 0.5 and 2 cm, shoe-lifts are beneficial to prevent limping and secondary scoliosis. Differences of greater than 2 cm are

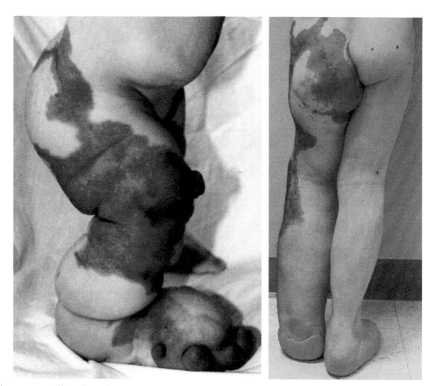

**Fig. 15.** Capillary-lymphaticovenous malformation (CLVM) of the lower extremity. (*Left*) CLVM of right lower extremity with soft-tissue overgrowth and characteristic lateral LM. (*Right*) CLVM of left lower extremity with notable small lymphatic vesicles on the surface.

often treated with epiphysiodesis at the distal femoral growth plate around 12 years of age. Grotesque enlargement of the foot requires selective ablative procedures (ie, ray, midfoot, or Syme amputation) to allow the child to wear proper footwear.[179] In selected patients, sclerotherapy can be used to obliterate incompetent superficial veins and to shrink focal VMs or lymphatic cysts. Lymphatic vesicle may be sclerosed. Persistent embryonic veins may be amenable to endovenous laser ablation or resection. Veins with direct connection to the femoral or iliac veins or inferior vena cava require preemptive ablation to prevent pulmonary embolism.

Debulking procedures can offer both physical and psychological benefits. Patients with intrafascial soft-tissue overgrowth are not candidates for debulking because of the risk of injury to major neurovascular structures and mobility concerns. Staged repair is often necessary, particularly when involving the trunk or thoracic region. Postoperative wound healing may require an extensive time period, given involved tissues possess poor lymphatic drainage and altered blood flow. Because of the increased risk of pulmonary embolism and deep venous thrombosis, placement of an inferior venous cava filter and preoperative anticoagulation may be necessary.[179]

CLOVES syndrome is characterized by congenital lipomatous overgrowth, vascular malformation, epidermal nevi, and musculoskeletal anomalies (scoliosis, skeletal and spinal anomalies, seizures).[180,181] This condition may be identified on prenatal imaging, with the combination of truncal cystic mass, body, and acral anomalies.[182]

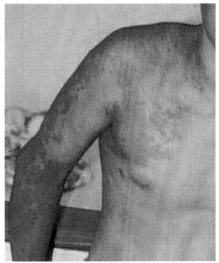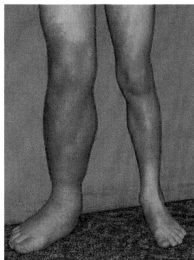

**Fig. 16.** Parkes Weber syndrome (PWS). (*Left*) PWS of left arm with pink, macular stain. (*Right*) Enlarged right lower extremity in PWS.

### Fast-flow anomalies

The Parkes Weber syndrome (PWS) shares many similarities with Klippel-Trenaunay syndrome, but should be distinguished by a component of an additional capillary-arteriovenous malformation/fistula (**Fig. 16**).[3] The lesions are obvious at birth and the involved, asymmetrically enlarged limb is covered by a geographic pink, warm, macular stain with an underlying bruit or thrill. There may be associated lymphatic abnormalities. Mutations in RASA1, an inhibitor of cellular growth, proliferation, and differentiation, are either inherited or occur de novo, and are responsible for PWS.[176] Large lesions may be associated with high-output cardiac failure. MRI/MRA complemented by angiography is important for diagnosis and anatomic delineation. Treatment is reserved is symptomatic patients, and may involve repetitive embolization to improve heart failure.[3]

### SUMMARY

The last 3 decades have witnessed remarkable forays into understanding the pathogenesis of vascular anomalies. Improved definitions based on this genetic-anatomic-histologic classification have allowed the development of multidisciplinary approaches toward disease treatment and management. As the appreciation of the embryonic and developmental contributions to disease increases, so does the ability to develop novel strategies for management of previously insurmountably complex lesions. Molecular and pharmacologic manipulation of vascular anomalies may hold promise.

### REFERENCES

1. Mulliken JB, Young AE. Vascular birthmarks: hemangiomas and malformations. Philadelphia: Saunders; 1988.

2. Vikkula M, Boon LM, Mulliken JB, et al. Molecular basis of vascular anomalies. Trends Cardiovasc Med 1998;8:281–92.
3. Mulliken JB, Fishman SJ, Burrows PE. Vascular anomalies. Curr Probl Surg 2000;37:517–84.
4. Mulliken JB, Glowacki J. Hemangiomas and vascular malformations in infants and children: a classification based on endothelial characteristics. Plast Reconstr Surg 1982;69:412–22.
5. Enjolras O. Vascular tumors and vascular malformations: are we at the dawn of a better knowledge? Pediatr Dermatol 1999;16:238–41.
6. Holmdahl K. Cutaneous hemangiomas in premature and mature infants. Acta Paediatr 1955;44:370–9.
7. Amir J, Metzker A, Krikler R, et al. Strawberry hemangioma in preterm infants. Pediatr Dermatol 1986;3:331–2.
8. Drolet BA, Swanson EA, Frieden IJ. Infantile hemangiomas: an emerging health issue linked to an increased rate of low birth weight infants. J Pediatr 2008;153: 712–5, 715.e711.
9. Cheung DS, Warman ML, Mulliken JB. Hemangioma in twins. Ann Plast Surg 1997;38:269–74.
10. Marchuk DA. Pathogenesis of hemangioma. J Clin Invest 2001;107:665–6.
11. Boye E, Yu Y, Paranya G, et al. Clonality and altered behavior of endothelial cells from hemangiomas. J Clin Invest 2001;107:745–52.
12. Haggstrom AN, Drolet BA, Baselga E, et al. Prospective study of infantile hemangiomas: demographic, prenatal, and perinatal characteristics. J Pediatr 2007;150:291–4.
13. Finn MC, Glowacki J, Mulliken JB. Congenital vascular lesions: clinical application of a new classification. J Pediatr Surg 1983;18:894–900.
14. Chiller KG, Passaro D, Frieden IJ. Hemangiomas of infancy: clinical characteristics, morphologic subtypes, and their relationship to race, ethnicity, and sex. Arch Dermatol 2002;138:1567–76.
15. Haggstrom AN, Drolet BA, Baselga E, et al. Prospective study of infantile hemangiomas: clinical characteristics predicting complications and treatment. Pediatrics 2006;118:882–7.
16. Horii KA, Drolet BA, Frieden IJ, et al. Prospective study of the frequency of hepatic hemangiomas in infants with multiple cutaneous infantile hemangiomas. Pediatr Dermatol 2011;28:245–53.
17. Boon LM, Enjolras O, Mulliken JB. Congenital hemangioma: evidence of accelerated involution. J Pediatr 1996;128:329–35.
18. Enjolras O, Mulliken JB, Boon LM, et al. Noninvoluting congenital hemangioma: a rare cutaneous vascular anomaly. Plast Reconstr Surg 2001;107:1647–54.
19. Berenguer B, Mulliken JB, Enjolras O, et al. Rapidly involuting congenital hemangioma: clinical and histopathologic features. Pediatr Dev Pathol 2003;6: 495–510.
20. Kulungowski AM, Alomari AI, Chawla A, et al. Lessons from a liver hemangioma registry: subtype classification. J Pediatr Surg 2012;47:165–70.
21. Gorincour G, Kokta V, Rypens F, et al. Imaging characteristics of two subtypes of congenital hemangiomas: rapidly involuting congenital hemangiomas and non-involuting congenital hemangiomas. Pediatr Radiol 2005;35:1178–85.
22. Razon MJ, Kraling BM, Mulliken JB, et al. Increased apoptosis coincides with onset of involution in infantile hemangioma. Microcirculation 1998;5:189–95.
23. Bowers R, Graham E, Tomlinson K. The natural history of the strawberry birthmark. Arch Dermatol 1960;82:667–80.

24. Bischoff J. Progenitor cells in infantile hemangioma. J Craniofac Surg 2009;20: 695–7.
25. Khan ZA, Boscolo E, Picard A, et al. Multipotential stem cells recapitulate human infantile hemangioma in immunodeficient mice. J Clin Invest 2008;118:2592–9.
26. Dadras SS, North PE, Bertoncini J, et al. Infantile hemangiomas are arrested in an early developmental vascular differentiation state. Mod Pathol 2004;17:1068–79.
27. North PE, Waner M, Mizeracki A, et al. A unique microvascular phenotype shared by juvenile hemangiomas and human placenta. Arch Dermatol 2001;137:559–70.
28. Leon-Villapalos J, Wolfe K, Kangesu L. GLUT-1: an extra diagnostic tool to differentiate between haemangiomas and vascular malformations. Br J Plast Surg 2005;58:348–52.
29. Huang SA, Tu HM, Harney JW, et al. Severe hypothyroidism caused by type 3 iodothyronine deiodinase in infantile hemangiomas. N Engl J Med 2000;343: 185–9.
30. Picard A, Boscolo E, Khan ZA, et al. IGF-2 and FLT-1/VEGF-R1 mRNA levels reveal distinctions and similarities between congenital and common infantile hemangioma. Pediatr Res 2008;63:263–7.
31. Bree AF, Siegfried E, Sotelo-Avila C, et al. Infantile hemangiomas: speculation on placental trophoblastic origin. Arch Dermatol 2001;137:573–7.
32. Kleinman ME, Tepper OM, Capla JM, et al. Increased circulating AC133+ CD34+ endothelial progenitor cells in children with hemangioma. Lymphat Res Biol 2003;1:301–7.
33. Jinnin M, Medici D, Park L, et al. Suppressed NFAT-dependent VEGFR1 expression and constitutive VEGFR2 signaling in infantile hemangioma. Nat Med 2008; 14:1236–46.
34. Yu Y, Varughese J, Brown LF, et al. Increased Tie2 expression, enhanced response to angiopoietin-1, and dysregulated angiopoietin-2 expression in hemangioma-derived endothelial cells. Am J Pathol 2001;159:2271–80.
35. Roberts DM, Kearney JB, Johnson JH, et al. The vascular endothelial growth factor (VEGF) receptor Flt-1 (VEGFR-1) modulates Flk-1 (VEGFR-2) signaling during blood vessel formation. Am J Pathol 2004;164:1531–5.
36. Fong GH, Rossant J, Gertsenstein M, et al. Role of the Flt-1 receptor tyrosine kinase in regulating the assembly of vascular endothelium. Nature 1995;376:66–70.
37. Jinnin M, Ishihara T, Boye E, et al. Recent progress in studies of infantile hemangioma. J Dermatol 2010;37:939–55.
38. Chang J, Most D, Bresnick S, et al. Proliferative hemangiomas: analysis of cytokine gene expression and angiogenesis. Plast Reconstr Surg 1999;103:1–9 [discussion: 10].
39. Tille JC, Pepper MS. Hereditary vascular anomalies: new insights into their pathogenesis. Arterioscler Thromb Vasc Biol 2004;24:1578–90.
40. Takahashi K, Mulliken JB, Kozakewich HP, et al. Cellular markers that distinguish the phases of hemangioma during infancy and childhood. J Clin Invest 1994;93: 2357–64.
41. Goldberg NS, Hebert AA, Esterly NB. Sacral hemangiomas and multiple congenital abnormalities. Arch Dermatol 1986;122:684–7.
42. Albright AL, Gartner JC, Wiener ES. Lumbar cutaneous hemangiomas as indicators of tethered spinal cords. Pediatrics 1989;83:977–80.
43. Kasabach H, Merritt K. Capillary hemangioma with extensive purpura: report of a case. Am J Dis Child 1940;59:1063–70.
44. Metry D, Heyer G, Hess C, et al. Consensus statement on diagnostic criteria for PHACE syndrome. Pediatrics 2009;124:1447–56.

45. Enjolras O, Gelbert F. Superficial hemangiomas: associations and management. Pediatr Dermatol 1997;14:173–9.
46. Sarkar M, Mulliken JB, Kozakewich HP, et al. Thrombocytopenic coagulopathy (Kasabach-Merritt phenomenon) is associated with Kaposiform hemangioendothelioma and not with common infantile hemangioma. Plast Reconstr Surg 1997; 100:1377–86.
47. Jones EW, Orkin M. Tufted angioma (angioblastoma). A benign progressive angioma, not to be confused with Kaposi's sarcoma or low-grade angiosarcoma. J Am Acad Dermatol 1989;20:214–25.
48. Osio A, Fraitag S, Hadj-Rabia S, et al. Clinical spectrum of tufted angiomas in childhood: a report of 13 cases and a review of the literature. Arch Dermatol 2010;146:758–63.
49. Hall GW. Kasabach-Merritt syndrome: pathogenesis and management. Br J Haematol 2001;112:851–62.
50. Rodriguez V, Lee A, Witman PM, et al. Kasabach-Merritt phenomenon: case series and retrospective review of the mayo clinic experience. J Pediatr Hematol Oncol 2009;31:522–6.
51. Seo SK, Suh JC, Na GY, et al. Kasabach-Merritt syndrome: identification of platelet trapping in a tufted angioma by immunohistochemistry technique using monoclonal antibody to CD61. Pediatr Dermatol 1999;16:392–4.
52. Martinez-Perez D, Fein NA, Boon LM, et al. Not all hemangiomas look like strawberries: uncommon presentations of the most common tumor of infancy. Pediatr Dermatol 1995;12:1–6.
53. Barnes CM, Huang S, Kaipainen A, et al. Evidence by molecular profiling for a placental origin of infantile hemangioma. Proc Natl Acad Sci U S A 2005; 102:19097–102.
54. Ryan C, Price V, John P, et al. Kasabach-Merritt phenomenon: a single centre experience. Eur J Haematol 2010;84:97–104.
55. Haisley-Royster C, Enjolras O, Frieden IJ, et al. Kasabach-Merritt phenomenon: a retrospective study of treatment with vincristine. J Pediatr Hematol Oncol 2002;24:459–62.
56. Fahrtash F, McCahon E, Arbuckle S. Successful treatment of kaposiform hemangioendothelioma and tufted angioma with vincristine. J Pediatr Hematol Oncol 2010;32:506–10.
57. Gidding CE, Kellie SJ, Kamps WA, et al. Vincristine revisited. Crit Rev Oncol Hematol 1999;29:267–87.
58. Chang E, Boyd A, Nelson CC, et al. Successful treatment of infantile hemangiomas with interferon-alpha-2b. J Pediatr Hematol Oncol 1997;19: 237–44.
59. Harper L, Michel JL, Enjolras O, et al. Successful management of a retroperitoneal kaposiform hemangioendothelioma with Kasabach-Merritt phenomenon using alpha-interferon. Eur J Pediatr Surg 2006;16:369–72.
60. Blatt J, Stavas J, Moats-Staats B, et al. Treatment of childhood kaposiform hemangioendothelioma with sirolimus. Pediatr Blood Cancer 2010;55:1396–8.
61. Hammill AM, Wentzel M, Gupta A, et al. Sirolimus for the treatment of complicated vascular anomalies in children. Pediatr Blood Cancer 2011;28:1018–24.
62. Gruman A, Liang MG, Mulliken JB, et al. Kaposiform hemangioendothelioma without Kasabach-Merritt phenomenon. J Am Acad Dermatol 2005;52: 616–22.
63. Enjolras O, Mulliken JB, Wassef M, et al. Residual lesions after Kasabach-Merritt phenomenon in 41 patients. J Am Acad Dermatol 2000;42:225–35.

64. Patrice SJ, Wiss K, Mulliken JB. Pyogenic granuloma (lobular capillary hemangioma): a clinicopathologic study of 178 cases. Pediatr Dermatol 1991;8: 267–76.
65. Boon LM, Fishman SJ, Lund DP, et al. Congenital fibrosarcoma masquerading as congenital hemangioma: report of two cases. J Pediatr Surg 1995;30: 1378–81.
66. Kirschner RE, Low DW. Treatment of pyogenic granuloma by shave excision and laser photocoagulation. Plast Reconstr Surg 1999;104:1346–9.
67. Hobert JA, Eng C. PTEN hamartoma tumor syndrome: an overview. Genet Med 2009;11:687–94.
68. Tan WH, Baris HN, Burrows PE, et al. The spectrum of vascular anomalies in patients with PTEN mutations: implications for diagnosis and management. J Med Genet 2007;44:594–602.
69. Chung KC, Weiss SW, Kuzon WM Jr. Multifocal congenital hemangiopericytomas associated with Kasabach-Merritt syndrome. Br J Plast Surg 1995;48: 240–2.
70. Margileth AM, Museles M. Cutaneous hemangiomas in children. Diagnosis and conservative management. JAMA 1965;194:523–6.
71. Greene AK, Rogers GF, Mulliken JB. Management of parotid hemangioma in 100 children. Plast Reconstr Surg 2004;113:53–60.
72. Hermans DJ, Boezeman JB, Van de Kerkhof PC, et al. Differences between ulcerated and non-ulcerated hemangiomas, a retrospective study of 465 cases. Eur J Dermatol 2009;19:152–6.
73. Waner M, Suen JY. The natural history of hemangiomas. New York: Wiley-Liss; 1999.
74. Morelli JG, Tan OT, Yohn JJ, et al. Treatment of ulcerated hemangiomas infancy. Arch Pediatr Adolesc Med 1994;148:1104–5.
75. Orlow SJ, Isakoff MS, Blei F. Increased risk of symptomatic hemangiomas of the airway in association with cutaneous hemangiomas in a "beard" distribution. J Pediatr 1997;131:643–6.
76. Leaute-Labreze C, Dumas de la Roque E, Hubiche T, et al. Propranolol for severe hemangiomas of infancy. N Engl J Med 2008;358:2649–51.
77. Leaute-Labreze C, Taieb A. Efficacy of beta-blockers in infantile capillary haemangiomas: the physiopathological significance and therapeutic consequences. Ann Dermatol Venereol 2008;135:860–2.
78. Buckmiller LM, Munson PD, Dyamenahalli U, et al. Propranolol for infantile hemangiomas: early experience at a tertiary vascular anomalies center. Laryngoscope 2010;120:676–81.
79. Bagazgoitia L, Torrelo A, Gutierrez JC, et al. Propranolol for Infantile Hemangiomas. Pediatr Dermatol 2011;28:108–14.
80. Storch CH, Hoeger PH. Propranolol for infantile haemangiomas: insights into the molecular mechanisms of action. Br J Dermatol 2010;163:269–74.
81. Sommers Smith SK, Smith DM. Beta blockade induces apoptosis in cultured capillary endothelial cells. Vitro Cell Dev Biol Anim 2002;38:298–304.
82. Zhang D, Ma Q, Shen S, et al. Inhibition of pancreatic cancer cell proliferation by propranolol occurs through apoptosis induction: the study of beta-adrenoceptor antagonist's anticancer effect in pancreatic cancer cell. Pancreas 2009;38: 94–100.
83. Zvulunov A, McCuaig C, Frieden IJ, et al. Oral propranolol therapy for infantile hemangiomas beyond the proliferation phase: a multicenter retrospective study. Pediatr Dermatol 2011;28:94–8.

84. Cushing SL, Boucek RJ, Manning SC, et al. Initial experience with a multidisciplinary strategy for initiation of propranolol therapy for infantile hemangiomas. Otolaryngol Head Neck Surg 2011;144:78–84.

85. Maisel AS, Motulsky HJ, Insel PA. Propranolol treatment externalizes beta-adrenergic receptors in guinea pig myocardium and prevents further externalization by ischemia. Circ Res 1987;60:108–12.

86. Harrison DC, Meffin PJ, Winkle RA. Clinical pharmacokinetics of antiarrhythmic drugs. Prog Cardiovasc Dis 1977;20:217–42.

87. Holland KE, Frieden IJ, Frommelt PC, et al. Hypoglycemia in children taking propranolol for the treatment of infantile hemangioma. Arch Dermatol 2010; 146:775–8.

88. Pope E, Chakkittakandiyil A. Topical timolol gel for infantile hemangiomas: a pilot study. Arch Dermatol 2010;146:564–5.

89. Garzon MC, Lucky AW, Hawrot A, et al. Ultrapotent topical corticosteroid treatment of hemangiomas of infancy. J Am Acad Dermatol 2005;52:281–6.

90. Enjolras O, Riche MC, Merland JJ, et al. Management of alarming hemangiomas in infancy: a review of 25 cases. Pediatrics 1990;85:491–8.

91. Greenberger S, Boscolo E, Adini I, et al. Corticosteroid suppression of VEGF-A in infantile hemangioma-derived stem cells. N Engl J Med 2010;362:1005–13.

92. George ME, Sharma V, Jacobson J, et al. Adverse effects of systemic glucocorticosteroid therapy in infants with hemangiomas. Arch Dermatol 2004;140: 963–9.

93. Boon LM, MacDonald DM, Mulliken JB. Complications of systemic corticosteroid therapy for problematic hemangioma. Plast Reconstr Surg 1999;104:1616–23.

94. Blei F, Chianese J. Corticosteroid toxicity in infants treated for endangering hemangiomas: experience and guidelines for monitoring. Int Pediatr 1999;14: 146–53.

95. Barlow CF, Priebe CJ, Mulliken JB, et al. Spastic diplegia as a complication of interferon alfa-2a treatment of hemangiomas of infancy. J Pediatr 1998;132: 527–30.

96. White CW, Wolf SJ, Korones DN, et al. Treatment of childhood angiomatous diseases with recombinant interferon alfa-2a. J Pediatr 1991;118:59–66.

97. Ezekowitz RA, Mulliken JB, Folkman J. Interferon alfa-2a therapy for life-threatening hemangiomas of infancy. N Engl J Med 1992;326:1456–63.

98. Greinwald JH Jr, Burke DK, Bonthius DJ, et al. An update on the treatment of hemangiomas in children with interferon alfa-2a. Arch Otolaryngol Head Neck Surg 1999;125:21–7.

99. Perez J, Pardo J, Gomez C. Vincristine—an effective treatment of corticoid-resistant life-threatening infantile hemangiomas. Acta Oncol 2002;41:197–9.

100. Hohenleutner S, Badur-Ganter E, Landthaler M, et al. Long-term results in the treatment of childhood hemangioma with the flashlamp-pumped pulsed dye laser: an evaluation of 617 cases. Lasers Surg Med 2001;28:273–7.

101. Sie KC, McGill T, Healy GB. Subglottic hemangioma: ten years' experience with the carbon dioxide laser. Ann Otol Rhinol Laryngol 1994;103:167–72.

102. Fishman SJ, Fox VL. Visceral vascular anomalies. Gastrointest Endosc Clin N Am 2001;11:813–34, viii.

103. Christison-Lagay ER, Burrows PE, Alomari A, et al. Hepatic hemangiomas: subtype classification and development of a clinical practice algorithm and registry. J Pediatr Surg 2007;42:62–7 [discussion: 67–8].

104. Christison-Lagay ER, Fishman SJ. Vascular anomalies. Surg Clin North Am 2006;86:393–425, x.

105. Limaye N, Boon LM, Vikkula M. From germline towards somatic mutations in the pathophysiology of vascular anomalies. Hum Mol Genet 2009;18:R65–74.
106. Brouillard P, Vikkula M. Genetic causes of vascular malformations. Hum Mol Genet 2007;16:R140–9.
107. Sadler TW. Langman's medical embryology. Philadelphia: Lippincott Williams & Wilkins; 2004.
108. Folkman J, D'Amore PA. Blood vessel formation: what is its molecular basis? Cell 1996;87:1153–5.
109. Wang HU, Chen ZF, Anderson DJ. Molecular distinction and angiogenic interaction between embryonic arteries and veins revealed by ephrin-B2 and its receptor Eph-B4. Cell 1998;93:741–53.
110. Ramsauer M, D'Amore PA. Getting Tie(2)d up in angiogenesis. J Clin Invest 2002;110:1615–7.
111. Karpanen T, Alitalo K. Molecular biology and pathology of lymphangiogenesis. Annu Rev Pathol 2008;3:367–97.
112. Rodriguez-Niedenfuhr M, Papoutsi M, Christ B, et al. Prox1 is a marker of ectodermal placodes, endodermal compartments, lymphatic endothelium and lymphangioblasts. Anat Embryol (Berl) 2001;204:399–406.
113. Oliver G, Srinivasan RS. Lymphatic vasculature development: current concepts. Ann N Y Acad Sci 2008;1131:75–81.
114. Banerji S, Ni J, Wang SX, et al. LYVE-1, a new homologue of the CD44 glycoprotein, is a lymph-specific receptor for hyaluronan. J Cell Biol 1999;144:789–801.
115. Hong YK, Harvey N, Noh YH, et al. Prox1 is a master control gene in the program specifying lymphatic endothelial cell fate. Dev Dyn 2002;225:351–7.
116. Karkkainen MJ, Haiko P, Sainio K, et al. Vascular endothelial growth factor C is required for sprouting of the first lymphatic vessels from embryonic veins. Nat Immunol 2004;5:74–80.
117. Jacobs AH, Walton RG. The incidence of birthmarks in the neonate. Pediatrics 1976;58:218–22.
118. Smoller BR, Rosen S. Port-wine stains. A disease of altered neural modulation of blood vessels? Arch Dermatol 1986;122:177–9.
119. Breugem CC, Alders M, Salieb-Beugelaar GB, et al. A locus for hereditary capillary malformations mapped on chromosome 5q. Hum Genet 2002;110:343–7.
120. Eerola I, Boon LM, Mulliken JB, et al. Capillary malformation-arteriovenous malformation, a new clinical and genetic disorder caused by RASA1 mutations. Am J Hum Genet 2003;73:1240–9.
121. Tan OT, Sherwood K, Gilchrest BA. Treatment of children with port-wine stains using the flashlamp-pulsed tunable dye laser. N Engl J Med 1989;320:416–21.
122. van der Horst CM, Koster PH, de Borgie CA, et al. Effect of the timing of treatment of port-wine stains with the flash-lamp-pumped pulsed-dye laser. N Engl J Med 1998;338:1028–33.
123. Chapas AM, Eickhorst K, Geronemus RG. Efficacy of early treatment of facial port wine stains in newborns: a review of 49 cases. Lasers Surg Med 2007;39:563–8.
124. Amitai DB, Fichman S, Merlob P, et al. Cutis marmorata telangiectatica congenita: clinical findings in 85 patients. Pediatr Dermatol 2000;17:100–4.
125. Fujita M, Darmstadt GL, Dinulos JG. Cutis marmorata telangiectatica congenita with hemangiomatous histopathologic features. J Am Acad Dermatol 2003;48:950–4.

126. Vogel AM, Paltiel HJ, Kozakewich HP, et al. Iliac artery stenosis in a child with cutis marmorata telangiectatica congenita. J Pediatr Surg 2005;40:e9–12.

127. McDonald J, Damjanovich K, Millson A, et al. Molecular diagnosis in hereditary hemorrhagic telangiectasia: findings in a series tested simultaneously by sequencing and deletion/duplication analysis. Clin Genet 2011;79:335–44.

128. McAllister KA, Grogg KM, Johnson DW, et al. Endoglin, a TGF-beta binding protein of endothelial cells, is the gene for hereditary haemorrhagic telangiectasia type 1. Nat Genet 1994;8:345–51.

129. Johnson DW, Berg JN, Baldwin MA, et al. Mutations in the activin receptor-like kinase 1 gene in hereditary haemorrhagic telangiectasia type 2. Nat Genet 1996;13:189–95.

130. Shovlin CL. Hereditary haemorrhagic telangiectasia: pathophysiology, diagnosis and treatment. Blood Rev 2010;24:203–19.

131. Govani FS, Shovlin CL. Hereditary haemorrhagic telangiectasia: a clinical and scientific review. Eur J Hum Genet 2009;17:860–71.

132. Florez-Vargas A, Vargas SO, Debelenko LV, et al. Comparative analysis of D2-40 and LYVE-1 immunostaining in lymphatic malformations. Lymphology 2008;41:103–10.

133. Bruder E, Perez-Atayde AR, Jundt G, et al. Vascular lesions of bone in children, adolescents, and young adults. A clinicopathologic reappraisal and application of the ISSVA classification. Virchows Arch 2009;454:161–79.

134. Malone FD, Canick JA, Ball RH, et al. First-trimester or second-trimester screening, or both, for Down's syndrome. N Engl J Med 2005;353:2001–11.

135. Graesslin O, Derniaux E, Alanio E, et al. Characteristics and outcome of fetal cystic hygroma diagnosed in the first trimester. Acta Obstet Gynecol Scand 2007;86:1442–6.

136. Marler JJ, Fishman SJ, Upton J, et al. Prenatal diagnosis of vascular anomalies. J Pediatr Surg 2002;37:318–26.

137. Puig S, Casati B, Staudenherz A, et al. Vascular low-flow malformations in children: current concepts for classification, diagnosis and therapy. Eur J Radiol 2005;53:35–45.

138. Fishman SJ, Burrows PE, Upton J, et al. Life-threatening anomalies of the thoracic duct: anatomic delineation dictates management. J Pediatr Surg 2001;36:1269–72.

139. Padwa BL, Hayward PG, Ferraro NF, et al. Cervicofacial lymphatic malformation: clinical course, surgical intervention, and pathogenesis of skeletal hypertrophy. Plast Reconstr Surg 1995;95:951–60.

140. Gorham LW, Stout AP. Massive osteolysis (acute spontaneous absorption of bone, phantom bone, disappearing bone); its relation to hemangiomatosis. J Bone Joint Surg Am 1955;37:985–1004.

141. Vinee P, Tanyu MO, Hauenstein KH, et al. CT and MRI of Gorham syndrome. J Comput Assist Tomogr 1994;18:985–9.

142. Venkatramani R, Ma NS, Pitukcheewanont P, et al. Gorham's disease and diffuse lymphangiomatosis in children and adolescents. Pediatr Blood Cancer 2011;56:667–70.

143. Gondivkar SM, Gadbail AR. Gorham-Stout syndrome: a rare clinical entity and review of literature. Oral Surg Oral Med Oral Pathol Oral Radiol Endod 2010;109:e41–8.

144. Connell FC, Ostergaard P, Carver C, et al. Analysis of the coding regions of VEGFR3 and VEGFC in Milroy disease and other primary lymphoedemas. Hum Genet 2009;124:625–31.

145. Karkkainen MJ, Ferrell RE, Lawrence EC, et al. Missense mutations interfere with VEGFR-3 signalling in primary lymphoedema. Nat Genet 2000;25:153–9.

146. Irrthum A, Karkkainen MJ, Devriendt K, et al. Congenital hereditary lymphedema caused by a mutation that inactivates VEGFR3 tyrosine kinase. Am J Hum Genet 2000;67:295–301.

147. Petrova TV, Karpanen T, Norrmen C, et al. Defective valves and abnormal mural cell recruitment underlie lymphatic vascular failure in lymphedema distichiasis. Nat Med 2004;10:974–81.

148. Mellor RH, Brice G, Stanton AW, et al. Mutations in FOXC2 are strongly associated with primary valve failure in veins of the lower limb. Circulation 2007;115: 1912–20.

149. Fang J, Dagenais SL, Erickson RP, et al. Mutations in FOXC2 (MFH-1), a forkhead family transcription factor, are responsible for the hereditary lymphedema-distichiasis syndrome. Am J Hum Genet 2000;67:1382–8.

150. Rezaie T, Ghoroghchian R, Bell R, et al. Primary non-syndromic lymphoedema (Meige disease) is not caused by mutations in FOXC2. Eur J Hum Genet 2008;16:300–4.

151. Orford J, Barker A, Thonell S, et al. Bleomycin therapy for cystic hygroma. J Pediatr Surg 1995;30:1282–7.

152. Niramis R, Watanatittan S, Rattanasuwan T. Treatment of cystic hygroma by intralesional bleomycin injection: experience in 70 patients. Eur J Pediatr Surg 2010;20:178–82.

153. Perkins JA, Manning SC, Tempero RM, et al. Lymphatic malformations: review of current treatment. Otolaryngol Head Neck Surg 2010;142:795–803, 803.e791.

154. Alqahtani A, Nguyen LT, Flageole H, et al. 25 years' experience with lymphangiomas in children. J Pediatr Surg 1999;34:1164–8.

155. Baskerville PA, Ackroyd JS, Lea Thomas M, et al. The Klippel-Trenaunay syndrome: clinical, radiological and haemodynamic features and management. Br J Surg 1985;72:232–6.

156. de la Torre L, Carrasco D, Mora MA, et al. Vascular malformations of the colon in children. J Pediatr Surg 2002;37:1754–7.

157. Kulungowski AM, Fox VL, Burrows PE, et al. Portomesenteric venous thrombosis associated with rectal venous malformations. J Pediatr Surg 2010;45: 1221–7.

158. Limaye N, Wouters V, Uebelhoer M, et al. Somatic mutations in angiopoietin receptor gene TEK cause solitary and multiple sporadic venous malformations. Nat Genet 2009;41:118–24.

159. Jones N, Iljin K, Dumont DJ, et al. Tie receptors: new modulators of angiogenic and lymphangiogenic responses. Nat Rev Mol Cell Biol 2001;2:257–67.

160. Maisonpierre PC, Suri C, Jones PF, et al. Angiopoietin-2, a natural antagonist for Tie2 that disrupts in vivo angiogenesis. Science 1997;277:55–60.

161. Suri C, Jones PF, Patan S, et al. Requisite role of angiopoietin-1, a ligand for the TIE2 receptor, during embryonic angiogenesis. Cell 1996;87:1171–80.

162. Vikkula M, Boon LM, Carraway KL 3rd, et al. Vascular dysmorphogenesis caused by an activating mutation in the receptor tyrosine kinase TIE2. Cell 1996;87:1181–90.

163. Calvert JT, Riney TJ, Kontos CD, et al. Allelic and locus heterogeneity in inherited venous malformations. Hum Mol Genet 1999;8:1279–89.

164. Boon LM, Mulliken JB, Enjolras O, et al. Glomuvenous malformation (glomangioma) and venous malformation: distinct clinicopathologic and genetic entities. Arch Dermatol 2004;140:971–6.

165. Brouillard P, Boon LM, Mulliken JB, et al. Mutations in a novel factor, glomulin, are responsible for glomuvenous malformations ("glomangiomas"). Am J Hum Genet 2002;70:866–74.

166. Oranje AP. Blue rubber bleb nevus syndrome. Pediatr Dermatol 1986;3:304–10.

167. Barlas A, Avsar E, Bozbas A, et al. Role of capsule endoscopy in blue rubber bleb nevus syndrome. Can J Surg 2008;51:E119–20.

168. Hofhuis WJ, Oranje AP, Bouquet J, et al. Blue rubber-bleb naevus syndrome: report of a case with consumption coagulopathy complicated by manifest thrombosis. Eur J Pediatr 1990;149:526–8.

169. Smithers CJ, Vogel AM, Kozakewich HP, et al. An injectable tissue-engineered embolus prevents luminal recanalization after vascular sclerotherapy. J Pediatr Surg 2005;40:920–5.

170. Berenguer B, Burrows PE, Zurakowski D, et al. Sclerotherapy of craniofacial venous malformations: complications and results. Plast Reconstr Surg 1999; 104:1–11 [discussion: 12–5].

171. Fishman SJ, Burrows PE, Leichtner AM, et al. Gastrointestinal manifestations of vascular anomalies in childhood: varied etiologies require multiple therapeutic modalities. J Pediatr Surg 1998;33:1163–7.

172. Fishman SJ, Smithers CJ, Folkman J, et al. Blue rubber bleb nevus syndrome: surgical eradication of gastrointestinal bleeding. Ann Surg 2005;241:523–8.

173. Fishman SJ, Shamberger RC, Fox VL, et al. Endorectal pull-through abates gastrointestinal hemorrhage from colorectal venous malformations. J Pediatr Surg 2000;35:982–4.

174. Liu AS, Mulliken JB, Zurakowski D, et al. Extracranial arteriovenous malformations: natural progression and recurrence after treatment. Plast Reconstr Surg 2010;125:1185–94.

175. Kohout MP, Hansen M, Pribaz JJ, et al. Arteriovenous malformations of the head and neck: natural history and management. Plast Reconstr Surg 1998;102: 643–54.

176. Revencu N, Boon LM, Mulliken JB, et al. Parkes Weber syndrome, vein of Galen aneurysmal malformation, and other fast-flow vascular anomalies are caused by RASA1 mutations. Hum Mutat 2008;29:959–65.

177. Jacob AG, Driscoll DJ, Shaughnessy WJ, et al. Klippel-Trenaunay syndrome: spectrum and management. Mayo Clin Proc 1998;73:28–36.

178. Liu NF, Lu Q, Yan ZX. Lymphatic malformation is a common component of Klippel-Trenaunay syndrome. J Vasc Surg 2010;52:1557–63.

179. Smithers CJ, Fishman SJ. Vascular anomalies. Philadelphia: Elsevier Saunders; 2004.

180. Alomari AI. Characterization of a distinct syndrome that associates complex truncal overgrowth, vascular, and acral anomalies: a descriptive study of 18 cases of CLOVES syndrome. Clin Dysmorphol 2008;18:1–7.

181. Sapp JC, Turner JT, van de Kamp JM, et al. Newly delineated syndrome of congenital lipomatous overgrowth, vascular malformations, and epidermal nevi (CLOVE syndrome) in seven patients. Am J Med Genet A 2007;143: 2944–58.

182. Fernandez-Pineda I, Fajardo M, Chaudry G, et al. Perinatal clinical and imaging features of CLOVES syndrome. Pediatr Radiol 2010;40:1436–9.

# Index

## A

Surg Clin N Am 92 (2012) 801–821
doi:10.1016/S0039-6109(12)00085-0
0039-6109/12/$ – see front matter © 2012 Elsevier Inc. All rights reserved.

surgical.theclinics.com

# Moving?

## Make sure your subscription moves with you!

To notify us of your new address, find your **Clinics Account Number** (located on your mailing label above your name), and contact customer service at:

Email: **journalscustomerservice-usa@elsevier.com**

**800-654-2452** (subscribers in the U.S. & Canada)
**314-447-8871** (subscribers outside of the U.S. & Canada)

Fax number: **314-447-8029**

**Elsevier Health Sciences Division**
**Subscription Customer Service**
**3251 Riverport Lane**
**Maryland Heights, MO 63043**

*To ensure uninterrupted delivery of your subscription, please notify us at least 4 weeks in advance of move.

Printed and bound by CPI Group (UK) Ltd, Croydon, CR0 4YY

03/10/2024

01040448-0009